REMOTE AS EVER

REMOTE AS EVER

The Aboriginal struggle for autonomy in the Western Desert

David Scrimgeour

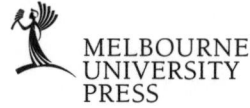

MELBOURNE UNIVERSITY PRESS
An imprint of Melbourne University Publishing Limited
Level 1, 715 Swanston Street, Carlton, Victoria 3053, Australia
mup-contact@unimelb.edu.au
www.mup.com.au

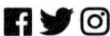

First published 2022
Text © David Scrimgeour, 2022
Images © David Scrimgeour, various dates
Design and typography © Melbourne University Publishing Limited, 2022

This book is copyright. Apart from any use permitted under the *Copyright Act 1968* and subsequent amendments, no part may be reproduced, stored in a retrieval system or transmitted by any means or process whatsoever without the prior written permission of the publishers.

Every attempt has been made to locate the copyright holders for material quoted in this book. Any person or organisation that may have been overlooked or misattributed may contact the publisher.

Cover design by Pilar Aguilera
Typeset by Megan Ellis
Cover image
Patju Presley has depicted the significant site of Piltjitjara and Karukali. These two sites are highly sacred and detail the movement of people as they traverse the country on initiation ceremony accompanying the young boys as they transform into men. This is set out by creation beings, those who shaped the landscape as they moved through it, leaving indelible physical reminders of their power and presence. This is Patju's country, situated to the west of present day Watarru, near the border between South Australia and Western Australia, and is country that he has the birthright and cultural authority to depict. Patju, who currently lives at Tjuntjuntjara and works with the Spinifex Arts Project, has been a friend of the author since 1978, when Patju lived at Pipalyatjara.

Printed in Australia by McPherson's Printing Group

 A catalogue record for this book is available from the National Library of Australia

9780522878974 (paperback)
9780522878981 (ebook)

Warning
This book contains references to deceased First Nations people. First Nations people should exercise care when reading the excerpts of historical sources.

To Margaret, Sophie, Laura and Callum

Contents

Preface		ix
1	Alice Springs and out bush: A time of Utopian idealism	1
2	The Pitjantjatjara and Ngaanyatjarra homelands	16
3	The Pitjantjatjara Home-made Health Service	43
4	The Strelley mob and the *Martu*	75
5	Pintupi country, Pintupi health	109
6	The Spinifex people	141
7	First contact, last contact	166
8	The reoccupation of the Western Desert and the counter-attack	183
9	Autonomy in Aboriginal health and the government response	208
	Conclusion	242
Notes		247
Bibliography		255
Index		265

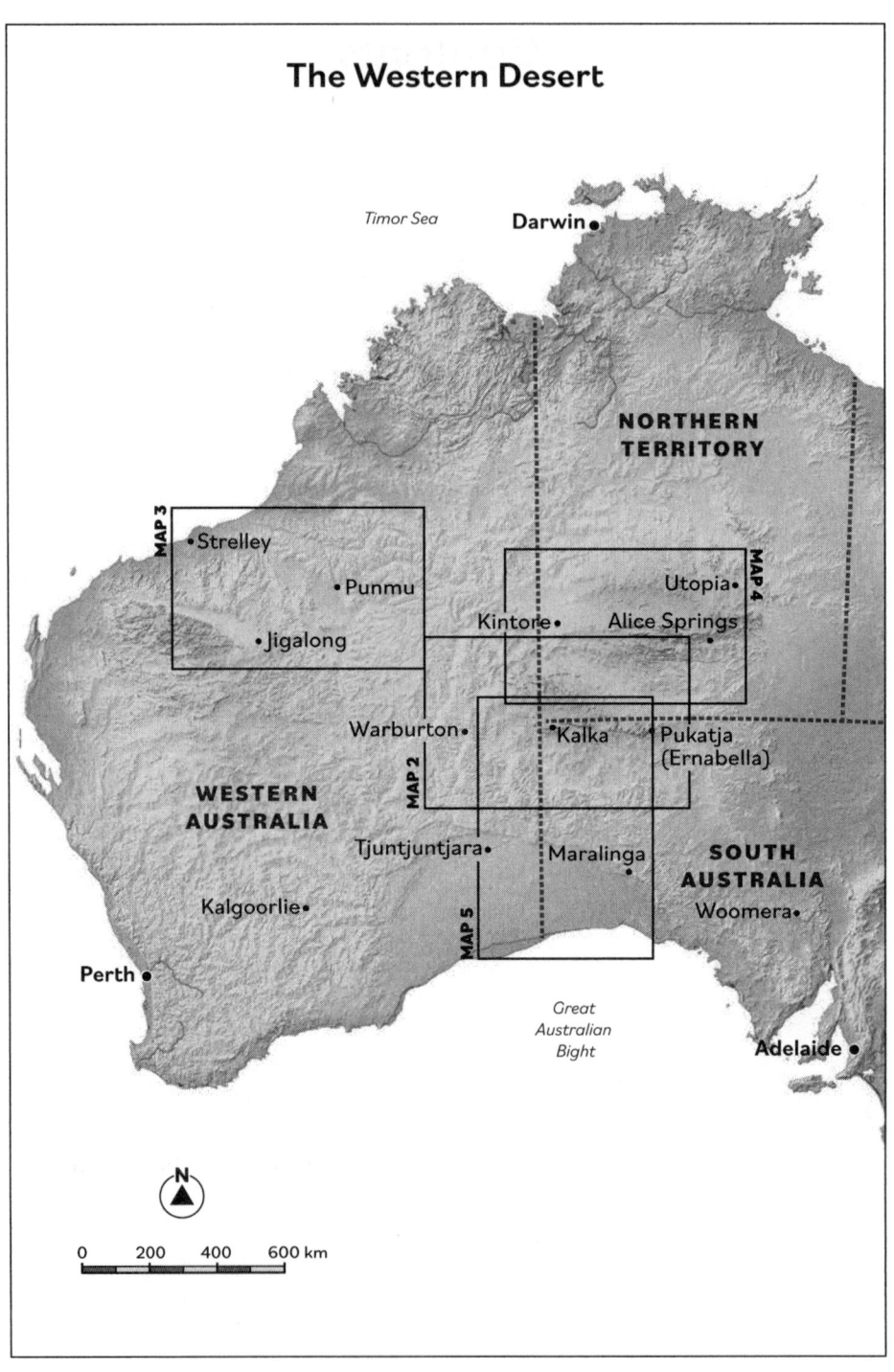

Preface

In the 1970s two significant Aboriginal social movements were gathering momentum across Australia. These movements reflected the aspiration to self-determination and autonomy that had probably always existed among Australian Aboriginal people since colonisation, but in the 1970s was leading to more effective collective actions. One of these was the Aboriginal community-controlled health-service movement, a remarkable and often successful attempt by Aboriginal people to take control of their own primary healthcare services. The other was the Aboriginal homelands movement (also known as the outstation movement) in which Aboriginal people relocated from missions and government settlements to live in more dispersed settlements on their traditional country.

From the late 1970s, I happened to find myself living and working in a number of remote communities where the homelands movement was occurring and where I was employed as a doctor within the newly developing Aboriginal community-controlled health services. By virtue of being in the right place at the right time, I became involved in both these movements. The communities in which I worked are located in Australia's Western Desert region, where people were in the process of reoccupying their homelands.

The Western Desert is a vast region, occupying a large part of inland Western Australia and adjoining parts of South Australia and the Northern Territory. It extends from the Great Australian Bight on the south coast of the continent to the southern edge of the tropical Kimberley region in northern Western Australia. It encompasses the Great Victoria Desert, the Gibson

Desert and the Great Sandy Desert. The Great Victoria Desert includes the dune-field homelands of the Spinifex people. Further north, ancient mountain ranges and surrounding grasslands constitute the homelands of the Pitjantjatjara and Ngaanyatjarra people. Further north again is the Gibson Desert, where the Pintupi people live, and west of the Gibson Desert the Great Sandy Desert, which are the homelands of the Manyjilyjarra and Kartujarra people. All these people have cultural and linguistic links; the anthropologists Ronald and Catherine Berndt used the term 'Western Desert culture bloc', and their languages constitute the 'Western Desert language group'.

I lived and worked with these four major groupings of Western Desert peoples. How to refer to the groups can be problematic as, from pre-contact times to the present, Western Desert groups have been fluid in composition. The boundaries between groups are blurred and permeable, with interconnections through ritual links and intermarriage. They are often referred to by linguistic characteristics (e.g. Pitjantjatjara, Ngaanyatjarra, Manyjilyjarra, Pintupi) but often these are terms that have been applied by others rather than used by group members themselves. In this book I often use the terms that the people used to refer to themselves (e.g. *Anangu, Yarnangu, Marrngu, Martu* meaning 'the people' in their own language). Sometimes I use the term 'mob' in the Aboriginal-English sense of a group of people of indeterminate size, without the connotation of unruliness that the word has in other countries. Robert Tonkinson named his book *The Jigalong Mob*, suggesting that this is a term people have attributed to themselves, which 'connotes a new form of local organization and indicates their feeling of common identity when contrasting themselves with outsiders'.[1]

The fact that each 'mob' was part of the Western Desert cultural and linguistic bloc eased my communication difficulties. Although distances between the different homelands was great, there were sufficient similarities in the languages that were spoken for me to adapt the Pitjantjatjara language I initially learnt to be able to also communicate in the Ngaanyatjarra, Manyjilyjarra, and Pintupi languages.

It is not uncommon to find various ways of spelling Aboriginal linguistic groups. I have followed the spelling generally adopted by the groups concerned, even though this makes the orthography sometimes inconsistent from region to region. The spelling adopted by any particular group is generally a function of the orthography used by the main linguists who worked with that particular language. For example, the spelling of the suffix '-tjara/-tjarra/-jara' (which has effectively the same sound, with the same meaning of 'having') uses one 'r' in Pitjantjatjara and Yankunytjatjara and two 'r's in Ngaanyatjarra and Manyjilyjarra. Further, the 'tj/j' sound is spelt tj in Pitjantjatjara, Yankunytjatjara and Ngaanyatjarra, and j in Manyjilyjarra. Pintupi, particularly in the past, was often spelt Pintubi, but this spelling is inconsistent because the bi-labial stop that starts the first and last syllable in the word 'Pintupi' is the same sound (half-way between a hard 'p' and a soft 'b' in English), so it is inappropriate to use a different consonant for the same sound in the one word.

Australian Indigenous people include Torres Strait Islander people as well as Aboriginal peoples. My experience is limited to working with Aboriginal peoples only. Therefore I use the term Aboriginal throughout, rather than Indigenous or Aboriginal and Torres Strait Islander—except occasionally when it may be appropriate. For people such as myself who are not Aboriginal, I use the somewhat clumsy but accurate term 'non-Aboriginal'.

Both Commonwealth and state or territory health departments inevitably appear in my narrative. Governments have an annoying tendency to continually re-structure and re-name their health departments so, to avoid confusion, I refer to these departments as 'health departments' throughout, regardless of what the actual departmental name may have been at the time.

I may appear presumptuous to be writing about Aboriginal affairs as a non-Aboriginal person. Like all non-Aboriginal Australians, I cannot escape complicity in the settler-colonial structures in which I am embedded. The social scientist Alissa Macoun cautions people like me to be conscious of what she calls 'colonising white innocence', and the tendency for 'white settlers to make ourselves the subjects and heroes of our own stories, even when our actual contributions may be experienced negatively or profoundly ambivalently by Indigenous peoples, as have been the bulk of white settler contributions to Indigenous peoples' lives and struggles'.[2] I would have liked to include more Aboriginal voices, but many of the protagonists have passed away and most did not leave written records. The stories I tell in the chapters that follow are partly the stories of those with whom I have worked (and their organisations and struggles), and partly my own story of my life and work while employed within these organisations, which are accountable to Aboriginal leadership. I have attempted to gain approval from relevant people for what I have written.

The book is divided into nine chapters, which constitute two parts. The first part, chapters 1–7, is based on my experiences in the Western Desert, with some contextual detail. In the second part, chapters 8 and 9, I describe subsequent political and policy developments that have impacted upon the social movements with which I was involved.

In chapter 1, I describe how I came to live and work in Central Australia; in chapter 2, I provide some of the historical background to events in Central Australia (with a particular focus on Pitjantjatjara and Ngaanyatjarra lands), which led to the reasons for my work in the area. Consequently, these chapters are in a sense an introduction to what follows.

Chapters 4–6 each give the story of a particular area and Aboriginal 'mob' I worked with. The structure of each of these chapters is similar: I start with a brief historical background of how this mob came to reoccupy their homeland, followed by a description of how I came to be involved with them and the development of healthcare that I was involved with in that area. I also give an account of developments after my departure in each case. Chapter 7 describes the events and implications of the last two Western Desert families to abandon a full hunter-gatherer lifestyle.

Chapter 8 focuses on the homelands movement, as well as recent government policy responses to this movement. The final chapter focuses on the Aboriginal community-controlled health-service movement, describing its development and positive aspects, as well as providing a critique of recent government policies with regard to this movement. In the Australian settler-colonial context, Aboriginal policies are frequently unruly and irrational, as Tess Lea eloquently describes in her book *Wild Policy*. It is in this wild policy space that Aboriginal communities and organisations struggle to survive.

The concept of 'settler colonialism' is one that I have found useful and that I use in this book, especially in the latter part. The concept refers to the form of colonialism in which the settler comes to stay, replacing the

Indigenous population in various ways, including through Indigenous deaths, land take-overs, cultural and linguistic loss, and marginalising assertions of Indigenous autonomy. Patrick Wolfe described settler colonialism as a structure, not an event and, within this ongoing structure, dispossession and settler domination take many forms. This reflects how I have come to understand my experiences in working with Aboriginal people and their organisations in the Western Desert and elsewhere, and it informs my discussion and analysis.

I have been privileged to be involved in both social movements I discuss in this book, which have shown me the strength of the Aboriginal struggle for autonomy. I am convinced that Aboriginal yearning for autonomy has been a key feature of Aboriginal community actions in the past and in the present. Too often, however, the struggle for autonomy has been beset by obstacles, frequently as a direct consequence of government policies. I have been a witness to both the struggle for autonomy and also the way this struggle has been undermined. The early chapters in this book are about my perspective on the struggle for autonomy in the Western Desert communities in which I lived and worked. The final two chapters describe how this struggle has continued while being too often undermined by recent Australian governments.

The homelands movement and the Aboriginal community-controlled health movement have not been without their own faults and weaknesses, and it might be argued that these do not get sufficient attention in this book. However, one of my main points is that often problems within these movements are due to external factors (especially government policies) and so this is where my emphasis lies. Inevitably, I bring a particular perspective to my account.

I am grateful to many people who provided information, documentation and memories, all of which have contributed to this book. They include Rob Amery, Ian Baird, Ben Bartlett, Suzanne Bryce, Mark Chambers, Mark Clendon, David Dunn, Tom Gara, Roger Hammond, Peter Lake, Peter McCaul, Fred Myers, Fiona Pemberton, Stephan Rainow, Inawantji Scales, Glendle Schrader, Anne Scrimgeour, Audrey Scrimgeour, Margaret Scrimgeour, John Sherwood, Adrian Sleigh, Greg Stubbs, Peter Tait, Graham

Townley, John Tregenza and Robyn Withnell. I thank them all, but I take full responsibility for any errors that may appear in the text. I also wish to thank Cathy Smith, my project manager at MUP, and Emma Fajgenbaum, my editor at MUP, for their support, and two anonymous reviewers for their very helpful comments and suggestions. Also, I thank Maggie Brady, Tim Rowse, Kerrie Nelson and Fred Myers for providing encouragement to persist with the writing and publication of this book. Finally, I thank Margaret for her ongoing support and many helpful suggestions.

Many wonderful people with whom I have worked over the four decades described in this book (Aboriginal and non-Aboriginal, but mostly Aboriginal) have since passed away, many before their time. This is due in part to ongoing high Aboriginal mortality rates, which reflect the ongoing injustice experienced by Aboriginal people in contemporary Australia. I sometimes mention names of those who have passed away some time ago, and I trust this will not cause undue offence to surviving relatives; if it does, I apologise. To those who have passed away, I pay my respects.

To those who are maintaining the struggle, I also pay my respects.

1

Alice Springs and out bush

A time of Utopian idealism

Introduction to Alice

When I was approaching the end of my six-year medical degree at the University of Melbourne in 1974, the issue of post-graduate employment and study began to arise. Hospital residency was mandatory for at least a year before being registered as a medical practitioner and, while most of my colleagues hoped for a position in one of the major teaching hospitals in Melbourne, I wanted to travel and see more of both Australia and the world. The idea of the tropical far north of Australia appealed to me. I wrote to the Royal Darwin Hospital expressing an interest and was offered a position there, as long as I passed my final exams. Fortunately, I passed.

After my graduation, I was due to fly to Darwin to commence work on 27 December 1974. On Christmas Day, however, Cyclone Tracy swept through Darwin, stopping all communications and flights. As the hospital was not contactable, all I could do was wait; it was over a week before I finally heard anything. I was told that it would be some time before the hospital in Darwin would be ready for junior resident medical officers. However, a temporary position had been created for me at Alice Springs Hospital—a hospital that normally did not have positions for first-year medical graduates, but that had agreed, under the circumstances, to make special arrangements.

A couple of days later I landed at Alice Springs airport, where I was met and driven to the hospital. I was provided with accommodation on the hospital campus and told that I had been allocated to the paediatric department. I was introduced to the paediatrician, Gregor Sutherland, and the paediatric registrar on a rotation from the Children's Hospital in Adelaide, and I soon found myself at work in the ward.

All my patients were Aboriginal children, mostly infants, and most of the mothers spoke little if any English. Although I must have realised that working as a doctor in the Northern Territory would involve working with Aboriginal people, I had not thought much about what this might entail. During my medical training, I had been given no introduction at all to any of the issues and insights that might be useful to a doctor providing healthcare to Aboriginal people.

I struggled through my first day as well as I could and in the evening met a couple of colleagues who also were staying in the hospital accommodation. Rick Hambour was a friendly young man who had recently graduated from Adelaide University and, like me, had expected to do his residency at Darwin Hospital but had also found himself in Alice Springs. He had arrived there a few days before me and had a friend who was a dental graduate who had just started working in Alice Springs. They had a car, so in the balmy January evenings we were able to drive around Alice Springs and nearby sites in the magnificent MacDonnell Ranges. I was smitten by the country. Under the big blue sky, the red earth, the rocky outcrops and the pale green foliage of eucalypts, mulga trees and desert grasses appealed to me in a way that was quite unexpected.

Alice Springs, referred to by locals as Alice, is in a valley within the MacDonnell Ranges and on the traditional lands of the Mpartnwe Arrernte people. Its origins as a non-Aboriginal settlement occurred when a telegraph station on the Overland Telegraph Line was established there in the 1870s. Over the ensuing one hundred years, it had become a service centre for the pastoral and mining industries of Central Australia and, more recently, had started to become a resource centre to meet the service needs of the widely dispersed Central Australian Aboriginal people, as Australian settler colonialism was evolving to a new phase that some people refer to as welfare colonialism.

My initial sojourn in Alice Springs was short. A couple of days after my arrival, Rick and I received a message explaining that the situation in

Darwin was such that the kind of experience required for a junior hospital residency was not going to be available that year. Consequently, we were to be provided with airfares back to our places of recruitment to look for positions elsewhere. My introduction to Alice Springs was brief but it was inspirational. As my flight took off from Alice Springs airport a few days after my arrival, I looked out at the MacDonnell Ranges and knew that I would return.

Three years later, I was working in country Victoria, considering a career in rural general practice, but with some doubts as to whether it was what I really wanted to do. Towards the end of the year I saw an advertisement for a position for a general practice trainee at a recently formed Aboriginal Health Service, which was part of an organisation called the Central Australian Aboriginal Congress in Alice Springs. As I had been wondering what my next career step would be, this seemed to be a good option, and it would also be an opportunity to get back to Alice Springs. I applied and flew to Alice Springs for an interview.

Congress

On arrival at the Alice Springs airport I boarded a shuttle bus to take me through Heavitree Gap, and I was met at the bus station by a wiry man with a dark beard, lively eyes and a welcoming smile, in his early thirties, who introduced himself as Trevor Cutter, the Senior Medical Officer with the Central Australian Aboriginal Congress (known locally as just 'Congress'). As I was to stay in Alice one night, he took me to book into the Melanka Lodge and then, for the rest of the day, under Trevor's wing, I had a whirlwind tour of Alice Springs and an insight into what the job entailed.

Trevor showed me around the Congress premises, an old house on the corner of Bath and Hartley streets near the centre of Alice Springs. The house had been modified and extended to operate as a clinic as well as offices for the various administrative and other support functions that Congress provided. Congress had been formed in June 1973 by local Aboriginal activists, including Neville Perkins, the nephew of the more well-known activist Charlie Perkins. It was one of the early manifestations of the Aboriginal civil-society organisations that were being formed at that time as an expression of self-determination, which I discuss further in chapter 9. The term 'Congress', I was told, had been suggested by Neville Perkins, who named it after Mahatma Gandhi's All-India Congress—a sign of Neville's respect for Gandhi's non-violent methods of achieving political change and self-determination.[1]

One of the pressing needs recognised by the early leaders of Congress was to address the lack of appropriate healthcare for Aboriginal people, so they approached Professor Basil Hetzel for assistance. Basil Hetzel was an eminent physician with an interest in nutritional medicine, who had recently moved from Adelaide to accept a position at Monash University in Melbourne as Australia's first Professor of Social and Preventive Medicine. Basil knew the ideal person to provide the help that was needed—a young protégé of his who had recently completed his specialist physician training and had worked with him in the Monash Department of Social and Preventive Medicine, Trevor Cutter. In 1975 Trevor moved with his wife and young family from Melbourne to Alice Springs to help start the Congress primary healthcare service, one of the early Aboriginal community-controlled health organisations in Australia.

Trevor was a very energetic person, constantly on the go. While he was known by most Aboriginal people as Dr Cutter, which in Aboriginal English was more like 'Takata-kata', I found out later that his Aboriginal colleagues at Congress called him 'Cyclone Cutter'. I experienced his cyclonic nature on that first day as we rushed from place to place as he showed me around. He was later to become an important mentor for me. He conveyed to me the concept of what was later coined the 'social determinants of health', and how this understanding relates to how healthcare should be structured. I once heard him say that 'dignity is more important than penicillin or toilets', and it was his concern for human dignity, and his recognition that dignity pre-supposed autonomy, which motivated his dedication to working with Aboriginal people and their organisations.

I soon met the acting Director of Congress, Janet Layton, and many of the staff, most of whom were Aboriginal. There was a definite sense of purposeful activity and optimism that impressed me. I also met, and immediately liked, the other two GPs employed at Congress, Helen Tom and Hugh Nelson.

In the afternoon I went with Trevor around the 'town camps' that were scattered around Alice Springs. These were areas where Aboriginal people lived, often with few or no facilities or amenities and certainly no houses. Trevor was warmly welcomed at all these places. In most cases there were particular people with illnesses needing review and re-assessment. Sometimes people presented with new health problems, in which case Trevor would provide treatment on the spot or arrange, via two-way radio, for a Congress vehicle to come to take them to Congress for further assessment and treatment.

In the evening, we went to a barbecue in honour of Neville Perkins. In addition to being one of the Congress's founders, Neville had just been elected to the position of deputy leader of the Labor Party in the Northern Territory. It was there that I met a number of Aboriginal leaders, among them Geoff Shaw, who was a Vietnam veteran, a member of the Board of Management of Congress, and an advocate for the rights of Aboriginal people living in town camps. Not long afterwards, Geoff was instrumental in the establishment of Tangentyerre Council, a council of town camps; he soon became its director. I don't recall having a formal interview on that day in Alice Springs, but I do remember sitting next to Geoff while he asked probing questions about my attitude towards Aboriginal people and self-determination. My responses may have been naive, but not so bad that my application to work at Congress was rejected. What I had seen that day excited me and on the following day, before returning to Victoria, I readily accepted the offer of a job.

Working at Congress

A few weeks later, on 8 December 1977, I returned to Alice Springs to start working at Congress. My initial impression of the organisation's vibrancy was reinforced. The staff gave me a friendly reception and I quickly felt that I was part of the team. There were a number of Aboriginal people who became not just my colleagues but long-term friends. Many of these people who worked at Congress then went on to become important Aboriginal leaders: examples include Vince Forrester, John Liddle and Tracker Tilmouth.[2] Kathy Abbott had recently moved from being a cleaner to becoming an Aboriginal health worker who showed a great propensity for her work and subsequently became a leading Aboriginal health worker in the Northern Territory and an advocate for the role of Aboriginal health workers.

I also found my medical colleagues—Trevor, Helen and Hugh—friendly and helpful. What I particularly learned from them was a different way of being a general practitioner (GP). We worked as part of a team with the aim of improving the health of a community. Individual medical consultations had an important role, but as part of a bigger picture of developing strategies for improving health. The health service was not centred on the GP; we were employees like everyone else, each with their role to play. The Aboriginal health workers, with their knowledge of Aboriginal culture, family and community dynamics and politics, made a major contribution to the healthcare of both individuals and groups.

One of my particular responsibilities was to provide medical care for the Aboriginal people undergoing rehabilitation from alcohol problems at the 'Congress Farm'. This was a property a little to the south of Alice Springs on the other side of Heavitree Gap. The rehabilitation program was run by a charismatic Aboriginal man, John Macumba, and an eccentric Canadian mental health nurse, John Hill. John and his partner Jo Wynter had arrived in Alice not long before me and we became good friends. The site of the Congress Farm is still used for alcohol rehabilitation work; in the 1990s, Congress transferred the title of the farm to the newly established Central Australian Aboriginal Alcohol Programs Unit (CAAAPU).

Congress provided me with subsidised rental accommodation. Initially I was in a flat in Palmer Court on the East Side, but soon ended up in a flat on Bradshaw Drive in the suburb of Gillen, with a beautiful view of Mount Gillen and a magnificent white gum tree just across the road in the foreground. Occasionally people who came to work with Congress and needed accommodation would share my flat. This was fine with me; I was happy to be there and happy that I was meeting so many interesting people.

The fact that Congress was an Aboriginal community-controlled organisation was a major contributor to its vibrancy and effectiveness. There was a sense of ownership and pride among the Aboriginal staff and the constant stream of patients was evidence of its acceptance by the community. To me this all seemed obvious. I was surprised, however, to find that among some of my medical colleagues working for the Northern Territory health department, views ranged from support for Congress to outright hostility. Not long after I started working with Congress, I attended an evening presentation for doctors at the Alice Springs Hospital. I found myself engaged in conversation with one of the doctors from the hospital. He said that Congress was just duplicating services already being provided by the health department and without the resources of the department the Congress service would inevitably be amateurish and second-rate.

I was somewhat taken aback at the time, but in the forty years since, I have heard many variations on this argument in opposition to the Aboriginal community-controlled health-service movement. It ignored the fact that health-department services, despite the efforts of well-meaning staff, clearly had not been meeting the needs of Aboriginal people over a long period of time. The response of the Aboriginal community itself to the unsatisfactory government service had been to develop its own services with greater Aboriginal involvement. It made sense to me that the effort should be supported.[3] Within the Aboriginal community itself, it certainly appeared to me that the momentum for greater self-determination was strong.

The Congress management board recognised that outside Alice Springs there was a need for improved health services. Its health staff, including the GPs, sometimes went 'out bush' to provide healthcare but this did not meet the ongoing needs of people living in the various remote Aboriginal communities around Central Australia. Consequently, the Congress board had in 1976 asked Trevor Cutter to undertake a study to investigate how Congress could support health-service development beyond Alice Springs. A decision was made to focus on the remote community of Papunya, 200 kilometres to the west of Alice Springs. Papunya had been established as a government settlement in 1960 and by the mid 1970s had a population of over a thousand Western Arrernte, Luritja and Pintupi people. (The story of Papunya is discussed in more detail in chapter 5.)

Trevor undertook a number of visits to Papunya to talk with people from the community and investigate their health needs. While he was undertaking the project, Congress Board was asked by people from Alyawarr and Anmatyerre country to the north-east of Alice Springs, centred around the

Aboriginal-owned cattle station of Utopia, for support to improve their health services. As a result, Trevor was asked to include this area in his study also.

The result was the 'Cutter Report', which recommended establishing two Aboriginal community-controlled health services; one at Papunya and one at Utopia. The report included a proposed budget for these health services. Congress submitted the report to the Commonwealth Department of Aboriginal Affairs (DAA) for consideration. Funding for such projects in remote communities would be a new development as, until that time, all such services were in urban areas. When I arrived to work at Congress, DAA was yet to make a decision about whether funding support would be provided for the Papunya and Utopia health services. I was informed by Trevor that another submission for a remote Aboriginal community-controlled health service was also being considered by DAA. The Pitjantjatjara Council, representing Pitjantjatjara, Yankunytjatjara and Ngaanyatjarra communities in the far north-west of South Australia and the adjoining Central Desert region of Western Australia had proposed a community-based health service for a number of communities that were not at the time receiving reliable healthcare.

Within a few weeks of my employment at Congress, news came through that the DAA had agreed to fund the health service at Utopia. The decision about the other two areas, Papunya and the Pitjantjatjara homelands, were still under consideration but it was expected that the applications would be successful and the announcement to this effect would soon be made. The plan for Utopia was that Congress would administer the funding and provide staff until the health service at Utopia was ready to become independent. Helen Tom had been asked, and had agreed, to relocate to Utopia to become the first GP for their service.

I continued to work in the Congress clinic in Alice Springs, learning much about the health problems experienced by Aboriginal people in Central Australia and how to deal with them. I admired Helen and envied her for taking on the role of working in the bush. I considered the possibility of doing something similar myself but thought that, for the time being at least, I had enough to do within the regional centre of Alice Springs, and much to learn. Little did I realise that it would not be too long before I too ended up out bush, in Utopia.

Utopia

Utopia is an Aboriginal-owned cattle station about 200 kilometres northeast of Alice Springs. In 1977, when the health service was funded, about 600 Anmatjerre and Alyawarr Aboriginal people lived in a number of small, dispersed communities on Utopia Station and on surrounding cattle stations. Three years earlier, in 1974, Utopia Station was purchased on behalf of the Aboriginal traditional owners, and a claim for land rights over the pastoral lease was successfully lodged in 1978. Prior to these developments, the pastoral lease had been held by a series of station managers. Aboriginal experiences of living and working on pastoral stations in remote Australia in the twentieth century have been mixed, with the disparity in power between the station owners and managers (with the support of the authorities and the police) on the one hand, and the Aboriginal traditional owners on the other. This often led to abuses of power. According to Geoff Shaw,

> No one was allowed to live on Utopia Station. Only people who were employed at Utopia Station were allowed to live there, like the stockmen and housemaids ... So you had a couple of hundred people living across the river at Mount Skinner Station. Jock Nelson [the Mount Skinner station-owner] had empathy for Aboriginal people, and he let them stay there. He got rations for them, so maybe him and Peg were the protectors of Aboriginal people there.[4]

Wanting to demonstrate a history of benign regimes on Utopia Station as a cause of future developments, Helen Anderson and Emma Kowal present an alternative narrative that is inconsistent with Shaw's account, suggesting that Utopia Station managers always allowed access to traditional lands. It appears that, at least for some of the time, it was not so much the situation on Utopia that allowed people to live in communal groups, but rather the neighbouring station of Mount Skinner. However, most of the stations in the area provided employment for many of the men and women and, at least on some stations, non-employed dependants were allowed to stay with the families. The nature of the work on cattle stations meant that there was ample opportunity for people to retain cultural activities and their attachment to the land, and many were able to live in small groups. When the Northern Territory Administration tried to establish a centralised settlement on Utopia Station in 1969/70, this was resisted by the people who preferred to continue living in smaller groups. In this struggle they had the support of the station managers at the time, Mac and Rose Chalmers, and the government backed down.

In 1977, with the Aboriginal people now in charge of the station, the government again planned the establishment of a resource centre for these Aboriginal people at a place called Three Bores, to which Aboriginal people, the government envisaged, were to relocate. This still was not, however, the vision of Aboriginal people themselves. By gaining control of their own cattle station they saw that this was a way to continue to maintain their culture and lifestyle on their own land. To them this meant continuing to live in small, dispersed groups.

In December 1977, Helen Tom, after accepting the role as the first doctor at Utopia, moved there and started work on health-service development. The people there had made it clear that a centralised service was not what they required; instead they had wanted a service that would support them in living the way they wanted to live. Helen and other non-Aboriginal people living and working with the people of Utopia were prepared to adapt the mode of service delivery to support this vision.

However, Helen was still employed by Congress and she was due six weeks of annual leave. Soon after commencing at Utopia she contacted me and asked whether I would be interested in moving out to Utopia to fill in for her during her absence. So, in January 1978 I found myself in Utopia. I travelled there the first time in a four-wheel-drive Toyota with two non-Aboriginal people also working at Utopia, Toly Sawenko and Julia Murray. Toly was an ex-teacher who was now providing administrative support for the Utopia people and Julia was working with women in developing an art industry. In later years Utopia would become a renowned centre for Aboriginal art.

On my arrival, Helen took me to some of the nearer small communities and introduced me around. At the time, the health-service staff consisted of Helen as the GP and a number of Aboriginal health workers. Administrative support was provided by Congress, as an interim measure, but once the service was established it was expected that the administrative function would be devolved to the local organisation.

Helen also introduced me to the work that was being done there. This included providing training and support for the Aboriginal health workers and ensuring that they had adequate medical supplies, as well as developing systems to ensure that the local health needs were met. It also involved frequent travel to the dispersed communities to provide the decentralised service that was required.

On the very first night that I was at Utopia there was a traditional ceremony with dancing and singing by the fire that went well into the night. I was entranced. I had found myself in another world.

Over the first few days I met other non-Aboriginal people living and working at Utopia. These included Jenny Green, who was working with Julia on the art project; Valentine Sawenko, Toly's brother, who provided maintenance support for various activities; Rod Horner, employed by DAA as the community advisor, and his wife Cusha. There was a primary school with a single teacher, Neil Bell, whom I had known at school in Melbourne and who was later to become a Labor Party member of the Northern Territory legislative assembly.

A week or so after I arrived, another non-Aboriginal worker returned from his Christmas leave. Tony Davies was a young engineer, a tall man with a ready smile and laugh, who installed and maintained the bores and windmills that supplied the water for each of the small camps scattered over the station. He was called by the local Aboriginal people El Punj, meaning 'tall man'. We were later to work together on the Pitjantjatjara homelands.

Another non-Aboriginal person I met was Roy Potter. Roy was a hard-bitten long-term Territorian and ex-stockman who had been in the Northern Territory since 1926. He lived with his Aboriginal wife Katie in a caravan and shack near a windmill at Goofy Bore, located on Utopia. Roy and his wife were dedicated to each other and had lived there for many years. Both had made compromises with their living arrangements. Roy had removed himself from white society and his wife had removed herself from being embedded in the Aboriginal community. However, they hospitably received any visitors,

Aboriginal or non-Aboriginal, and were always ready to provide a large mug of strong tea and good conversation.

After a couple of days of handover, Helen left on her annual leave and I worked as the locum GP. The work was challenging but I enjoyed it and developed a sense of satisfaction that I was working in a situation that had the potential to achieve significant gains for the local Aboriginal people.

I enjoyed working with the Aboriginal health workers. In particular, I remember Michael Ngwarraye and his wife Gloria Pitjara, who became my friends. Michael's brother, Kutadji, who was not a health worker, also became a friend and we spent a number of hours together in which Kutadji attempted to teach me the Anmatjerre language while telling me many stories about the life and history of the people of Utopia.

Since my first visit to Central Australia some years prior, the landscape in the area around Alice Springs, with its big blue sky, red earth, rocky outcrops and sun-bleached green foliage, had induced in me a strong emotional response. Whereas Alice Springs was dominated by the spectacular MacDonnell Ranges, parallel mountain ranges running east and west from Alice, the Utopia area was arid-zone subtropical savannah country, with some areas quite thickly wooded with mulga and eucalyptus trees. It was different country but, once again, I was drawn to it. There were many evenings when I sat outside my accommodation unit, sometimes alone and sometimes with company, after a hot and busy day, with the sun going down and casting a gentler light among the lengthening shadows. I understood why the place might be called Utopia. Sometimes, in the background, I would hear Valentine, an accomplished guitarist, playing his guitar and softly singing George Gershwin's 'Summertime'. It was summertime, and although the living might not best be described as easy, it was good.

As the days went past, I began to think that I would like to continue to do this kind of work, and spend more time in this wonderful kind of country. I wondered whether I should consider applying for a position with one of the two other remote Aboriginal community-controlled health services, which were likely to be commencing in the next few months, either at Papunya or in the Pitjantjatjara homelands in the border region of the Northern Territory, South Australia and Western Australia.

One day, a visitor arrived. Glendle Schrader was a man about my age, born and raised in the Midwest and west coast of the United States. He had come to Australia as an adventurous young traveller, and found employment with an Aboriginal arts and crafts organisation in Alice Springs and then had become the community advisor for the Aboriginal community of Pipalyatjara on the Pitjantjatjara lands in the north-west of South Australia. He was now undertaking work for the Pitjantjatjara Council, which had now been advised by the DAA that it would receive funding for its proposed Aboriginal community-controlled health service in that area. Glendle had been asked to work on the development strategy for the health service and had come to Utopia for research.

Glendle and I quickly became good friends. He stayed for two or three days, and I showed him around the area and explained how the health service was developing. We discussed the plans for the health service proposed for the Pitjantjatjara area. On one occasion, we visited Roy Potter and Katie, and spent a couple of hours drinking tea with them and talking. We discussed what kind of person should be recruited, and agreed that the right person would be somebody who not only knows the theory but knows how to put it in practice. Roy's comment was that 'theory without practice is ratshit'.

By the time Glendle left Utopia I had decided that I would apply for the position as medical officer with the incipient health service on the Pitjantjatjara lands. Glendle soon sent me the Pitjantjatjara Council's recruitment advertisement in the mail; they were seeking a medical officer, a nurse and an administrator to set up their new health service. The ad included a note that read, 'in the words of the great bush philosopher Roy Potter, theory without practice is ratshit'. The newspaper, however, had changed the term 'ratshit' to 'rat faeces'. With some reticence I considered applying. I was not convinced that I had enough experience—neither in theory nor in practice. However by this stage I wanted to continue the trajectory on which I had found myself.

After six weeks, Helen returned to Utopia and I soon returned to Alice Springs to start work again in the Congress clinic.

Health services at Utopia continued to develop. It was originally named Angarappa Health Service, after the land on which the main clinic was based.

Later, in recognition of the fact that the health service covered a large area of dispersed communities, it was named the Urapuntja Health Service, after the Alyawarr name for the Sandover River, the usually dry riverbed that runs through Utopia Station.

Helen continued to work as doctor for the health service. After a couple of years she left and was replaced by Toby McLeay, who stayed there as the Urapuntja GP for eight years. In the first year of operation, Congress transferred the administration to the health service itself, so Toly Sawenko, already living at Utopia, was employed as the administrator, and continued in the role for a number of years. It also became clear that nursing support was required, so initially one, and later two, nurses were employed. Several nurses who worked at Utopia in the early years, including Annie Dixon (with whom I later worked at Kintore), Pip Duncan and Lizzie McLeay, continued working for many years in Aboriginal primary healthcare. The service continued to employ Aboriginal health workers in most of the small communities, which with the support of the health service, continued to exist.

Bureaucratic pressures to centralise services and facilities persisted. In 1990 the Aboriginal and Torres Strait Islander Commission (ATSIC), which had been established by the federal Labor Government, ostensibly as a vehicle for self-determination, applied pressure for Urapuntja Health Service to establish a base at the site of the central store, effectively establishing a large service centre. With the support of their health service, the community resisted and once again were successful in maintaining a dispersed structure. From its inception, Urapuntja Health Service has supported this structure, not only in the way it has provided healthcare through outreach visits, but by advocating for the community.

In 1994 the largest community serviced by Urapuntja Health Service, Ampilatwatja, separated to establish its own health centre. This was achieved by a man from Ampilatwatja who was at the time chairperson of the local ATSIC Regional Council, and hence had access to the instruments of power within ATSIC. The Ampilatwatja Health Centre now employs a doctor and nurse and provides a service for a population of about 400 people, while Urapuntja Health Service employs a doctor, two nurses and an administrator, as well as several Aboriginal health workers, and provides a service to a widely dispersed population of about 600 people.

A health survey conducted at Utopia in the mid-1980s showed that the people of the Utopia area had more favourable health outcomes with respect to mortality, hospitalisation, hypertension, diabetes and injuries than those people living in larger settlements.[5] A follow-up survey ten years later showed that better health outcomes persisted: there was lower overall mortality, cardio-vascular disease mortality, and hospitalisation for cardio-vascular disease compared to the statistics for the Aboriginal population of the Northern Territory as a whole.[6] The authors attributed these benefits at least in part to the nature of Urapuntja Health Service, 'which provided regular outreach to outstation communities, as well as the decentralised mode of outstation living (with its attendant benefits for physical activity, diet and limited access to alcohol), and social factors, including connectedness to culture, family and land, and opportunities for self-determination'.

2

The Pitjantjatjara and Ngaanyatjarra homelands

I had heard about the Pitjantjatjara people since childhood. Growing up as the son of a Presbyterian minister, I often heard about the Presbyterian mission at Ernabella and the Pitjantjatjara people in South Australia, so the idea of living and working with Pitjantjatjara people had a special appeal for me. I had also heard about the Pitjantjatjara people during my stay at Utopia when one day Michael Ngwarraye informed me, with concern written on his face, that Pitjantjatjara Red Ochre lawmen were in the area. He said that the Pitjantjatjara people had strong traditional law with severe punishment, even death, for contraventions of the law. Consequently, the whole camp at Three Bores on Utopia where I was living went into hiding. The lawmen did not arrive; it appeared that it was just a rumour. However, the level of awe and respect with which the Pitjantjatjara people were held by the very traditional Alyawarr and Anmatyerre people impressed me. A year or two later I was to learn that among all traditional groups there was often a similar fear and respect for other groups from further afield: there was similar nervous anticipation among Pitjantjatjara and Ngaanyatjarra people in 1978 when the 'Strelley mob' were bringing a Rain-Making ceremony and their 'strong Law'. It appeared that people with a strong hold on traditional law and who were based at a far enough distance to mean that there was not regular contact, often had an exaggerated reputation for the severity with which the distant group maintained the law. In all these areas the law was strong, but usually not as severely punitive as rumour suggested.

Early contact history

The Pitjantjatjara, Yankunytjatjara and Ngaanyatjarra people come from desert country south of the Alice Springs area. The MacDonnell Ranges and associated smaller ranges extend east and west of Alice Springs. To the south of the ranges is an extensive, generally flat, depression with large salt lakes, the largest being Lake Amadeus, and with occasional rocky outcrops, particularly the spectacular Uluru (Ayers Rock) and Kata Tjuta (the Olgas). Further south, around the border of what is now the Northern Territory and South Australia and extending into Western Australia, is another large system of ranges running mostly east–west, and extending further west than the MacDonnells. Around these ranges—the Everard, Musgrave, Mann, Tomkinson, Petermann, Rawlinson, Blackstone, Jamieson and Warburton ranges—and in the surrounding plains, extending north to include Uluru and Kata Tjuta and south into spinifex country, is the country of the Pitjantjatjara, Yankunytjatjara and Ngaanyatjarra people. These terms used to identify them refer to mutually intelligible linguistic variations of the Western Desert languages, which are used in different parts of their country. They all refer to themselves as *Anangu*, or *Yarnangu*, meaning 'the people'.

The first non-Aboriginal explorations into the Pitjantjatjara and Ngaanyatjarra homelands were in 1873, when two separate expeditions, one led by William Gosse and the other by Ernest Giles, attempted to cross from the Overland Telegraph Line to the west coast. Gosse set off from Alice Springs, travelling south-west, where he 'discovered' and named Ayers Rock and Mount Olga, and then travelled through the Mann and Tomkinson ranges and on to the Cavenagh Range south-west from Blackstone Range. Attempts to travel further west were stymied by the apparently waterless desert, and the expedition returned to the Northern Territory. Giles and his team travelled from Peake Telegraph Station, near Anna Creek in South Australia, through the Musgrave, Mann and Tomkinson ranges as far as Warburton Range, and then north to Rawlinson Ranges, from where they struck out into desert country that Giles named Gibson's Desert after one of his men who died of thirst, also leading to an abandonment of the attempt to reach the west coast. In 1875 John Forrest travelled in the other direction, from the west coast across Gibson's Desert to the Warburton Range, and then followed the tracks of Gosse and Giles through the Tomkinson and Mann ranges to the Overland Telegraph Line. On these expeditions, the explorers reported 'skirmishes' with *Anangu*.

The next wave of non-Aboriginal intrusion into the homelands followed the discovery of gold in Western Australia at Coolgardie in 1892 and Kalgoorlie in 1893. A number of prospectors set off for the West Australian goldfields from Oodnadatta in South Australia or from Alice Springs, prospecting as they went. In 1894 a party led by William Earle, having travelled through the Musgrave and Tomkinson ranges, claimed to have found a rich gold reef near Mount Davies in the Tomkinson Range, and brought back a sample of gold-bearing quartz that he said came from a cave within the reef. This claim led to expeditions into the area looking for 'Earle's Cave of Gold'. On some of these expeditions, *Anangu* sometimes helped prospectors to find water, but also, particularly as time went on, conflict and sometimes spearings and deaths occurred. These incidents led to the *Anangu* from the area gaining a reputation for being hostile and dangerous, and in the early years of the twentieth century the intrusions by prospectors declined.[1]

In 1920 the West Australian government gazetted a large area of Ngaanyatjarra lands, including the Warburton, Rawlinson and Blackstone ranges, as an Aboriginal reserve, and in 1921 the South Australian government did the same for the Pitjantjatjara and Yankunytjatjara lands in the north-west of the state, and the Australian Government declared a reserve in the Pitjantjatjara country in the south-west corner of the Northern Territory. The three adjoining reserves together formed the Central Australian Aboriginal Reserves. In theory, non-Aboriginal people now had to apply to the state or Commonwealth authorities for permission to enter, but there was little policing of this.

While the intrusion of prospectors had declined by the 1920s, there were by this time other non-Aboriginal people with quite different motivations for entering the reserves—'doggers' and missionaries. The doggers, non-Aboriginal people mostly based in Alice Springs, Oodnadatta or Laverton, were usually experienced bushmen who travelled extensively through the area trading flour, sugar, tobacco and clothes with *Anangu* for dingo scalps, for which there was a government bounty. Doggers sometimes developed good relations with *Anangu*, and many had Aboriginal wives. Missionaries travelled from Oodnadatta through the Musgrave and Tomkinson ranges in 1926, 1928 and 1929, hoping to convert the desert people to Christianity. In the early 1930s, one of these missionaries, Bill Wade, known as *Aliluya-nya* to the *Anangu* due to his frequent exclamation of 'Halleluiah!', travelled from Mount Margaret Mission in Western Australia to the Warburton Range to start the United Aborigines Mission at Warburton.[2]

According to anthropologist A.P. Elkin, who undertook fieldwork in the area in 1930, while non-Aboriginal people were encroaching on their country, a severe drought in the 1920s had caused some *Anangu* people to drift away from their country towards areas of non-Aboriginal settlement. Elkin thought that over time the desert people 'lose their desire to return to their own comparatively inhospitable country'.[3] I believe Elkin underestimated the attachment to country that drew people back to their homelands, and he did not perhaps sufficiently appreciate that movements in and out of the Western Desert had probably always occurred in times of drought—a movement that led Peter Sutton to liken the Western Desert to a 'pulsating heart'. However, concern about the deleterious effect on *Anangu* of contact with non-Aboriginal people on the settlement fringes, expressed by people such as the Scottish-born Adelaide-based surgeon Charles Duguid, was one of the motivating factors that led to the establishment of the Ernabella Mission.

The Ernabella Mission

In the 1930s, Duguid undertook three extensive trips into the outback of South Australia and the Northern Territory, and this opened his eyes to the plight of Aboriginal people and the pervasive discrimination that existed in the areas of non-Aboriginal settlement throughout the outback. Duguid was active in the Presbyterian Church and became the first lay moderator of that church in South Australia in 1935. He used this position to assist him in his advocacy for the rights of Aboriginal people. In his inaugural address as moderator, he stated that, 'My plan is for the Presbyterian Church to start a mission in the vicinity of the Musgrave Ranges.' Although in his autobiography, Duguid implied that his idea for a mission arose from his experiences when visiting the Musgrave Ranges, his biographer Rani Kerin points out that the speech in which the mission was proposed was given before he travelled to the area. Rather, it appears that he was influenced by the ideas of, among others, A.P. Elkin. Elkin was a professor of anthropology at Sydney University and an ordained Anglican priest. He had been advocating reform of missions in the outback where Aboriginal people were still living a hunter-gatherer lifestyle, to be run by missionaries with 'training in social anthropology … the functional and comparative study of religion, the study of population-problems, cultural contact and mission methods … [and] medicine'.[4] With this in mind, Duguid initially proposed the establishment of a 'Christian anthropological mission' but, reflecting his medical interests, he subsequently decided on a 'medical mission'.

While he had not at this stage visited Pitjantjatjara lands, Duguid's vision for a medical mission was influenced by his experiences during a journey he made to Alice Springs in 1934. He had formed an impression that Aboriginal people, prior to contact, had led healthy lives. This impression was consistent with the historical record of early contact, and also with my own experience later (which will be discussed in chapter 6). Duguid saw evidence that the health status of Aboriginal people who have been living a traditional hunter-gatherer lifestyle was adversely affected by contact. He envisaged a medical hostel on the Pitjantjatjara lands, staffed by two nurses 'trained in infant welfare and general medical work', as well as a 'medical missionary patrol', which would involve a doctor travelling out to provide medical care while allowing Aboriginal people to remain on their homelands. 'My idea,' he wrote, 'is to have a fixed point, out near the Reserve, and a patrol (medical) from it.'[5]

After he visited the Pitjantjatjara and Yankunytjatjara lands in the northwest of South Australia in June 1935, Duguid proposed that the Presbyterian Church should purchase the outermost sheep station, named Ernabella, so as to establish the Ernabella Mission on the lands. In the following year, the general assembly of the Presbyterian Church agreed to establish the mission and negotiations to buy Ernabella were completed in April 1937. The Presbyterian Board of Missions sent Rev. J.R.B. Love, an experienced missionary, and Dr Lewis J. Balfour to report on the situation. Balfour concluded that the health of the Aboriginal people was generally good and that a full-time doctor was not needed. The emphasis changed from being a medical mission to that of being a 'buffer' between the people still leading a traditional lifestyle and the encroaching doggers, pastoralists and other non-Aboriginal people, who were gradually moving into the area.

Duguid's advocacy for the rights of Aboriginal people brought him into conflict with many establishment figures, including some in his own church. The Presbyterian Church had a considerable amount of money available in the Smith of Dunesk bequest, which was meant to be for 'the education and evangelisation of the Aborigines of South Australia'. However, until Duguid intervened, the money was being used for the Australian Inland Mission (AIM), founded by the Rev Dr John Flynn, which was exclusively for non-Aboriginal people living in the outback, and which had nothing to do with Aboriginal people. Flynn is better known as the founder of the Royal Flying Doctor Service, which was originally a part of the AIM but later became an independent organisation. After Duguid's journey to Alice Springs in 1934, when he found that the AIM medical facility refused to treat Aboriginal people, he met with Flynn. According to Duguid, Flynn told him that 'the AIM is only for white people—you are only wasting your time among so many damned, dirty niggers'.[6] Despite Flynn's opposition, Duguid was able to get some of the Smith of Dunesk bequest diverted to the Ernabella Mission.

I had the privilege of meeting Charles Duguid in 1978. He told me that he had insisted on four principles that the mission should follow: first, that the culture of the local people should be respected; second, that all non-Aboriginal people working at the mission should learn to speak Pitjantjatjara as this would be the language used for mission activities; third, that there was to be no coercion, including religious coercion; and finally that mission staff should work towards handing over control of the mission to local people as soon as was feasible. This made it a progressive institution for its time. The mission was actually on Yankunytjatjara country but the majority of people who used it came from nearby Pitjantjatjara country to the west, and the Pitjantjatjara language became the language studied and learnt by the missionaries. When I met Duguid in 1978, he was very interested in and supportive of the plans for the Pitjantjatjara Homelands Health Service. He suggested that this was, in a way, the realisation of his original vision for a 'medical patrol', forty years earlier.

The Warburton Ranges Mission

Further west from the Pitjantjatjara lands, from which people moved into the Ernabella Mission, the country merged into Ngaanyatjarra country. Ngaanyatjarra-speaking people come from the country along the ranges extending west from the Tomkinson Ranges, along the Blackstone and Jamieson Ranges and further on to the Warburton Ranges and north around the Rawlinson Ranges. Ngaanyatjarra people refer to themselves as *Yarnangu*, rather than *Anangu*, as used by the Pitjantjatjara and Yankunytjatjara people.

The Ngaanyatjarra people had links with the Warburton Mission, which was established by a non-denominational evangelical Christian group called the United Aborigines Mission (UAM) in 1933, under the leadership of Bill Wade (or '*Aliluya-nya*'), initially as an outpost of the Mount Margaret Mission. In 1937 it became a separate mission. The Warburton Mission was always in a more financially precarious position compared to the Ernabella Mission. In comparing the two missions, Brooks and Plant made the following observation:

> It is perhaps worth noting for comparative purposes that unlike their counterparts at Ernabella, the Warburton missionaries had no middle- or upper-class links in metropolitan society, and government correspondence shows that as people they were viewed by many bureaucrats almost with contempt, and certainly with none of the respect that someone like Dr. Duguid of the Ernabella Mission commanded in Adelaide circles.[7]

Not only did the Warburton Mission lack the institutional support of a large mainstream Christian denomination but there was also less support from the state government. It appears the West Australian government was always hostile to the mission and refused to assist it in any way for about the first twenty years of its existence. This led to a situation where the Ngaanyatjarra people continued to spend significant amounts of time on their country as well as at the mission, as *Yarnangu* were encouraged to hunt dingoes to make money by dingo-scalp trading in order to support the mission.

It appears that for quite different reasons, the missions at Ernabella and Warburton played an enabling role in allowing Aboriginal people to maintain connection with their homelands away from the mission sites. Ernabella Mission had a relatively enlightened attitude to Pitjantjatjara culture and actively supported *Anangu* to make trips back to their country and maintain their language and culture. The Warburton missionaries, on the other hand, believed that Aboriginal people should adopt Christianity exclusively, and this meant rejecting the old ways. Children were housed in dormitories and discouraged from speaking Ngaanyatjarra. However, financial pressures meant the mission supported opportunities to spend considerable amounts of time in the homelands areas. Also there was always a degree of resistance to efforts to interfere with cultural activities, and to avoid mission interference these activities were more likely to happen on the homelands. Both South Australian and West Australian governments supported a policy of assimilation that entailed a transition from Aboriginal to 'western' culture, but the Ernabella Mission resisted these policies and Warburton was too far away from government interference.

The Cold War and the Western Desert

In the 1950s and 60s, there were a number of motivations that led people to spend increasing amounts of time at Ernabella and Warburton missions, including the availability of food, water and basic medical care. After World War II, geo-political developments meant more people were encouraged to leave their homelands and gravitate towards Ernabella and Warburton missions, and to other missions and settlements around the Western Desert. The British government, having observed with concern the development of German V1 flying bombs and the V2 rockets used against Britain during the war, and the development and use of nuclear weapons by the US, wanted to develop similar weaponry. Australia with its vast outback seemed the ideal place to develop a testing program. As a result, the British and Australian governments entered into a joint partnership, with the Australians allocating an immense area in South Australia and Western Australia as a rocket range. There was, of course, no consultation with Aboriginal people who lived in their desert homelands affected by this development. The township of Woomera, 450 kilometres north of Adelaide, was the base for the rocket tests, but the area in which the planned long-range rockets might fall extended thousands of kilometres through the Western Desert to the north-west as far as the West Australian coast. The Woomera Prohibited Area occupied one-eighth of South Australia.

The surveyor for the rocket range was the bushman and raconteur Len Beadell, who established the 'centre-line', a virtual 3900-kilometre corridor across Aboriginal homelands in the Musgrave and Rawlinson ranges, the Gibson Desert and the Great Sandy Desert. In 1991 he said that the 'centre-line, although I didn't know it at the time, was going to govern the whole of the future of Central Australia forever'.[8] It certainly had an impact on the Western Desert people.

The Anglo-Australian negotiations to develop the Weapons Research Establishment (WRE) were initially held in secret but some information, including rumours that testing atomic weapons may be included, was leaked to the media. In 1946 the Adelaide *Advertiser* published around thirty letters and editorials on the subject, many expressing opposition. In the immediate postwar years there was some opposition for pacifist reasons, but there was also concern about the impact on the Aboriginal people living in the outback. Charles Duguid emerged as, once again, a passionate advocate for the Aboriginal people and an opponent to the activities of the WRE. He argued:

> What curse is on a civilisation, that, while the anguish of millions is still in our hearts, it should already be trying to devise a method of wiping out whole nations … Having driven [the Aboriginal people] from all the good country are we now to sit back and allow them to be treated as human guinea pigs in atomic tests?[9]

Duguid tried for some time to learn more about the plans for the WRE. When he was eventually able to see a map, he was very concerned to find that the firing range went right across the South Australian North-west Reserve and the West Australian Central Reserve—the homelands of the Pitjantjatjara and Ngaanyatjarra people—and then across the Great Sandy Desert (the homelands of the Manyjilyjarra people), as far as the Eighty-mile Beach on the Indian Ocean between Port Hedland and Broome. In a letter to the newspaper on 7 August 1946, Duguid wrote, 'I refuse to see them and their country offered in sacrifice to the moloch of militarism.'[10] On the same day, he was the principal speaker at the first protest against the WRE, organised by a social reform group called 'Common Cause'.

According to a secret Army intelligence report, reflecting the hysterical anti-Communism of the early Cold War years, Common Cause had been infiltrated by communists and the protesters were either duped or were fellow travellers:

> Although not officially affiliated with the Australian Communist Party Common Cause is known to have many Communist supporters in its midst ... There are many close ties between the two organisations ... Communist interest in the aborigine is evidenced in reports from Western Australia where a Communist agitator DW McLEOD was recently jailed for inciting the aborigines to strike. The true reason for Communist interest in the aborigine can be seen in the following note from McLeod to an unknown addressee that was produced during McLeod's trial: 'Each and every one of these natives are potential communists.'[11]

Charles Duguid was not a communist. In fact, he had anti-communist leanings and in 1961 he resigned as president of the Aborigines Advancement League of South Australia due to what he described as the 'communistic tendencies displayed by several members'. It is interesting, however, that in the Cold War paranoia of the time, he was compared to Don McLeod, who was for three years a member of the Communist Party, and with whom I would later work (see chapter 4). Common Cause was also not a communist organisation, although there were three members who were also members of the Communist Party. The fact was that in the 1940s, churches and the Communist Party where the main institutions advocating for the rights of Aboriginal people, and sometimes this made for strange bedfellows.

In October 1946, when it was becoming clear to Duguid that the government was firmly committed to the establishment of the rocket range, he proposed moving the firing point from Woomera to Eucla on the Great Australian Bight. This would have allowed for the potential rocket-landing sites to avoid the South Australian North-west Reserve and the West Australian Central Reserve. If this proposal had been followed, it might have had a much greater impact on the Spinifex people in the Great Victoria Desert north of Eucla, with whom I later worked. As it happened, Duguid's proposal was ignored.

However, in early 1947, the government recognised that it could not totally ignore someone of Charles Duguid's stature, and he and the anthropologist Donald Thomson were invited to present their case to the federal government's Guided Projectiles Committee. Duguid stated, with Thomson's support, that the problem was not the danger from the rockets themselves but from the impact of inevitable encroachment into the lives and culture of the Aboriginal people. The committee, however, took the attitude that 'detribalisation' was inevitable and that the rocket testing should proceed. They agreed, however, to appoint 'native patrol officers' to be responsible for the welfare of the Aboriginal people affected by the weapon tests.

Maralinga

The British were not only interested in developing long-range rockets but also in developing their own nuclear-weapons capability. In 1946 the US Government passed the McMahon Act, which forbade co-operation with any foreign powers, including US allies such as Great Britain, in the development of nuclear capacity for both peaceful and military purposes. Britain decided to establish its own nuclear program and approached then prime minister Robert Menzies for co-operation with a testing program. The Anglophile Menzies agreed, without even discussing it with his cabinet.

The first atom-bomb test conducted by the British in Australia occurred on the Monte Bello Islands, off the Pilbara coast of Western Australia, in 1952. A report by a British scientist on the potential impact on the human population, which used the *Encyclopaedia Britannica* as its main source, noted that there was a population of 715 people living within 240 kilometres of the Monte Bello Islands, 'excluding full-blooded Aboriginals, for whom no statistics are available'. A subsequent royal commission was able to establish from West Australian government records that there were about 1700 Aboriginal people living in the Pilbara at the time of the test.[12]

With the development of the Woomera Range, and the allocation of a large tract of land to the WRE, it was decided that this area could also be used for atom-bomb testing. A site in spinifex country south of the Everard Ranges, named Emu Field by Len Beadell, was identified for the initial tests on the Australian mainland. Emu Field is on the southern edge of Yankunytjatjara homelands, less than 200 kilometres from Wallatinna, where a number of *Anangu* were living. Two tests, Totem 1 and Totem 2, were conducted at Emu Field in October 1953. After the first, in which a 9.1-kilotonne atomic device was detonated from a 30-metre tower, *Anangu* at Wallatinna reported a black mist settling over the area, causing eye and skin irritation, vomiting and diarrhoea. Yami Lester, a blind Yankunytjatjara elder who died in 2017, recalled this event and attributed his blindness to the black mist.

Soon, it was decided that another site in South Australia was needed for nuclear tests, not due to concern for *Anangu* but because Emu Field was deemed too remote. Len Beadell identified a site closer to the Transcontinental Railway, west from Woomera, within the rocket range area in South Australia but near the West Australian border. This was called Maralinga, which means 'thunder' in Garik, an extinct Aboriginal language from the Cobourg Peninsula in the Top End of the Northern Territory. An Aboriginal mission at Ooldea, not far south from Maralinga, had recently closed. While some have suggested that it was the imminent nuclear testing at Maralinga that led to the closure, it was in fact worsening environmental conditions, particularly a diminishing water supply due to excessive use by the steam trains on the Transcontinental Railway, which led to the decision by the South Australian Aborigines' Protection Board to close Ooldea Mission in 1952.

Ooldea was a significant Aboriginal site, a permanent source of water that had always been a meeting-place for desert Aboriginal people in times of drought. It had become more settled when the Transcontinental Railway was constructed in 1912–17. It had been the base of the eccentric anthropologist Daisy Bates from 1918 to 1934 and, in 1933, the United Aborigines Mission was invited by the government to establish a mission there. When the Ooldea Mission closed in 1952, some of the residents moved westward to Cundeelee Mission, but the majority were moved further south to a government-owned sheep station named Yalata, where a Lutheran mission was established. Ooldea, Cundeelee, Yalata and the impact of the nuclear tests on the Spinifex people will be discussed further in chapter 6.

While Maralinga was being developed, the British were keen to continue testing. The agreement between the British and Australian governments excluded the possibility of testing a thermo-nuclear weapon (hydrogen bomb) but the British government wanted to test a device that could operate as a trigger for an H-Bomb. For this, they returned to the Monte Bello Islands for two tests in May and June of 1956. The second test was the largest nuclear device ever detonated in Australia, although the exact size continues to be shrouded in secrecy: the British government claimed it was 60 kilotonnes, but some commentators have suggested that it was as large as 98 kilotonnes. The mushroom cloud spread east across the entire Australian continent, attracting media attention and causing significant public concern.

These public concerns alerted those developing Maralinga to the need for information about meteorological conditions and prevailing winds, in order to minimise the risk of radioactive fallout from atom-bomb testing. This led to another government intervention in the Western Desert in 1955, which also interfered with Aboriginal people's access to their homelands and sacred sites. In July of that year the British Atomic Weapons Research Establishment decided it should establish a meteorological station. The Meteorological Branch of the Australian Department of the Interior excised a large area of land in Ngaanyatjarra country in the Rawlinson Ranges for the Giles Weather Station, again without any attempts at consultation with the traditional owners. The British government provided the initial funding for the weather station. The area in the Rawlinson Ranges was chosen because there was a source of ground water readily available—Sladen Waters, which was of course also important to the Ngaanyatjarra people as a water-source, as well as its proximity to sacred sites.

The appointment of native patrol officers that had been agreed to at the meeting of the Guided Projectiles Committee in 1947, when Duguid and Thomson had expressed their concerns, at least gave the appearance that an attempt was being made to minimise the risks of the Woomera rockets and the Maralinga nuclear tests on local Aboriginal people. In reality, it would never be sufficient, although it was not through want of trying by the individuals concerned. The first patrol officer, appointed in November 1947, was Walter MacDougall, a tall redheaded man who had previously worked at Ernabella and spoke Pitjantjatjara. He was based at Woomera but was constantly travelling through the Aboriginal areas affected by the rocket range and, later, the Maralinga atom bomb testing site.

I would hear stories about Walter MacDougall years later, when I was living and working with Pitjantjatjara people. They regarded him well and said he knew many of their stories and sites but always kept them to himself. He was known to the bureaucracy as an advocate for the rights of Aboriginal people. MacDougall's reports, which were kept in a confidential file by the government, were critical of the government for its neglect of the needs and safety of Aboriginal people. The chief scientist of Woomera, Alan Butement, described MacDougall as having a 'lamentable lack of balance (in) placing the affairs of a handful of natives above the British Commonwealth of Nations'.[13]

MacDougall was appointed 'Protector of Aborigines' by the South Australian government in November 1947, allowing him to be in the presence of Aboriginal people within Aboriginal Reserves without breaking the Crimes Act; he was later awarded the same authority in Western Australia. He continued in this role until he retired in 1972. He travelled extensively throughout the area potentially affected by the Maralinga nuclear tests and in 1955 estimated that there were about 1,000 Aboriginal people in the area. As we shall see in chapter 6, he was mistaken in considering the Spinifex country west of Maralinga uninhabited.

MacDougall campaigned against the siting of the Giles Weather Station in the Rawlinson Ranges. In a memo written in 1956, he claimed:

> The result ... is certain to be a degradation from self-respecting communities to pathetic and useless parasites—it has happened so often before that surely we Australians have learnt our lesson ... [the land] belongs to the tribe ... However we propose to take it away from them and give nothing in return—we might as well declare war on them and make a job of it.[14]

The second patrol officer appointed by the Australian Government, although not until 1956, was Robert Macaulay. Macaulay, only 23 years of age, was a recent anthropology graduate from Sydney University with no practical experience with Aboriginal people or knowledge of an Aboriginal language. Macaulay was based at the Giles Weather Station and he continued working as patrol officer for nine years until 1965, when he was replaced by Bob Verburgt, who had previously worked as a bores and stock overseer at the government settlement of Amata on the Pitjantjatjara lands.

The patrol officers' task of finding Aboriginal people over such a vast area of South Australia and Western Australia seemed an impossible one. It was, however, facilitated by an extensive network of bush tracks built by Len Beadell for the Woomera Rocket Range to allow access to the desert so as to retrieve rockets after firing. These roads were used in the early years to assist with the removal of Aboriginal people from their homelands to missions and settlements but would later prove useful when people started moving back to reoccupy their homelands. Even with the roads, however, the patrol officers' ability to find all those Aboriginal people who would be potentially affected by the tests was doomed to failure. As we shall see in chapter 6, one family was found in 1957 close to a crater left by a nuclear test a few months earlier. The patrol officers were also hampered by inadequate supplies. On the day of the first Maralinga test, Macaulay sent a cable from Giles: 'Unable to satisfy myself no natives south of mentioned line. Have not been there. Unable to penetrate without vehicle and radio ... Shall remain in Giles until vehicle and instructions arrive.'[15] The appointment of the patrol officers, it seems, was more of a public relations exercise and a sop to critics such as Duguid rather than a genuine attempt to ensure that the tests did not cause harm to Aboriginal people. A secret cable from Woomera in 1956 read '[MacDougall] is an insurance policy ensuring that the Department [of Supply] does not come under public criticism for interfering with tribal natives.'[16]

Seven nuclear-bomb tests were carried out at Maralinga in 1956 and 1957. After the seventh and final test, international concerns about the spread of radioactive fallout led to an agreement in 1958 by the then three nuclear powers—the US, the USSR and Britain—to implement a moratorium on atmospheric nuclear-weapons testing. Thus, the so-called 'major trials' came to an end. However, 'minor trials' continued until 1963 with innocent-sounding names like Kittens, Tims, Rats, Vixen A and Vixen B. These 'minor' trials did not involve the detonation of atom bombs, but they were deadly (and secretive) experiments that led to far more radioactive contamination of the Maralinga area than the major trials. The Vixen B trials, at the Taranaki site on Maralinga, ran for three years and involved blowing up plutonium-239 (with a half-life of 24,000 years) with conventional explosives, leading to the wide spread of plutonium.

The moratorium on atmospheric testing only lasted three years until the Soviet Union resumed testing in 1961 but, two years later, the Partial Test Ban Treaty banned atmospheric tests of nuclear weapons by all signatories, which included the UK and Australia. In preparation for a ban on atmospheric testing, the British had been investigating their options for underground testing. There were no sites within a 300-kilometre radius of Maralinga that were geologically suitable, but the place that appeared most suitable was Watarru (Mount Lindsay) on the Pitjantjatjara homelands, south of the Tomkinson Range and 400 kilometres north of Maralinga. The fact that it was on an Aboriginal Reserve was considered an inconvenience that could be overcome, but increasing public concerns about the nuclear arms race was also an issue. The British High Commission in Canberra cabled London: 'Some notice in gazette will be legally necessary before any excavation took place and there would be problem in devising a suitable cover story.'[17] The area around Watarru has sites of significant importance for *Anangu* but this was apparently not a consideration in itself. The Menzies government, concerned about its re-election chances, asked the British to delay any decisions about an underground site until after the next federal election in 1958. While awaiting the outcome of the election, the British reached an agreement with the US Government to use the underground testing sites in Nevada, and so Watarru remained intact.

I visited Watarru with some *Anangu* in 1978, and they showed me a site where, they said, MacDougall had established a base with a small hut. I was not aware at the time, and I doubt that my *Anangu* friends were aware, that this was the place where there had been discussions about underground nuclear-weapons testing about twenty years earlier. MacDougall had spent some time at Watarru with his fellow native patrol officer Robert Macaulay, the anthropologist Norman Tindale, and some Pitjantjatjara guides, in 1957. It is possible that MacDougall and his colleagues were visiting Watarru to survey the area in order to contribute to plans for the underground test site, but there is no evidence for this, and given MacDougall's strong advocacy for the rights of Aboriginal people, it is likely that he would have objected to the proposal. The hut that I had been told MacDougall had used may have been connected with a 'mobile weather station' that was used to augment information from Giles about weather patterns prior to the nuclear tests. In 1963 MacDougall visited Watarru and complained about beer cans and other rubbish around the hut, apparently left by Maralinga personnel for whom the area had become a popular recreation site. It would have been a long way to travel for recreation from Maralinga to Mount Lindsay, 400 kilometres over a rough bush track, but it is a particularly scenic area.

The 10-year agreement allowing the British to use Maralinga was not renewed when it expired in 1966. This ended the testing of nuclear devices at Maralinga but not the residual radioactive contamination. According to the terms of the agreement, the British government was obliged to clean up what had been left behind, a task that many allege was never adequately completed.

There was a flurry of external interest in the Warburton area around 1956 and 1957. After the Australian Government announced the pending nuclear-bomb tests at Maralinga, a West Australian politician, Bill Grayden, sought reassurances from the Australian Government that Aboriginal people in the Warburton area would not be adversely affected. Not being reassured, he then called for a parliamentary select committee to inquire into the health and wellbeing of, and future plans for, the Aboriginal people in the Warburton Reserve. The select committee, with Grayden as chairman, undertook an expedition to the area. While at Warburton, a group of nineteen Aboriginal people arrived in a 'starving and emaciated condition' from the country north of the Rawlinson Ranges. They may have been Pintupi people from their country in the Gibson Desert. From this and other experiences the select committee concluded that the 'the plight of the Aborigines in the Warburton-Laverton area is deplorable in the extreme'.[18]

The report made a number of recommendations, including establishing a pastoral industry at Warburton, and proposed that the Australian Government (which at that time, prior to the 1967 referendum, did not have constitutional responsibility for Aboriginal affairs, but had nonetheless affected the lives of Aboriginal people in the area by the excision of land for the Maralinga tests and the Giles Weather Station) should contribute funds to implement the recommendations. The reports received media attention across Australia and, in early 1957, the media mogul Rupert Murdoch—at that time the young publisher of the Adelaide *News* and the Perth weekly *Sunday Times* with a much smaller media empire than today—flew to the area and published his findings in his newspapers. He claimed that Grayden's report was 'hopelessly exaggerated' and that in fact Aboriginal people 'had never enjoyed better conditions'.[19] Murdoch's *Sunday Times* in Perth accused Grayden of providing ammunition for 'Communists and colour-conscious fanatics in our near North and at the United Nations ... to smear the good name of this country'.[20]

Other reports, including one by the anthropologists Ronald and Catherine Berndt, and a report of a medical survey led by the West Australian Deputy Commissioner of Public Health, W.S. Davidson, also suggested the situation was not as dire as that portrayed in the select committee report. The Commonwealth showed no interest in contributing funds, the media lost interest and the Ngaanyatjarra people, the majority of whom were unaware that they had been the subject of controversy, returned to the *status quo ante* of being ignored by most of Australia.

Grayden was no doubt well meaning. He may have overstated his case concerning the hardship suffered by Aboriginal people in the area but, despite Murdoch's somewhat fatuous statement that they 'had never known better conditions', there was a severe drought in Central Australia in the late 1950s, and Grayden cited a report in which Charles Duguid attributed an increase in infant deaths in Ernabella in 1957 to the drought.[21]

The select committee's recommendations, if implemented, would have brought more resources to the area. One of Grayden's few supporters was H.E. Green, the superintendent of the Warburton Mission, who presumably hoped that the days of financial hardship for the mission might be ending. More resources, however, can be a mixed blessing. A pastoral property on the mission may have led to meaningful employment but, on the other hand, without sufficient support in such a remote location, it may not have been successful and would have damaged the fragile ecology of the region. The select committee did appear to have had one beneficial effect: at the time of the report there were plans to take all the children away from the families in the Warburton area and relocate them to dormitories in Cosmo Newberry Mission. Grayden's committee opposed this plan for humanitarian reasons and the plan did not go ahead.

This episode, as described by Grayden, foreshadowed some aspects of Aboriginal affairs to come. This was an early example of state and federal governments disagreeing as to which jurisdiction had the funding responsibilities, an issue that continues to this day. It was also one of the first forays of Rupert Murdoch into Aboriginal affairs: half a century later, his newspapers continue to play a significant role.

Occupying the homelands

Despite the pressures from the Australian Government for people to leave their homelands and settle in missions, Pitjantjatjara and Ngaanyatjarra people continued to move throughout their homelands west of Ernabella and east of Warburton; this was not opposed by either mission. The Ngaanyatjarra people with links to the Warburton Mission maintained connections with their land to the west and north of Warburton. This was facilitated in the 1950s by mining activity in the Blackstone Ranges and at Wingellina, which led to an ongoing availability of windmill-pumped borewater; relations between Aboriginal people and miners were sometimes tense but generally accommodating. At the Giles Weather Station the relations between Aboriginal people and the weather station personnel were not always cordial, particularly in the early days of the station, but over time a number of Ngaatjatjarra people settled in the area.

In 1957 the native patrol officer Macaulay noted that there were about forty Aboriginal people living near the Giles Weather Station, and that 'contact between the personnel of the weather station and natives is almost non-existent'. In the same year he visited the Blackstone mining camp and made the following report:

> Natives are now discouraged from remaining in close vicinity to the mining camp. No employment will be available in the future. However, parties in transit will have water made available to them by the company ... With the inducement of employment removed, I doubt if natives will frequent the mining camp nearly as much as before, and this is to be desired ... [as] at this stage of contact employment of a few tends to parasitism by many ... This follows some trouble with officials of the South Australian Aborigines Department over the unauthorised cartage of natives, but seen also from the health angle. Several employees and children have contracted trachoma.

Macaulay was also concerned about the potential for the mining camp to introduce epidemic infectious diseases:

> People who fly to Blackstone or come from South Australia do not require a West Australian permit of entry to a reserve ... They may come into contact with fully tribalized natives ... Visitors may easily introduce diseases which would attain epidemic proportions, such as the measles epidemic which recently killed thirteen babies at Ernabella and at least two at Mulga Park. Further, such an epidemic could be spread to the Warburton and Rawlinson Ranges.[22]

At Ernabella, Charles Duguid had stated that one of the aims of the mission was to show that *Anangu* were better off living on their own country than 'sitting down at a cattle station in rags', and he advocated for the establishment of depots west of Ernabella to discourage eastward migration during times of drought. In a letter written from Ernabella to the South Australian Aborigines' Protection Board in June 1957, Victor Coombes, the General Secretary of the Presbyterian Board of Missions, claimed there were three to four hundred *Anangu* living in the Tomkinson and Blackstone ranges area who had only occasional contact with either the Ernabella or Warburton missions, and perhaps another one hundred or so who had had no contact with either mission. He proposed that a new mission, with an associated sheep station, be established at the western end of the Tomkinson Range (perhaps near Irrunytju).[23]

According to Bill Edwards, who arrived to work at Ernabella in 1958, Victor Coombes invited him to work at Ernabella as assistant to the mission superintendent. Coombes, 'concerned at the pressure on water and firewood supplies as the Ernabella population increased, proposed that a series of outstations be established to the west to enable some residents to return to their traditional homelands', and suggested that Bill could commence the process of establishing these outstations.[24] The South Australian Government Aborigines' Protection Board, however, rejected Coombes' proposals to establish a mission or outstations. Concerned that the Ernabella Mission was not assimilating Pitjantjatjara people quickly enough and critical of the respect for language and culture shown by the mission, the Protection Board opened its own settlement on South Australia's North-West Aboriginal Reserve at Amata in 1961. A nursing sister, employed by the South Australian health department, was posted to Amata in 1962 and a school was opened in 1967. The Ernabella Mission remained under the control of the Presbyterian Board of Missions until the end of 1973, and in January 1974 control was transferred to Ernabella Community Council Inc., and the South Australian health department took over the nursing post from the mission.

Meanwhile, further west, towards the West Australian border, a mining company undertook exploration of nickel deposits at Mount Davies, 200 kilometres west of Amata, and at Wingellina, a further 40 kilometres west. Bores were sunk at these sites, which assisted Pitjantjatjara people wanting to spend time visiting their country. When Bob Verburgt arrived in Amata to work as a bores and stock overseer in 1961, there were 180 *Anangu* camping in the area of Mount Davies.²⁵ It was not a permanent single camp at that stage; the people shifted camp regularly, living in *wiltjas*, the temporary structures made of logs, tree branches and grasses that had always been the traditional shelters of the nomadic Western Desert people. In the mid-1960s, a small scale chrysoprase mine near Mount Davies commenced as an employment project for *Anangu* who travelled to and from Amata, staying in temporary camps near the mine.

Concerns about nickel-mining operations potentially disturbing important sacred sites led to a more permanent camp being established, initially at Puta Puta, not far to the east of Mount Davies. By 1975 another community was established in the area at Pipalyatjara, closer to Mount Davies and close to *malu tjukurrpa* (kangaroo dreaming) sites. In that year, exactly 100 years after the first white explorers, William Gosse and Ernest Giles, had passed through and described the area, the anthropologist Peter Brokensha spent time there doing fieldwork for his book *The Pitjantjatjara and their Crafts*. His cook, mechanic and helper was Glendle Schrader (who, as mentioned in the previous chapter, I was to meet three years later in Utopia). The only facility was a hand-pump over an artesian borehole but it was home to about thirty-five people when Peter and Glendle arrived—a significant decrease from the 180 people who had been living there in 1962. Presumably the facilities at Amata such as the school, the clinic and the store had attracted people to relocate to Amata, at least until facilities could be established at Pipalyatjara.

Glendle was struck by the sense of autonomy and cultural freedom that existed among the people living at Pipalyatjara. There was, he has written in an unpublished account, 'a swagger of defiance and pride'. During 1975, there was a steady influx of people back to Pipalyatjara and the population had increased to over one hundred by the time Peter and Glendle left. Everybody still lived in *wiltjas* but now sometimes augmented with other available materials such as corrugated iron sheets and tarpaulins.

Later in 1975, a community advisor for Pipalyatjara and chrysoprase miner, Tom O'Flynn, was appointed by the DAA with the aim of further developing a community-based chrysoprase mining operation in the area. A few months after his arrival, Tom asked Glendle, who had returned to Alice

Springs, if he could come to live at Pipalyatjara and develop the community store. In late 1975, Tom O'Flynn left and Glendle moved into the one and only caravan—which doubled as a home and the community office—and became community advisor. A school was opened in 1976 with a young teacher named Paul Eckert, who was later to become a linguist and Bible translator. By 1977, the population was around 150 people.

Around the same time, people moved out from Amata to establish the community at Irrunytju, near the old mining site of Wingellina, where they were joined by others who moved east from Warburton Mission. John ('Tungku') Tregenza, who had been employed as a welfare officer by the South Australian Department of Community Welfare at Amata, was appointed as community advisor in 1976. A West Australian education department single-teacher school commenced in Irrunytju in 1977. By then, like Pipalyatjara, the population was between one and two hundred people.

Several smaller communities with less permanent populations were also established west of Amata, but still on the South Australian side of the border, in the 1970s—at Puta Puta, near *malu tjukurrpa* (kangaroo dreaming) sites in 1973; Kunamata, an important *ili tjukurrpa* (wild fig dreaming) site, in 1976; Aparatjara near the Mann Ranges; Kunytjanu, south of Pipalyatjara in 1977; Kanypi in 1977, and nearby Nyapari in 1979. Just across the border in Western Australia, a small community at Kata Ala, a *nyinyi tjukurrpa* (zebra finch dreaming) site south of Wingellina, was established early in 1978. Just over the Northern Territory border, north of Pipalyatjara, Walytitjata became another small community.

By the 1960s there was a more permanent settlement at Warburton Mission, after the fluid movement of *Yarnangu* between the mission and their country in the earlier years. The dingo-scalp trade was dying and the mission continued to have financial problems. Many Ngaanyatjarra people continued to spend much of their time on their country. By the 1970s permanent communities were developing on the homelands: Irrunytju (near the old Wingellina mining site, as discussed above), Papulangkatja (near the old mine in the Blackstone Range), Marntamaru (also called Jamieson, near the Jamieson Range west of the Blackstone Range) and Warakurna (to the north, near the Giles Weather Station and the Rawlinson Ranges).

During the 1970s, as the homelands movement was developing momentum, so did the political awareness about ensuring Aboriginal control of the land. A 'Pan-Pitjantjatjara' meeting of Pitjantjatjara, Yankunytjatjara and Ngaanyatjarra people met at Ernabella in 1975 to discuss land rights and other matters. A meeting at Amata the following year established the Pitjantjatjara Council, with recognition that it included all the groups from across the area and was to be the voice for land rights and other issues of concern.

Health in the homelands

With the development of the homelands movement into the Pitjantjatjara and Ngaanyatjarra homelands, the South Australian and West Australian education departments responded by establishing small one-teacher schools at Pipalyatjara, Irrunytju, Papulangkatja, Marntamaru and Warakurna. However, there was less support from the respective departments of health. The South Australian Department of Health employed nurses at nursing posts in Amata, Ernabella, Fregon and Indulkana, but there was little support for the decentralisation movement from within the department, and appeals for services to be provided to the growing communities west of Amata went unheeded.

Across the border at Warburton, the clinic, staffed by the Aborigines' Inland Mission, provided services only within Warburton. In 1977 the Royal Flying Doctor Service (RFDS) based in Kalgoorlie started fortnightly clinic flights to Warburton, Warakurna, Irrunytju, Papulangkatja and Marntamaru. This entailed visiting all the communities for two days—the RFDS pilot, doctor and nurse would stay overnight at the Giles Weather Station—and providing short clinics of one or two hours at each community. In addition, the West Australian Department of Health employed two Kalgoorlie-based community-health nurses, who made occasional outreach visits into the homelands communities in Western Australia. The only permanent health providers in all the communities between Warburton and Amata were Aboriginal health workers who did a remarkable job despite limited training. Often, community advisors or other non-Aboriginal people working in the communities in both states would assist with providing medical services and, in the case of medical emergencies, liaise with RFDS doctors over the two-way radios.

When Glendle was at Pipalyatjara, initially as Peter Brokensha's assistant and later as storekeeper and then as community advisor, he found he was being frequently asked to provide basic healthcare. He made efforts to maintain a supply of medical equipment and pharmaceuticals to support the local Aboriginal health workers. Although he asked the RFDS based in Alice Springs for a medical box, this was refused on the basis that Pipalyatjara was not a cattle station. The RFDS base in Kalgoorlie was more sympathetic and despite the fact that Pipalyatjara was slightly outside their area of operations, they offered to provide a monthly clinic flight to the community but the airstrip was not suitable. The Kalgoorlie RFDS base did, however, provide a medical box. Andy Barr, the chief pharmacist at Alice Springs Hospital, was also supportive and, whenever Glendle visited, Andy would put together a box of medical stores. Glendle approached Congress in Alice Springs to ask about the possibility of providing a medical service to the area. Congress was sympathetic and did provide a couple of medical visits, but did not have the resources to provide the sustained service that was required.

In 1976 Fred Hollows visited the Pitjantjatjara and Ngaanyatjarra lands with his trachoma team. Hollows was Professor of Ophthalmology at the University of New South Wales and had developed an interest in Aboriginal eye health, particularly trachoma. He had obtained funding through the Royal Australasian College of Ophthalmologists to travel around Australia visiting Aboriginal communities, undertaking surveys of eye health and providing much-needed services including field surgery. Through his experience, he became an effective advocate for improved health services for Aboriginal people and particularly for the nascent Aboriginal community-controlled health service movement. When Hollows was at Pipalyatjara, Glendle discussed with him the need for health services in the area. He suggested putting together a submission and sending it to both the South Australian and federal governments.

In 1977 Glendle wrote a submission for a community-controlled health service, which would provide healthcare to all the communities between

Warburton and Amata. The newly formed Pitjantjatjara Council supported this proposal and agreed to act as the incorporated body, which would sponsor the submission. There was a negative response from the South Australian health department but there was a more sympathetic response from the federal government, which at the time was led by Malcolm Fraser, and had continued with the policy of self-determination that had been implemented by the previous Whitlam government. Under Fraser, however, the term 'self-determination' had been replaced by 'self-management'. The notion that Aboriginal community organisations should be involved in service delivery was supported and, as it happened, the submission for a health service on the Pitjantjatjara and Ngaanyatjarra lands arrived not long after Congress in Alice Springs had lodged their submission, based on the Cutter Report, for funding for Aboriginal community-controlled health services at Papunya and Utopia. Consequently, early in 1978 the Pitjantjatjara Council was advised that funding would be made available for their health service.

After my experience at Utopia, and my discussions with Glendle, I was hoping to be the first doctor to work with the service. The outcome of this aspiration is discussed in the next chapter.

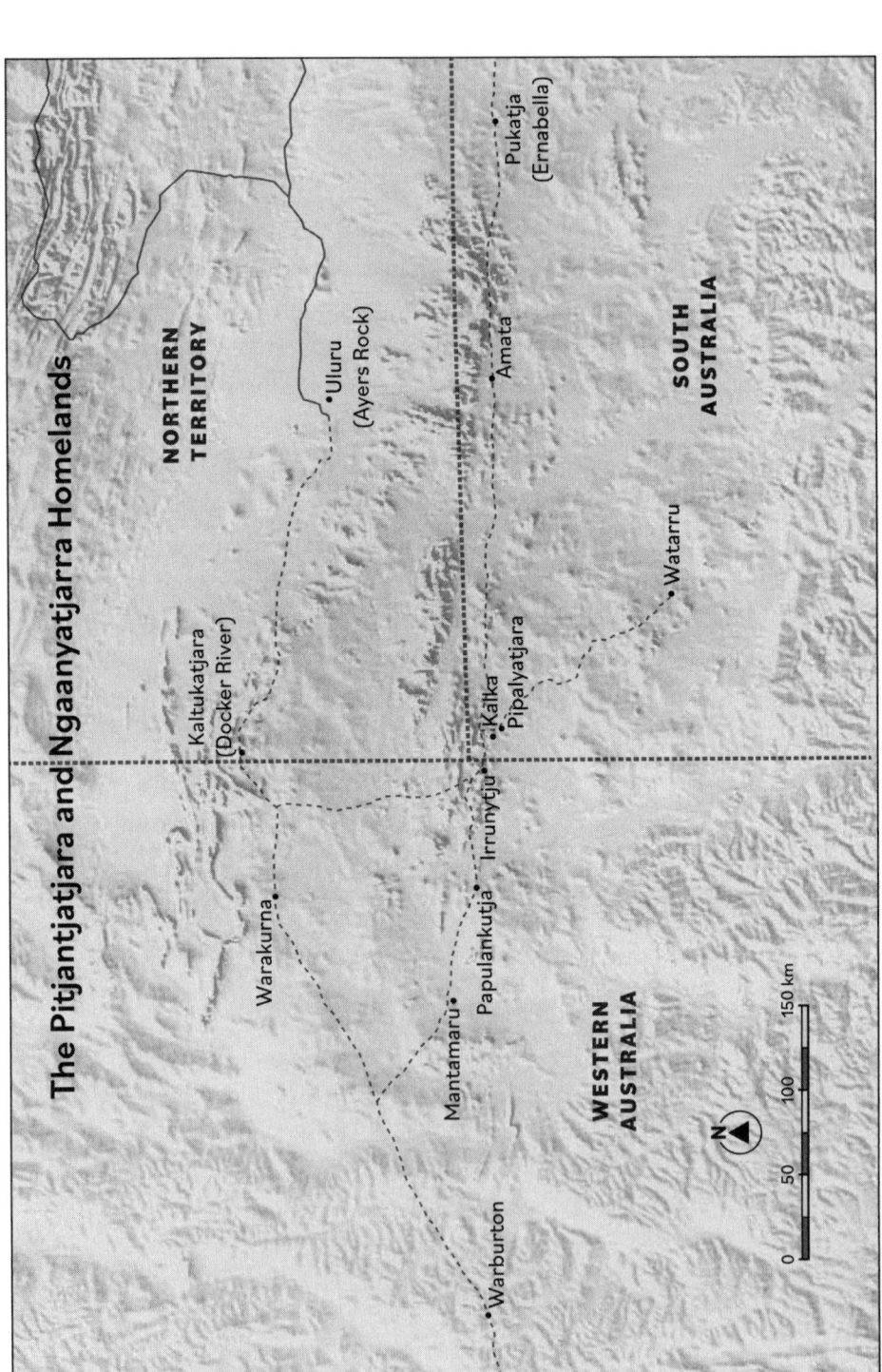

3

The Pitjantjatjara Home-made Health Service

Encountering the homelands

When my employers at Congress learned that I was interested in applying to work with the forthcoming health service on the Pitjantjatjara homelands they were encouraging, as this was consistent with Congress's support for the development of community-controlled health services throughout Central Australia. Consequently, while still an employee of Congress, it was arranged for me to go on a 'bush trip' in February and March 1978 to provide clinical services and to get a better understanding of the area and the people's health needs.

Soon afterwards, I found myself driving out towards the Pitjantjatjara lands with Leo Williams, a senior Arrernte man and an employee of Congress, as my companion and guide. We drove south down the Stuart Highway from Alice Springs and then west along the Lasseter Highway towards Uluru or, as it was more commonly referred to in those days, Ayers Rock. We stopped at the roadhouse on Mount Ebenezer Station, where we were informed that a site had been selected to be excised from the station and granted to the local Aboriginal people, and that the people had already settled there, even though the process for the excision had not been completed. We drove a short distance to the north of the roadhouse to a camp of about fifty Pitjantjatjara/Luritja people, and we spent some time there while I consulted with various people about a number of medical issues. This site would eventually become the community of Imanpa.

We continued west past Uluru but we did not stop there, as the Northern Territory administration had subsidised private companies to develop tourism around the base of the rock and actively discouraged the presence of Aboriginal people, despite the fact that it was the place of a number of significant sacred sites for *Anangu*. A few years later in 1984, this would change when, with considerable resistance from the Northern Territory government, *Anangu* would be granted land title to the area around Uluru with joint management of the national park.

We continued travelling westward to the Aboriginal community of Docker River near the beautiful Petermann Ranges. Docker River was established as a government settlement in 1967 and, at the time we visited, had a community of about 500 Pitjantjatjara, Ngaanyatjarra and Pintupi people. The Northern Territory government provided a primary healthcare centre staffed by a single nurse. As it was after working-hours when we arrived, I sought out the nurse's accommodation to introduce myself and to offer my assistance if any medical emergencies arose. It was not hard to find the accommodation. It consisted of a large silver metal caravan, which in those days were commonly used for non-Aboriginal accommodation in remote communities and known as 'silver bullets'. I met the nurse—a rather eccentric Englishwoman known as Sister Pat. She made it clear that she had doubts about the viability of the imminent Pitjantjatjara Homelands Health Service, and I had the impression she considered me a naive newcomer—which, of course, I was. About twenty years later, when I worked for a time as an Alice Springs–based district medical officer, providing fortnightly clinic visits to Docker River, Sister Pat was still there and, by that time, she considered me an old-timer and we became good friends.

Leo and I camped in Docker River community overnight and the next morning travelled west across the West Australian border and then south until we reached the community of Irrunytju. When we pulled up, an Aboriginal man walked over to meet us. He introduced himself as Wilton Foster and said, 'You must be the doctor.' I was pleased to note that the bush telegraph was working and that I was expected. Although still a young man, Wilton was an emerging leader who had been involved with Glendle in the development of the submission for the health service. He said that I was expected in Pipalyatjara and told me who I should contact on arrival.

From Irrunytju we travelled east across the border between Western Australia and South Australia and soon reached Pipalyatjara. Leo introduced me to the people who Wilton had mentioned, particularly Arthur Richards, the secretary of the Pitjantjatjara Council. Arthur was a Ngaanyatjarra man who had been educated at the Warburton Mission and due to his obvious intelligence had been selected by the missionaries to go away to Bible College, in the hope that he would return as a local pastor. He had gratefully received his education but decided against a career as a Christian pastor, having instead decided to use his education to support the political aspirations of his people. He lived in Pipalyatjara because his *waputju* (father-in-law) was one of Pipalyatjara's senior men. I came to know Arthur well while I lived on the homelands; sadly, he died a few years later, while still a relatively young man, in a motor-vehicle accident.

I met other leaders of the Pipalyatjara community over the next few days, most of whom have now passed away. I was shown the clinic at Pipalyatjara, which consisted of a shed with three walls and a roof and a medical kit that was carefully and conscientiously tended by the two Aboriginal health workers, Roma Peterman (now Roma Butler) and Nelly Mick (now known as Josephine Mick). I was also shown the silver bullet, which was similar to the accommodation I had seen at Docker River, that was to be my accommodation while staying at Pipalyatjara.

I also met the non-Aboriginal people living at Pipalyatjara. The community advisor Patrick Morgan, who had taken over the role from Glendle, lived with his wife Marie and their three-year-old son in a small caravan. The schoolteacher was Annie Davis, who had replaced Paul Eckert, and had only recently arrived with her husband Bill, a musician, to start work at the Pipalyatjara School as her first remote area posting. Annie and Bill resided in another small caravan. The Pipalyatjara community had maintained the small-scale chrysoprase mining operation and the mining advisor was now Ray Glastonbury, who lived with his Aboriginal wife Mercy and her two young children.

About 20 kilometres to the east of Pipalyatjara was a small homeland community called Puta Puta. The senior man here was a wise old man, custodian of nearby *malu tjukurrpa* (kangaroo dreaming) sites, called Tjutjupayi. There were also two non-Aboriginal men of around my age who, with Tjutjupayi's approval, had recently set up their base at Puta Puta, Ushma Scales and Stephan Rainow. I had met Ushma and Stephi in Alice Springs a month or two earlier as they were on their way out to the Pitjantjatjara country to commence work as gardening advisors to the small homeland communities. Both had worked previously at Amata. Ushma and his wife Eva had commenced work as art advisors in Amata in 1972 and had lived there with their three young girls. Stephi was Eva's brother, and had visited them in Amata and, due to his useful building and maintenance skills, had stayed on for some time to provide assistance on community projects. They had all left Amata the previous year and headed home to the east coast, but were drawn back to the Pitjantjatjara country. Ushma and Stephi had successfully applied for a position to support the development of vegetable gardens in the small homelands communities west of Amata. At this stage, the two of them were living at Puta Puta in a dwelling that they had constructed, which was similar to a Bedouin tent. They both had studied anthropology as undergraduates at university and had a profound respect for Aboriginal culture which, combined with their experience in the alternative lifestyle and self-sufficiency movement of the 1960s and 70s, found a good fit on the homelands. They were also both decent human beings and their respect for *Anangu* was clearly reciprocated. Ushma and Stephi became good friends and I learnt a lot from their experience.

Ushma, in particular, had developed a deep involvement in Pitjantjatjara life and culture. In the summer of 1978/79, Ushma was involved in some men's ceremonial business near Irrunytju and, on one occasion, took time off from the activities to go hunting with some men. They happened across a vehicle with some miners who were illegally prospecting, who were subsequently told to leave. Before they left, the miners saw that one of the men, covered in red dust and with ceremonial markings still visible, was a white man. When they heard somebody call him by his name, they mistook the name Ushma for Ishmael. Subsequently, an article appeared in a West Australian newspaper about a white man named Ishmael who has become the 'king of the desert Aborigines'. In fact, it was my friend Ushma.

I was visiting Ushma and Stephi one balmy evening when we saw a Ford F100 ute coming along the road from the east. When it arrived, it stopped and from the cabin emerged John Tregenza. I had heard about John. A month or two previously while in Alice Springs, I had seen an ABC documentary about John and his family and their life in Irrunytju where John was the first community advisor. He had initially come to the Pitjantjatjara lands from Adelaide as a social worker working with the South Australian Department of Community Welfare at Amata. When people had moved out to reoccupy Irrunytju they had asked John to be their community advisor, so he had moved there with his wife Bronnie and their two young children, Yolonde and Julian. John was a nuggetty man, full of energy and enthusiasm. Like his friends Ushma and Stephi, he had become immersed in Pitjantjatjara life and culture, and he was also a grass-roots political activist. Inspired by Third World liberation movements and their theorists such as Paolo Freire, he always saw his role as supporting the aspirations of *Anangu* for self-determination. He was usually referred to as Tungku, meaning 'short fellow' but in many ways John was, and continues to be, a big man. On this occasion, when I met him at Puta Puta, he was returning from his annual leave over the summer and had brought with him his brother-in-law Simon Thompson. Bronnie, Yolonde and Julian were to follow later. Like Ushma and Stephi, Tungku became a good friend.

I spent a week or so in Pipalyatjara working with the Aboriginal health workers Roma and Nelly, getting to know the people and learning how to provide healthcare with limited facilities. Leo stayed for a few days in Pipalyatjara to ensure that I had settled in before he returned on a mail plane to Alice Springs.

I was keen to see the other communities and to meet the people living in those communities that constituted the area to be covered by the impending Pitjantjatjara Homelands Health Service. Nelly's brother Ginger Mick offered to drive with me to the communities in Western Australia. So, for about four days we drove through Irrunytju to Papulangkatja, to Linton Bore, to Marntamaru and across to Warburton Ranges Mission, north-east to Warakurna and then south to Walypa Pulka, back to Irrunytju, and finally back to Pipalyatjara.

These communities that we visited were all on the West Australian side of the border. Warburton had its own primary healthcare service—staffed by nurses employed by the Aborigines' Inland Mission—and so wasn't intended to be part of the incipient Pitjantjatjara Homelands Health Service. The other communities west of Warburton—Irrunytju, Papulankatja, Marntamaru and Warakurna—each had a rudimentary clinic, usually an old caravan, with one or two people from the community employed as health workers. The Royal Flying Doctor Service, based in Kalgoorlie, provided a fortnightly clinic flight to each of these communities and was available for evacuation when necessary. As I travelled round these communities for the first time with Ginger, I met the Aboriginal health workers and worked with them in their clinics.

I particularly remember two wonderful Aboriginal health workers at Jamieson, both mature women, Belle Davidson (who passed away in 2017) and Thelma McLean (also now deceased). In Warakurna, Molly Porter, a senior woman from the community, and Judith Golding, a younger woman being nurtured into the role by Molly, worked as Aboriginal health workers. These health workers did a remarkable job in quite difficult circumstances. In emergencies they were usually supported by the non-Aboriginal community advisor, who would liaise by two-way radio with the RFDS base in Kalgoorlie. It was hoped that, with the development of the Pitjantjatjara Homelands Health Service, primary healthcare and health outcomes in these communities would improve.

On the South Australian side of the border, I visited the smaller communities as well as Pipalyatjara. These included Walytitjata, Puta Puta, Kunytjanu, Aparatjara, Nyapari and Kunamata. The population of these small homeland communities varied. Usually there were up to twenty or thirty people but occasionally they would be empty when people had commitments elsewhere. Unlike on the West Australian side of the border, Piplayatjara and these communities did not have regular RFDS clinics but the South Australian health-department nurse based in Amata, Chris McCall, would sometimes drive out to provide support and deliver clinical services as required. This, however, was done surreptitiously as her superiors in Adelaide actively discouraged these outreach visits.

After four weeks living at Pipalyatjara and travelling round the other communities, I thought that I had made the right decision in applying for the position as medical officer with the Pitjantjatjara Homelands Health Service. I liked the people and the country and I was aware of challenge ahead in developing the Pitjantjatjara Homelands Health Service. I hoped, with some trepidation, that I was up to the challenge.

Growing the Pitjantjatjara Homelands Health Service

Just before my initial visit to the Pitjantjatjara and Ngaanyatjarra homelands was over, I attended a Pitjantjatjara Council meeting at Jamieson, where the appointments to the new Pitjantjatjara Homelands Health Service were to be made. The meeting continued for two days, with land rights as the main agenda item. There was much activity related to land rights happening at that time and both men and women, young and old, were very involved in the discussions about strategies to achieve political and legal recognition of their ownership of the land.

The Health Service was also included in the discussions and, at the conclusion, I was appointed as their medical officer. Tungku Tregenza had thrown his hat in the ring to be the administrator and was appointed. An Aboriginal nurse from North Queensland, Glenis Grogan who, about two years previously, had worked with Congress and visited the Pitjantjatjara lands, had applied for the nursing position. She was known and liked by the *Anangu* and was appointed. After we had received confirmation of our employment, Tungku introduced me to a senior Aboriginal man named Ivan Baker. He explained that Ivan had been a strong supporter of moves to get a community-controlled health service in the Pitjantjatjara homelands and he had put his name forward to be the trainee administrator of the service.

So the team had been appointed and we were due to start a few weeks later. In the submission to obtain funds, Glendle had proposed that the staff for the health service be based at Pipalyatjara. However, Tungku and Ivan proposed that a separate base should be established. There were two main reasons for this: first, an influx of non-Aboriginal staff based at Piplayatjara would have a significant impact on the community. Second, and more importantly, it was recognised that the Pitjantjatjara Homelands Health

Service was a regional service that was to provide primary healthcare support to all the communities constituting the Pitjantjatjara and Ngaanyatjarra homelands. If the service was seen to be based in one community, there could have been a centralising tendency, which would have been in opposition to the spirit of the proposed health service.

There was an unused borehole near Pipalyatjara at a site named Kalka and, after discussions with the traditional owners of this area, it was agreed that Kalka would become the residential base for the Pitjantjatjara Homelands Health Service.

In the meantime, I needed to prepare for my new position. I returned to Alice Springs and gave my notice to Congress. My new appointment received full support from Congress but I continued to work in the clinic until my resignation took effect, and I continued to live in my flat on Bradshaw Drive. At one stage, for a week or so, I shared the flat with Myrna Tonkinson, a Jamaican-born anthropologist who was visiting from Perth for a short-term consultancy. We had many interesting and useful conversations that alerted me to the importance of cultural considerations in providing healthcare to Aboriginal people. She directed me to some useful resources, particularly an article on 'Socio-cultural aspects of health amongst the Pitjantjatjara people' by the anthropologist Annette Hamilton, and a cultural-training handbook by O'Brien and Plooij at Flinders University, written specifically for health professionals working with Pitjantjatjara people. As a result of my discussions with Myrna and my exposure to these resources, I am sure that the number of cultural mistakes I subsequently made were fewer than they otherwise would have been.

I enrolled in a Pitjantjatjara language course in Adelaide. This ran for two weeks over the school holidays in April. Bill and Ann Davis from Pipalyatjara, on their first school holidays, also attended the course. Glendle was in Adelaide for a short time while I was there, and we arranged to visit Charles Duguid at his home on Dequetteville Terrace in Kent Town, as mentioned in the previous chapter. He was ninety-four years old at the time and, although physically rather frail, he still had a definite presence, and his mind was still active. He was a tall man with a kindly demeanour and was delighted to hear about the development of the new health service, which he suggested was, in a way, the realisation of his original aspiration for a 'medical mission' on the lands. He wished us well with our efforts.

I also went on a trip to Perth and Kalgoorlie with Glendle and Teddy Porter, a Ngaanyatjarra man from Warburton who had been appointed by the Pitjantjatjara Council to travel with us and to discuss with relevant stakeholders the new developments east of Warburton Mission. We had, at best, a mixed reception. Both the West Australian Department of Health and the RFDS were decidedly cool on the idea of a Commonwealth-funded health service in the West Australian Central Reserve—particularly as it seemed to be coming across the border from South Australia.

At the beginning of May 1978, I returned to Pipalyatjara to begin work officially as medical officer with the Pitjantjatjara Homelands Health Service. Tungku was already there, working to establish our base at Kalka. The 'silver bullet' was moved from Pipalyatjara to Kalka and a windmill was established over the bore. More silver bullets were on their way but initially we all had to share the one. We consisted of Tungku, his wife Bronnie, their two children Julian and Yolonde, Simon (Bronnie's brother), who had been employed to help with the establishment of Kalka, Glenis Grogan and her young son Brad, and myself. As we were often travelling, it was not as difficult as it might have otherwise been and, within a couple of months, the new accommodation had arrived. For a while Glenis's caravan was based at Puta Puta and mine was based at Pipalyatjara while Kalka was being developed. Eventually we were all based at Kalka.

We envisaged that the new health service would be mobile with an accommodation base. The decision was made that, to avoid the risk of centralisation, no clinic should be constructed at Kalka. This meant that both Glenis and I were travelling most of the time. In an attempt to achieve as much reach as possible, we usually travelled separately. We travelled to each community, usually staying a day or two in each place, providing clinical services and support and training for Aboriginal health workers and restocking the clinics. We carried swags, consisting of a foam mattress and bedding rolled up in a tarpaulin for sleeping. Most nights were spent somewhere in the area, sleeping under the stars and next to a small campfire. This was no hardship as the desert nights, under the canopy of myriad stars, always provided a very pleasant end to the day. Even when back at Kalka, I usually slept outside in my swag.

The overall population of the area was around 1,000 people, spread across a number of communities. We tried to ensure that each of the major communities was visited at least every two weeks but, for various reasons, this was not always possible. We were also guided by the movement of people. There were frequent gatherings of people in a particular community for reasons including ceremonial business, funerals or sporting events, and on these occasions we often made ourselves available. As people often needed lifts to these events, and there was always a shortage of privately owned vehicles, our transport was appreciated. Our vehicles were frequently full with adults, children and, not uncommonly, dogs. This flexibility, in itinerary and the use of vehicles, would have been more difficult within a larger bureaucracy and was thus a strength of the community-controlled health service model.

Developing the PHHS was a daunting task. With such a small team covering such a wide area, and with limited resources, it was always going to be difficult. The service developed as we went along and we kept learning and adapting. I settled into the life of a travelling doctor, which was to be my life for the next three years and, in general, I found the experience rewarding and enjoyable.

I made an effort to learn to speak Pitjantjatjara. The two-week course I had undertaken in Adelaide provided the scaffolding to assist with learning the language, without providing fluency. Once I was on the lands and immersed in the language I was able to develop my linguistic ability. The Pitjantjatjara people, with their exposure to the Ernabella Mission where language learning was expected among mission staff, continued to have an expectation that non-Aboriginal people working on the lands should speak their language. A<u>n</u>angu would speak Pitjantjatjara to me even if they had a reasonable knowledge of English. They would, however, speak slowly and clearly and helped correct my frequent mistakes. In the Ngaanyatjarra communities, after the Warburton Mission experience where speaking Aboriginal languages had been discouraged, there was less of an expectation that non-Aboriginal people would learn the language. However, I was conscious that, while I was learning to speak Pitjantjatjara and using it in my interactions, the language in these communities was not quite the same. Consequently, I made an effort to learn to speak Ngaanyatjarra as well. Herbert Howell was a missionary-linguist who lived with his family in a caravan at Warakurna, and he kindly agreed to help with my language development. Usually when I visited Warakurna, I would spend an hour or so with Herbert learning to speak Ngaanyatjarra.

Traditional medicine

At Marntamaru, I was introduced to a *ngangkari* (traditional healer), a man about my age named Ernie Mitchell. He became a friend and I usually camped with his family when I visited Marntamaru, and while I was there we worked together. Over time I met other *ngangkaris* (for example, Mr Yates at Papulankatja, Dickie Minyintiri who lived for a while at Kalka, Andy Tjilari at Nyapari) and we frequently worked together, and sometimes travelled together. There was also a *ngangkari* with lively sparkling eyes whom I met in the last year or so on my visits to Warakurna. He was a Pintupi man known as Doctor George. We were to resume our close working relationship a few years later at Kintore.

I discovered that there were two levels of traditional healthcare on the homelands, and in the Western Desert generally. Most adults were able to treat common conditions through using various techniques or by preparing 'bush medicine' from readily available materials, usually plants, sometimes to be taken orally, or more often applied to the skin, for various common complaints.

On a higher level there were certain people who are recognised as having healing powers: the traditional doctor or *ngangkari*. Most *ngangkaris* were recognised in childhood as having the potential to develop these powers and, after reaching adulthood and taking a period of development and initiation, they would be sought out to use their healing powers when required. Most were men, although there were some women. Most practised a form of massage, which would result in the apparent withdrawal of an object—a piece of wood, a stone, or even a bullet—from the affected part of the body. Others used suction rather than massage and, after putting a mouth to the affected part and applying suction, they would spit blood with black specks into any available container, usually a tobacco tin. These procedures would be conducted in public, often with a small crowd who would provide comment and support throughout. There were variations. One Ngaanyatjarra *ngangkari* man I knew used an unusual piece of quartz that he held to his eye to view the patient, so as to enable him to make a diagnosis. Another *ngangkari*, a woman, used song and dance rather than working on the body.

The use of *ngangkaris* was widespread and there did not appear to be any conflict in the use of both Western medicine on the one hand, and the healing powers of the *ngangkaris* on the other. In most cases, both systems were sought out, often together. Consequently, I often found myself working alongside a *ngangkari* colleague. Frequently, after the *ngangkari* had completed the procedure, he would indicate to me that it was the right time to give some medicine. I had the impression that whereas I was treating the superficial manifestations of a bodily disorder, the *ngangkari* was seen to be addressing the underlying spiritual disorder. Certainly, from the patient's perspective, the combination appeared to be desirable. In the PHHS, it was accepted practice that *ngangkari* consultations were supported.

Consolidating the Pitjantjatjara Homelands Health Service

A few months into the position, I returned to Kalka after travels around the communities in Western Australia, when Glenis informed me she was concerned about a baby named Rosie Daniels who had become ill that day. When I examined Rosie I saw she was clearly unwell, with a fever and a tense raised fontanelle. I recognised that she had meningitis. I raised the RFDS on the two-way radio and informed the doctor on-call, who agreed to send a plane to transfer Rosie to Alice Springs Hospital. While waiting for the plane I wanted to start treatment with antibiotics, but doing this before collecting a specimen of cerebrospinal fluid (to allow the causative organism to be cultured) would mean that it would be difficult to identify the correct antibiotic to use. As we did not have a clinic at Kalka, I performed a lumbar puncture on the dining table in my caravan. I successfully obtained cerebrospinal fluid, and labelled the tube to send to hospital with Rosie and then commenced the antibiotics.

Rosie's parents were present with me and we drove together to the Pipalyatjara airstrip; then the RFDS aircraft arrived to collect Rosie and her mother. I drove Rosie's father, Bobby Jakamarra Daniels, back to Pipalyatjara to drop him off at his *wiltja*. On the way, Bobby, clearly impressed with my dining table technique, said he would like to work with me. He subsequently talked to Ivan about this and he was employed by the PHHS as an Aboriginal health worker. For the rest of the time of my employment with PHHS, Bobby was my *malpa* (friend), cultural mentor and fellow driver. Bobby was a Warlpiri man who had married a Pitjantjatjara woman and had moved from Yuendumu to Pipalyatjara.

The core funding for the running of the PHHS came from the Commonwealth Department of Aboriginal Affairs. The PHHS was not an incorporated body, so the funding was officially held by the Pitjantjatjara Council. Consequently the PHHS reported to the Pitjantjatjara Council and we attempted to attend the quarterly meetings that were held somewhere on the Ngaanyatjarra, Pitjantjatjara and Yankunytjatjara lands. In reality, the PHHS administration had a large degree of control over the use of the budget, with the assistance of an accounting firm in Alice Springs, and with the support of two experienced and supportive DAA project officers, Chris Marshall and Richard Preece—both of whom made a significant contribution to Aboriginal affairs and particularly the governance of Aboriginal organisations over many years.

As administrator of the health service, Tungku Tregenza had the responsibility for its day-to-day management. Tungku, with his knowledge of the people, the language, the culture and the political dimensions of the homelands movement, provided me with useful guidance. Unfortunately, at the beginning of 1979 he left for Adelaide with his family for the sake of his children's education. Bill Davis, the husband of Annie Davis the Pipalyatjara schoolteacher, who had been employed by the PHHS as a health worker educator in 1978, stepped into the role for a while until, after an interim short term by Glendle, Glenis Grogan resigned her nursing position to take up the role of administrator.

Ivan Baker originally had the role as trainee administrator but he was a natural leader and quickly emerged as the effective and overall boss of the health service. Within the first year or so, his title was changed to Director of PHHS. He chaired our staff meetings, most of which were conducted in Pitjantjatjara. I remember an occasion where a recently employed nurse attended a meeting and asked whether the discussion could be translated into English for her benefit. Unfortunately, these days I doubt there are any Aboriginal health services where staff meetings are held in an Aboriginal language.

At staff meetings Ivan would always show a good grasp of issues and he had the ability, after ensuring he had canvassed everybody's opinions, to make appropriate decisions. When a criticism needed to be made, he would do it in an Aboriginal way, avoiding direct confrontation, but talking in general terms about a principle that may have been contravened. Sometimes the principle he raised was related to staff making decisions that should have involved discussions with the Aboriginal leadership. I realised, on more than one occasion, that Ivan was referring to a decision I had taken. As a doctor I was used to making decisions but I gradually came to realise that when working in an Aboriginal organisation, I was not always the right person to make non-clinical decisions. I tried to be *Anangu kulilpayi* (one who listens to Aboriginal people) but became aware that sometimes, perhaps too often, I am *watarrku* (oblivious to my surroundings, including what I am being told). I learned a great deal about working under community control from Ivan and I always appreciated the gentle way in which he conveyed these messages.

The PHHS was an Aboriginal community-controlled health organisation and consequently became part of the Australia-wide network of ACCHOs, called at that time the National Aboriginal and Islander Health Organisation (NAIHO). The ACCHO movement was still in its early years, and NAIHO was a very active organisation with some notable Aboriginal activists and intellectuals who had been involved in establishing the earliest ACCHOs—people such as Gary Foley, Naomi Meyers, Sol Belair, Dennis Walker and Bruce McGuinness.

NAIHO was dedicated to the principle of community control, and tried to ensure that all the ACCHOs were kept informed of national issues and had the opportunity to be involved in the decision-making processes. NAIHO meetings were held once or twice a year and all ACCHOs were encouraged to send representatives. I attended one such meeting in Perth in 1980 with some *Anangu*. I remember one evening, towards the end of a restaurant dinner for all the delegates, Gary Foley called me aside and suggested we go for a walk around the block. He produced a joint, which we smoked while we walked and talked about community control. He was checking my commitment but also, I think, signalling my acceptance into the exhilarating world of Aboriginal politics. Or perhaps I was just high.

The PHHS model of healthcare, which entailed a mobile doctor and nurse (later expanded to two nurses) moving between communities, placed a lot of responsibility on the Aboriginal health workers who lived and worked in the communities. The nurses and I tried to ensure that, as far as possible, we imparted knowledge and skills to the Aboriginal health workers. The Northern Territory health department had recently started an Aboriginal health worker training program, based on one-week modules in Alice Springs. A number of PHHS health workers went to these courses, which for some was an effective means of learning, but not for all. For a few, the problems associated with availability of alcohol in Alice Springs outweighed the benefits of attending courses there. Each Aboriginal health worker brought a particular set of skills and aptitude to the job, with some having more of a clinical role than others, but all played an important role.

The pay structure of the Aboriginal health workers within the PHHS was a difficult issue. In the larger communities, health workers effectively worked full-time and so were justified to full-time pay. In smaller communities (some of which were occasionally unoccupied when people had temporarily moved elsewhere) the role and the appropriate method of remuneration was less clear, and was sometimes a cause of conflict. We did, however, encourage all Aboriginal health workers to maintain a stocked medical box (made from metal toolboxes) that they could carry with them wherever they went. With high levels of mobility in the population generally, including among health workers themselves, this was important. We encouraged the idea that Aboriginal health workers should be recognised as such wherever they went, including when attending ceremonies, funerals, sporting events and so on, and that they should have the wherewithal to justify this recognition. In some cases it worked, but not in all.

This issue of remuneration was complicated by the introduction of the Community Development Employment Program (CDEP). This program was introduced into the Pitjantjatjara and Ngaanyatjarra lands at about the same time that the PHHS commenced. The concept behind CDEP was that, instead of each adult living in remote communities receiving individual welfare payments, each community would have control over the bundled welfare funds, based on the number of people who would be eligible for unemployment benefits, with the addition of a percentage for administration and equipment. These funds could be used at the community's discretion to pay people for community-related employment. The concept was a good one and, in general, it was a successful program until it was unfortunately closed down about twenty-five years later by the Howard government (see chapter 7). During the early days of both the PHHS and CDEP in the Pitjantjatjara and Ngaanyatjarra communities, the PHHS paid Aboriginal health workers by providing 'top-up' to their CDEP income. However, because each community administered their CDEP in a different way, CDEP incomes varied and made it difficult to ensure a standardised wage for Aboriginal health workers across the region.

One of our early tasks was to establish a health-record system. Glenis and I spent many hours at the clinics in Amata and Warburton, going through the records of people who usually lived in the homelands communities and transcribing relevant details into our records. We used a system developed and marketed by the Royal Australian College of General Practitioners, with information written by hand onto pages within a folder for each person. As we were a mobile service and could not take all our medical records with us, we carried special writing pads that allowed us to write the details of any consultation at the time. On returning to Kalka where the permanent records were based, this was pasted into the main record. It obviously had disadvantages, but it was the best we could do in the circumstances and it sufficed. In each clinic, a card system of records was maintained, but due to the frequent travel between communities, we recognised that we also needed a centralised health information system.

We needed to ensure that we had a source of medical supplies including pharmaceuticals. We also needed a method of getting them to where they were needed. The Alice Springs Hospital Pharmacy, under the chief pharmacist, Andy Barr, helped with the provision of pharmaceuticals. A commercial medical supplier provided other goods, but we also needed to get the supplies out from Alice Springs. When Glendle and Tungku were community advisors at Pipalyatjara and Irrunytju respectively, they had implemented an arrangement with a company called Northern Transport for the regular transfer of supplies by light aircraft and freight truck out of Alice Springs. The PHHS was able to get its supplies by using this system out to Kalka, and we then distributed the supplies to the various clinics. The weekly Northern Transport aircraft, a Cessna 210, which brought in perishable goods for the community store as well as needed medical supplies, was also the mail plane. With no telephone or internet, mail was an important way of keeping in touch with the rest of the world, so the weekly batch of mail was always eagerly awaited.

The other means of communication was two-way radio. The RFDS in Alice Springs maintained a radio base with regular 'sked' (a scheduled time to use the radio), where telegrams could be sent and received. As these had to be read out and transmitted over the radio, it was not a particularly private form of communication. The RFDS radio station was available for medical consultations. When we had a patient who needed evacuation to Alice Springs or Kalgoorlie, we could press an emergency button on our radio, which would then allow a discussion with a doctor based in Alice Springs or Kalgoorlie who could then arrange retrieval. Once again, there was little confidentiality.

So by way of the external radio network our links with the medical system outside the area was already well established. What we did not have when PHHS started was an easy way to communicate among clinics within the PHHS. However, through the Pitjantjatjara Council, we applied successfully for a high-frequency radio channel for our use. This meant we could set up a regular 'sked', through which the Aboriginal health workers could seek advice from Glenis or myself about patients they were dealing with. The radio channel became very popular. It was the first time that Aboriginal people had their own channel and soon it was constantly occupied by a cacophony of voices talking over each other in Pitjantjatjara, Ngaanyatjarra and

Yankunytjatjara. Although this meant the radio channel had clearly met a need, it made medical discussions very difficult.

As a mobile health service we were very reliant on our vehicles. The Japanese company Toyota was dominant in remote Australia and four-wheel-drive LandCruisers were ubiquitous. We designed, and had custom-built, a mobile clinic constructed from a Toyota LandCruiser with a cabin on the back with drawers for supplies, a small refrigerator and an examination area. While this had its uses, we eventually realised that the cost involved was probably too great. The vehicles were for transport and it was better to have well-stocked fixed clinics in the communities and work from them, rather than trying to maintain a mobile clinic.

The vehicles did have their problems. More often than not, their air-conditioners had broken down, so we had to drive in the hot desert summers with the windows open. I always tried to have a couple of two-litre plastic bottles full of frozen water when I left for a drive, allowing frequent swigs of cold water as the ice evaporated. Mechanically, the Toyotas were generally sound, although there were often electrical problems. Often the starter motor would not work and a vehicle would require a push, with a driver clutch-starting the vehicle. Sometimes there were two vehicles in this condition, so the first would rely on manpower for its initial push, and then when the vehicle was running, it would line up in front of the bull-bar of the second and push that one backwards, to allow a clutch-start. And then we were off for the day.

Tyres were another frequent problem. I became adept at changing tyres but probably not quite so adept at fixing punctures. *Anangu* often placed more importance on fresh meat than tyres, so a kangaroo sighted off the road would lead to a cross-country chase, which might result in a kangaroo shot, cooked and eaten, but often at the expense of a mulga stake through the tyre. At quite an early stage we introduced a rule that our vehicles were not to be used for hunting.

While the vehicles in which we travelled presented certain challenges, so did the roads over which we drove. They were dirt tracks requiring more frequent maintenance than was possible, given the remoteness and the limited resources available. With the increased support into the area, there was starting to be a concomitant influx of road travel in and out of the area by staff from government and other agencies. The increase in traffic, particularly near communities, led to severe corrugations of the roads, resulting in bone-jarring rides. Rains also caused much road damage. Rain in the desert is unpredictable and infrequent but especially in the summer months, when cyclonic activity near the West Australian coast turns into rain-bearing depressions moving inland, heavy downpours sometimes occur. My first year on the Pitjantjatjara homelands was a particularly wet year and the water-logged roads were sometimes impassable. The nature of my work, which necessitated frequent travel between communities, meant that I was frequently driving through long stretches of water over roads and, on several occasions, the vehicle I was using became bogged, sometimes for a day or two. As the stretches of water and the underlying mud were drying, traffic resumed but often created deep ruts in the roads that were further challenges to drivers, until the roads could be graded.

We often considered the possibility of using light aircraft to overcome the challenges of road travel, as well as saving unproductive time spent on the road. Tungku had a private pilot's licence and we lobbied the DAA to provide funds to purchase a single-engine aircraft for the PHHS. On a couple of occasions we believed our lobbying was on the verge of success, but it did not happen.

Health problems

We had to deal, of course, with all kinds of health problems. In particular, we were often managing sick infants and children. Infants were, fortunately, almost universally breastfed and tended to gain weight satisfactorily for the first six months or so of life. However, in the second six months, with the introduction of solids and often inadequate nutritional intake, combined with frequent infections, weight gain stalled, often until after the second birthday. Gastroenteritis was common and the combination of failure-to-thrive, gastroenteritis and respiratory infections led to quite frequent evacuations to the hospitals in either Alice or Kalgoorlie. Sometimes diarrhoea persisted for several days, and the babies were kept hydrated with oral rehydration salts dissolved in water, but eventually muscle tone would decrease, indicating that potassium levels were depleted, leading to evacuation for intravenous fluids in hospital. On occasion, the child would be severely dehydrated and a life-saving technique would be required to deliver fluid by intra-peritoneal infusion through a needle in the abdominal wall.[1]

Another common childhood problem that proved difficult to manage was chronic suppurative otitis media, or chronic discharging ears. It was not a condition I had learnt about in medical school or in my hospital experience and guidelines for treatment were not available. Consequently despite our efforts, it was not managed well and many children ended up with a degree of deafness. Similarly many children developed chronic suppurative lung disease and, apart from treating exacerbations with antibiotics, this condition was also not managed well. Forty years later, there are greater opportunities for medical interventions to have an impact. Evidence-based standard treatment protocols and electronic health-information systems provide automatic reminders, allowing systematic management of chronic conditions. In those early days, a lot of what I did was trial and error, and it often seemed like groping in the dark.

Another intractable problem was 'petrol sniffing'. There was a small core group of young teenagers who were habitually intoxicated with petrol fumes inhaled from a can held over the face. Most young people grew out of it but some became chronically addicted and, with the lead-based petrol used in those days, some young people developed major neurological disabilities.

As the homelands were sufficiently distant from alcohol outlets alcohol use was not a chronic problem. From time to time, however, a vehicle would arrive with a load of alcohol and this would usually cause mayhem for the short period in which it was consumed; not infrequently, it resulted in trauma requiring medical treatment. Sometimes, people would have drinking binges for days or weeks in Alice Springs or Kalgoorlie. They would return, looking sick and bedraggled, and would often present themselves for treatment with signs of alcohol withdrawal, alcoholic gastritis and often with sexually transmissible infections (STIs) that I soon came to recognise as an alcohol-related (or petrol-sniffing-related) disease. The common STIs were gonorrhoea, which is still quite common today, and what was then called non-specific urethritis, but is now recognised as chlamydia, which is also still common. The test for bacterial STIs involved taking a swab that, for men particularly, was uncomfortable and made widespread screening of people without symptoms impractical. These STIs do not always cause symptoms; it was generally in those who were symptomatic (if the patient presented for treatment) that diagnosis and treatment were possible, and that contacts could be identified. Undoubtedly, many cases went undiagnosed, leading to high rates of pelvic inflammatory disease and infertility in women. These days, with better testing techniques, screening is easier, allowing greater opportunities to reduce the prevalence of these diseases.

Syphilis was common, but generally it was easy to diagnose with a blood test and easy to treat with long acting penicillin injections. As we tested regularly for syphilis we were already starting to see a decline in the incidence. In subsequent decades, syphilis became quite rare in Aboriginal communities, and there was talk of its eventual eradication, but in 2014 a new outbreak in remote Aboriginal communities in northern Australia began. Another STI that did occur in those early days and now appears to be eradicated was lympho-granuloma venereum, or donovanosis, which presented with warty genital lesions that were sometimes quite extensive and, back then, difficult to treat. A new and easy-to-administer antibiotic, azithromycin, became available in the 1990s, leading to the apparent eradication of donovanosis in Aboriginal communities.

The chronic diseases that are now so prevalent in contemporary Aboriginal communities were less common in those days. Some people were started on treatment for hypertension and a few older people were prescribed tablets for diabetes. Occasionally there was a case of kidney disease leading to renal failure but, in those days, dialysis was not available outside major metropolitan hospitals, and it was not considered an option for Aboriginal people from remote communities. There would undoubtedly have been more cases of chronic diseases if we were actively looking for them but the chronic disease epidemic was only just beginning and, even when we found them, we did not have good systems in place for the ongoing monitoring and review that is required for effective management. It became clear over time that developing such systems was a priority.

We were aware of the need to support preventive activities. Ushma and Stephi had been supporting the development of vegetable gardens and fruit trees in the homelands communities until their funding ran out in mid-1978. The PHHS applied for funding to allow these activities to continue. Some initial funding was made available by the DAA and later we received a grant from the Australian Freedom from Hunger campaign.

We recognised that nutrition was a key to many of the health problems that we were dealing with: under-nutrition in infants, carious teeth in children, and the emerging chronic diseases in adults. The families who lived in the area were hunter-gatherers with skills in finding and preparing their own foods, but in recent years had commenced the transition to a more sedentary lifestyle, replacing much of their traditional nutrient-dense foods, which they previously had to move around to find, with a diet dominated by flour, tea, sugar and tinned meat. This transition was having an adverse impact on health. Suzanne Bryce, who moved to Kalka when she and Stephi developed a relationship, was engaged by PHHS to work with local women, and particularly with the Aboriginal health workers from Pipalyatjara, Kalka and Irrunytju to gain a better understanding of nutritional practice so as to help us develop our approach to nutritional-health promotion.

The high prevalence of infectious diseases in children, including skin infections, also led to us looking at preventive approaches. We obtained funding from Community Aid Abroad to build shower blocks in each community and Bill Davis, with support from Suzanne Bryce and Tungku, composed the iconic and catchy 'Shower-block Song',[2] with words in Pitjantjatjara that encouraged children to go to the shower block.

Developing Kalka

Kalka was originally envisaged as a small accommodation and administrative base for PHHS staff. However, over time, the population increased, both with other non-Pitjantjatjara workers involved in homelands development and gradually with *Anangu* as well. Ivan Baker, as trainee administrative officer and then as Director of PHHS, moved with his family to Kalka. During the first year of PHHS operations the challenges of vehicle maintenance led to the employment of a Pitjantjatjara man, Frank Young, as the PHHS mechanic and he also moved to Kalka from Amata.

As there was a significant amount of work required to develop Kalka, Tungku's brother-in-law, Simon Thompson, was retained as works manager to oversee the development. When it became clear that a clerical assistant was required to assist with the administrative tasks, a Kaidetj woman with whom I had worked at Congress, Maria Hayes, was appointed to the position, and she moved to Kalka from Alice Springs. Simon and Maria became partners and eventually married.

During 1978 it had become clear that there was a major need for a bore mechanic to install and maintain bores, hand-pumps, windmills and water tanks at the various homelands communities. I remembered Tony Davies or El Punj, the 'tall fellow' whom I had met at Utopia, and suggested that he apply for the position. He moved to Kalka in August 1978. In Pitjantjatjara he was called Watiwara, also meaning 'tall fellow'. By the following year, it was clear that the amount of work warranted the employment of another bore mechanic and Roger Hammond, who had also been working at Utopia, moved to Kalka with his dog Lije to take up the second position.

Stephi and Ushma moved from Puta Puta to Kalka in 1978. When Suzanne Bryce, an arts and craft advisor with the Institute of Aboriginal Development in Alice Springs, developed a relationship with Stephi, her employer allowed her to move to Kalka to be with Stephi and to continue her art and craft work there. Later, as mentioned, she was employed by PHHS as a nutrition-project worker.

It also became clear that there was a need for a homelands community advisor to support the small communities around Pipalyatjara and further east towards Amata, as the Pipalyatjara community advisor had sufficient work in the growing community of Pipalyatjara itself. A tall thin Maori man named Alec Henry, who had already been doing some support work with the Kunytjanu community, was appointed to the position and was based at Kalka. Alec has lived on the Pitjantjatjara lands continuously since then and is now a respected pastor.

Inevitably, *Anangu* also moved to Kalka as facilities were established. The main traditional owners were the Cooper family, with the two brothers

Ikuta and Tjapalyi as the patriarchs. They and their extended families were established at Kalka by the end of 1978. Other *A<u>n</u>angu* PHHS employees, such as Albert Fox who became a trainee administrator, also moved there with their families.

I considered it a great privilege to have had the opportunity to live and work on the Pitjantjatjara and Ngaanyatjarra homelands. I was fortunate in having a professional skill that was valued and appreciated—all the more so as I was the first doctor to live and work there, employed by the community organisation. People would often introduce me to visitors to their communities as 'our own doctor'—an indication that my presence was valued. This also applied to many other non-Aboriginal people who were part of that early Kalka contingent. They were hard-working, dedicated people and they became good friends with whom I spent many treasured times.

While there were hard times, we all experienced the good-humoured warmth that is a characteristic of Western Desert people. Anthropologists such as Fred Myers have referred to *kanyininpa* (meaning nurturance, holding or caring for) as an essential component of Western Desert sociality and culture. There was a strong sense that we, the non-Aboriginal people employed by the local organisations, were being nurtured in this way and incorporated into the local social networks. This sense may not be as strong these days, now that the desert communities are more established and there's an ongoing turnover of non-Aboriginal staff. In those earlier days, however, when Aboriginal people were re-establishing themselves on their country, there was a strong nurturing environment for non-Aboriginal people who were willing to listen to and work with the people. Another factor was that the limited infrastructure led inevitably to closer contact. In contemporary remote communities, with both Aboriginal and non-Aboriginal people able to withdraw inside the confines of houses, there are fewer opportunities for bonds to develop around a campfire.

I believe that a stronger community spirit existed when people were feeling empowered and were taking control of their own lives by reoccupying their country. Subsequent government policies have tended to crush this sense of agency, which has contributed at least in part to many of the problems in contemporary remote communities, now receiving a lot of media attention.

I think these are among the reasons why so many non-Aboriginal people who lived and worked in those communities in the 1970s and 80s have continued to work with Aboriginal people. These non-Aboriginal people, many but not all of whom are mentioned in this book, were part of my life when I lived in the Western Desert, and many are still friends. It is quite amazing to consider that, forty years on, so many of that group of people who worked in and around Kalka continue to work in Aboriginal affairs at a community level: Glenis Grogan, Stephi Rainow, Tungku Tregenza, Anne and Bill Davis, Glendle Schrader, Suzanne Bryce, Simon Thompson, Tony 'Watiwara' Davies, Alec Henry and Roger Hammond. Sadly, Ushma Scales passed away and is buried at Kalka.

In my research, I have come across some of Ushma's hand-written notes from 1983, that were intended to be developed into an article about the early development of services operating out of Kalka, with the purpose of assisting with orientation for new non-Aboriginal staff in the area. It captures, I believe, what was special about that period. An excerpt follows:

> The one thing that stood out was the desire of the *Anangu* to maintain control at whatever level necessary. It was of such strength that the major guiding principle of community development seemed to be just: 'Don't forget who is the boss.'
>
> There was no precedent, no ideology or dogma for the theory and pragmatics of *Anangu* control and community development within this framework. This can only be formulated through first-hand experience and trial and error. It was a learning process shared by both the employees and employers; hence the '*malpa*' system prevalent at Kalka.[3]
>
> Four major tasks occupied staff in the early days:
> 1. learning language;
> 2. establishing the base at Kalka—both service and domestic;
> 3. delivering the services, program, etc. i.e. health service became responsible for health and welfare of over 1,000 *Anangu*, and the bore mechanics had over twenty-five new windmills and tanks to erect and many more to maintain;

4. encouraging, stimulating, and supporting *A*n*angu* efforts to establish suitable infrastructure for meaningful *A*n*angu* control.

As far as the first is concerned, it has been characteristic of the staff of both Pipalyatjara and Kalka to make real sustained efforts at learning the language. From 1978 to 1981, 80% of staff had varying degrees of skills in language. From 1981 onwards this trend has persisted but to a lesser degree due to staff turnover and short-term workers. It takes time to learn a language but the benefits are indisputable. In fact in the Radford Report,[4] special note is made of the language skills of the staff and that there is no recognition outside the area of this fact.

A few other non-Aboriginal people who were employed in support roles for the homelands for varying lengths of time came and went, and were usually based at Kalka. One particularly colourful character was Artie Hearn, who was employed as a heavy-equipment contractor to help with road making and maintenance. He came with his own bulldozer and also his own aircraft, a small Cessna 152, a 'tail-dragger' that looked as if it had seen better days. He graded an airstrip at Kalka and based his aircraft there. While aviation fuel ('Avgas') was generally available, Artie did not bother with this. He would land his plane on the road near Pipalyatjara, taxi up to the petrol bowser, re-fuel directly from the bowser and then taxi the plane around and take off. Artie offered the use of his services as a pilot with an aircraft if ever it was needed to the PHHS. While keen on the idea of getting an aeroplane, we were a little cautious about Artie's casual approach towards air safety. However, on one occasion I needed to get to Warakurna and there was no Toyota available. So, with some trepidation, I approached Artie in his caravan and he agreed to fly me there and back. He pulled a map from his drawer, cast a cursory glance at it and then returned the map to the drawer.

After we departed, I realised the map in his caravan was his only map; he did not have one in the aeroplane. I hoped he knew the way. However as we were flying north-west, I could see what looked like the Rawlinson Ranges out to the right and, after a while, I suggested to Artie that we were off course. 'You are probably right', he said and, after a sharp turn to the right, he made a beeline for Warakurna. I sometimes wonder what would have happened if

I had not spoken up. The direction in which we had been heading was desert all the way to the Indian Ocean.

After three years living and working on the Pitjantjatjara and Ngaanyatjarra homelands, I decided it was time to have a break and tendered my resignation, and helped with the appointment of a replacement doctor. There was one major issue that had been concerning me and that I thought should be addressed: the issue of the distinction between the Pitjantjatjara and Nagaanyatjarra communities over the area covered by the PHHS. In a report I prepared to the Pitjantjatjara Council in January 1981, not long before I left the PHHS, I discussed this issue, and it is worth quoting in full:

> One of the major problems that has prevented the PHHS from developing as a truly effective community-controlled health service has been due to the fact that the area covered includes two distinct populations. The communities in these two areas are as follows:
> 1. Papulangkutja, Marntamaru, Warakurna, Linton Bore, Walpa Pulka, Pintur Mulal, Ngatur, Paltikara.
> 2. Wingellina, Pipalyatjara, Kalka, Murray Bore, Anamara Piti, Kantarangutjara, Kunatjara, Kunytjanu, Walytitjata, Inarki, Aparatjara, Kanpi, Nyapari, Angatja and Kunamata.
>
> There are a number of reasons why these two areas represent distinct populations:
> 1. Different languages are spoken in the two areas;
> 2. Since the formation of regional councils, one area is covered by the Ngaanyatjarra Council and the other by the Pitjantjatjara Homelands Council. For true community control, these regional councils should be the decision-making bodies for health and other services within their areas;
> 3. The movement of people is backwards and forwards from Warburton in one area, and backwards and forwards from Amata and other communities in the other area. For adequate follow-up of patients and keeping of records, continual liaison needs to be kept up with these communities;

4. The people from the Western area prefer to go to Kalgoorlie and Perth when hospitalisation is required, whereas in the eastern area Alice Springs and Adelaide are preferred;
5. The borderline between the two areas corresponds roughly with the state border; hence different state authorities are concerned with health and other issues in the two areas.

It was suggested late in 1980 that the PHHS budget be divided to provide a health service for each area. It is now apparent that sufficient money is not available for this to happen but it is definitely a goal that should be worked towards. The European medical staff now consists of a doctor and two sisters. With each sister responsible for one area and preferably living in each area, and with the doctor providing cover for the whole area, the operation of the health service should be more effective. The regional councils should be seen as the governing bodies for the health services in each area.

The Pitjantjatjara Council should be actively working towards a situation where there is a Ngaanyatjarra health service covering the Ngaanyatjarra area including Warburton and its outstations, a Pitjantjatjara Homelands health service including Amata, Cave Hill and Ulkiya; a Pitjantjatjara and Yankunytjatjara health service for Ernabella, Fregon, Mimili, Indulkana and outstations, and possibly a northern Pitjantjatjara health service for Docker River, Ayer's Rock, Mount Ebenezer and Areyonga.

Subsequent health-service developments

The PHHS was not immediately divided into two parts as I had proposed but, in 1981, after I had left, the name was changed from the Pitjantjatjara Homelands Health Service to the Pitjantjatjara-Ngaanyatjarra Health Service (PNHS), operating over the same terrain.

In 1982 the Aboriginal health section of the South Australian health department, the Aboriginal Health Organisation, was under its first Aboriginal director, Elliot MacAdam. He decided to investigate the possibility of community, rather than government, control for all the other health services for Pitjantjatjara and Yankunytjatjara communities in South Australia. Trevor

Cutter and Tungku Tregenza were appointed as consultants to undertake a review and, after extensive community consultation, released the Cutter-Tregenza Report. The report proposed that the communities of Amata, Ernabella, Fregon and Indulkana-Mimili each have their own community-controlled health service for the main communities and surrounding outstations, under a confederation to be called Nganampa Health Council (meaning 'our health council' in both Pitjantjatjara and Yankuntjatjara). The PHHS (now renamed the PHNS) was not initially to be part of Nganampa Health Council. As it already had a functioning structure and extended across the border into Western Australia, the advice was that the organisation could decide at a later date whether or not, and how, to become part of the Nganampa Health Council.

In 1983 the South Australian government, with the agreement of the Commonwealth DAA, agreed to provide funding to implement the findings of this report and to establish Nganampa Health Council (NHC). Glendle Schrader, along with two Yankuntjatjara leaders, Donald Fraser and Yami Lester, was given the task of organising the transfer from the South Australian health department to the Nganampa Health Council.

In September 1983, I arrived back in Alice Springs after working with the Strelley mob (chapter 4), to work with Glendle, Donald and Yami to provide medical advice on the transfer. A large number of positions were to be appointed—one coordinator, four administrators, four doctors and about a dozen registered nurses. We advertised the positions and subsequently produced a short-list of applicants from all over Australia. In December, we flew them to Alice Springs and then bussed them *en masse* to Indulkana where a large group of *Anangu* from across the lands interviewed the applicants and chose the team. The successful applicants returned to Alice Springs in January 1984 and, after a one-week orientation course there, which I helped to organise, they travelled out to the respective communities and Nganampa Health Council became a functioning reality.

In 1981 the Ngaanyatjarra people formed the Ngaanyatjarra Council, as *Anangu* on the South Australian side of the border had by then been granted freehold title to the Anangu Pitjantjaraku Yankunytjatjaraku (APY) Lands and there was a need for an organisation to concentrate on the land-rights struggle on the West Australian side. The Ngaanyatjarra Council decided to establish the Ngaanyatjarra Health Service to provide primary healthcare across the West Australian Central Reserve, involving all the communities west of the border previously served by the PNHS, with the Eastern Goldfields RFDS contracted to provide a fortnightly visiting doctor. It also included Irrunytju which, being predominantly Pitjantjatjara, I had suggested remain as part of the old PHHS; ultimately, however, the pragmatic decision was to observe state borders rather than the somewhat blurry cultural boundaries. Other Ngaanyatjarra communities (Tjukurla, Tjirrkali and Wannan, and later Patjarr) were established in the 1980s and 90s and these were also provided with a resident nurse. In 1989 the West Australian health department contracted the Ngaanyatjarra Health Service to take over the provision of health services to the Warburton community. The Pintupi community at Kiwirrkurra, in Western Australia north of the Ngaanyatjarra lands, became part of the Ngaanyatjarra Health Service in 1990. Kiwirrkurra had previously been serviced by the Pintupi Homelands Health Service based in Kintore, as discussed in chapter 5.

The formation of the Ngaanyatjarra Health Service left a smaller health service based at Kalka, once again called the PHHS and now limited to providing healthcare to the South Australian communities between Amata and the border of Western Australia. In 1985, with Nganampa Health Council up and running, an appropriate decision was made for the PHHS to be absorbed into the NHC. The NHC continues to provide primary healthcare to the communities on the Anangu Pitjantjatjaraku Yankunytjatjaraku (APY) Lands of North-West South Australia and the Ngaanyatjarra Health Service continues to be the primary healthcare service for the Aboriginal communities covered by the Ngaanyatjarra Council.

The Pitjantjatjara Homelands Health Service was the forerunner of these developments. I was there for the first three years of its existence, working with Pitjantjatjara, Ngaanyatjarra and non-Aboriginal colleagues to build a primary healthcare service, with a structure that attempted to allow control by the community of the process and support the aspiration for autonomy and to live in dispersed homelands communities, in challenging circumstances. We did not have much in the way of precedents to follow, and mistakes were made, but we did manage to ensure that primary healthcare was provided where it was needed. Geoff Crack, a community health nurse in Kalgoorlie who occasionally did outreach visits into the homelands, jokingly termed it the Pitjantjatjara Home-made Health Service. In retrospect, it did have a bit of a rickety feel to it, but it was a fascinating time to be in a very special part of the world. I learned a lot and was proud to have been there.

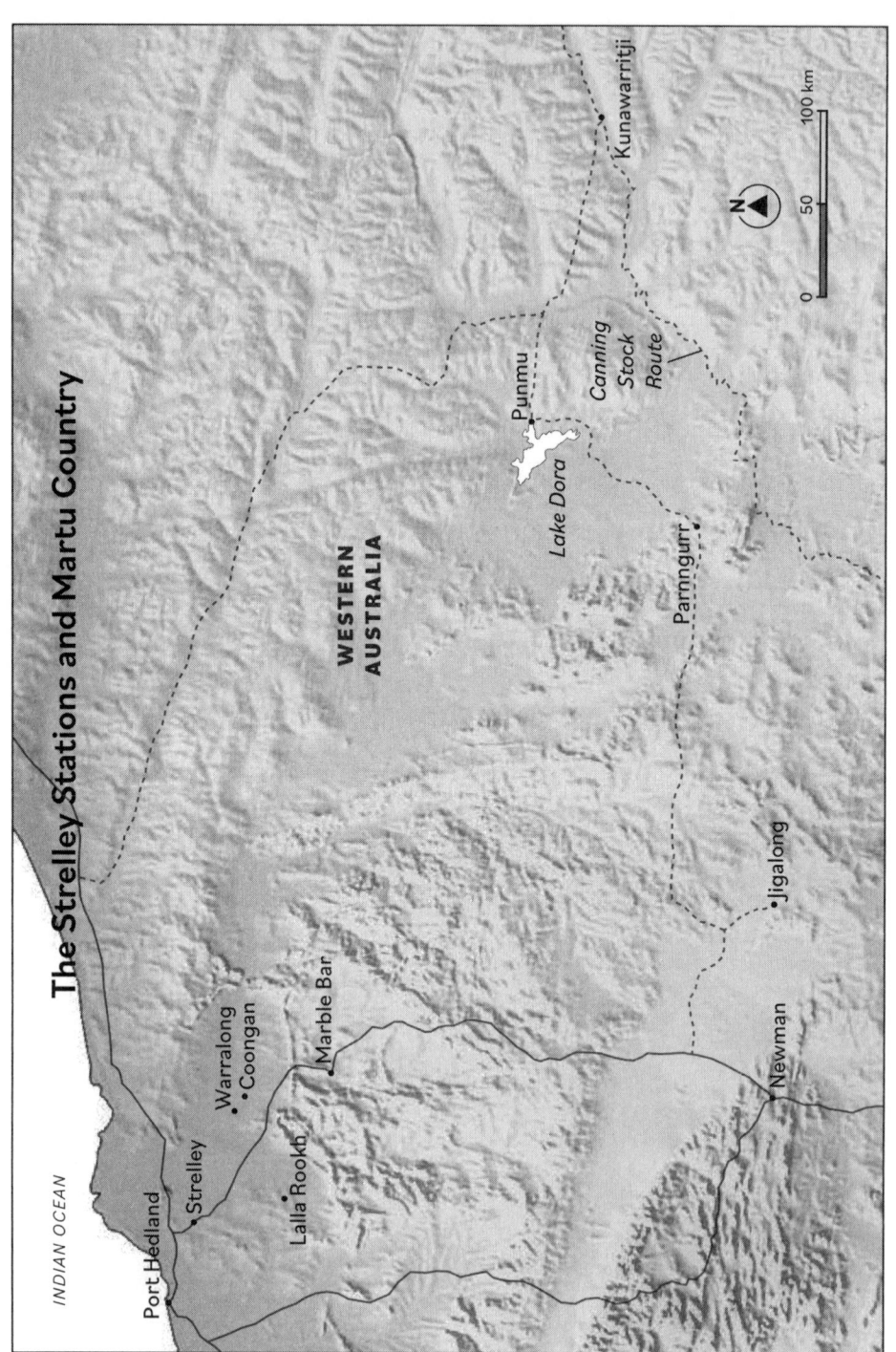

4

The Strelley mob and the *Martu*

In 2016 the ABC produced a documentary to mark the fiftieth anniversary of the Gurindji Strike of Aboriginal workers at Wave Hill cattle station in the Northern Territory. The announcer proclaimed that the Gurindji Strike was 'the first Aboriginal strike in Australian history'. This was not correct, and the fact that Australia's national broadcaster could make such a mistake is indicative of the fact that significant events in the history of settler-colonial relations in Australia do not receive the attention they deserve. There was an earlier, and largely successful, Aboriginal pastoral strike in the Pilbara in the 1940s. This strike was the catalyst for a social movement that led to a unique Aboriginal organisation. In the early 1980s, after my three years living and working on the Pitjantjatjara and Ngaanyatjarra lands, I had the privilege to work with it.

The story of the so-called Strelley mob, the Aboriginal organisation that arose out of the Pilbara pastoral strike seventy years ago, is a fascinating tale in itself. There is, however, another interconnected story that has received even less attention—that of the Manyjilyjarra people, or *Martu*. Originally from the Great Sandy Desert, the *Martu* migrated into Jigalong Mission, then left Jigalong to throw their lot in with the Strelley mob, enabling them to move back to reoccupy their homelands, and subsequently to reconnect with the Jigalong mob. I worked with these people on two occasions, 1982–83 and 1994–95, and in this chapter I tell the story of both the Strelley mob and the *Martu*; I recount my involvement with health-service development on both these occasions.

Early contact history

The Pilbara is in the hot north-west of Western Australia, an arid region with flat-topped mountains and river systems that are dry for much of the year; with cyclonic activity in the summer months, however, the rivers can flow for days or weeks. Non-Aboriginal settlement in the Pilbara began in the 1860s when land grants were given by government to pastoralists. Convict labour was not permitted in the north of the state, so Aboriginal labour became essential to the pastoral industry.

Discovery of minerals in the Pilbara in the late 1800s led to the development of a mining industry as well as the pastoral industry. An Aboriginal innovation at this time—the use of a traditional wooden dish, called a 'yandy' for winnowing and separation of minerals—contributed to opportunities for small-scale mining among Aboriginal people that was to prove useful many years later after the strike. In the early days of mining in the Pilbara, the use of the yandy by independent small-scale Aboriginal miners permitted a degree of economic independence that was actively discouraged by the authorities: there were periodic attempts by the police to round up Aboriginal people involved in their own mining activities to return to servitude on the pastoral stations.

After white settlement, the coastal Aboriginal people, such as the Nyamal people, suffered depopulation, due to epidemic diseases and infertility related to sexually transmissible infections. Aboriginal labour was replenished by people moving in from the desert, particularly Nyangumarta people but also Pijikarli, Ngurlipatu and Warnmun people, all of whom called themselves *Marrngu*. This movement meant that the traditional culture was constantly being replenished as people from the desert brought their traditions with them and developed ritual links with the land on which they settled. They also maintained linkages with the desert people further inland, the *Martu*.

Martu is the self-referential term used by a group of Western Desert language-speaking people from the Great Sandy Desert—the Manyjilyjarra, Kartujarra, Kurajarra and Putijarra peoples, in the same way the Pitjantjatjara people refer to themselves as *Anangu* and the Nyangumarta people, *Marrngu*. Although remote from non-Aboriginal settlement, the lives of *Martu* were impacted in the early 1900s with the construction of the Canning Stock

Route, linking pastoral areas in the Kimberley in the tropical north of Western Australia to a railhead at Wiluna. The Stock Route was a vague track extending through the Great Sandy Desert and involved wells being dug at strategic points, generally using water holes that were essential to the *Martu* lifestyles.

In 1907, around the same time the Canning Stock Route was being imposed through *Martu* country, a rabbit-proof fence was constructed on the margins of the pastoral areas of Western Australia to protect pastoralists from the plague of rabbits extending across from the eastern part of Australia. The rabbit-proof fence required maintenance patrols operating out of small depots, including one at Jigalong on the edge of the Great Sandy Desert, which attracted local Aboriginal groups. In the 1930s, the Jigalong Depot superintendent was made a 'Protector of Natives'. Many of the original inhabitants of Jigalong, such as the Nyiapali, drifted west to work on pastoral stations and through the 1930s, 40s and 50s, desert Aboriginal people, particularly Kartujarra and Manyjilyjarra people, moved in to Jigalong.

Maintenance of the rabbit-proof fence ceased in 1945. The ration depot also closed but the state government offered it as a mission site to the Apostolic Church of Australia, a 'small Protestant fundamentalist sect'.[1] Construction of the Jigalong Mission commenced in December 1945.

The strike

Meanwhile, on the Pilbara pastoral stations, Aboriginal people continued to provide labour in return for food and access to their land but they also maintained their traditional rituals. Although a situation of mutual dependence had developed, it was unequal, with the power very much on the side of the pastoralists and backed up by the police. In the 1940s, Aboriginal workers had begun to talk to each other about the situation and discussed it with a sympathetic non-Aboriginal ally, Don McLeod.[2]

Don McLeod was born in Meekatharra, in rural Western Australia in 1908. He left school at the age of fifteen and eventually became a prospector. He was also an avid reader and an autodidact. Through his reading and his observations of the racial prejudice suffered by Aboriginal people, he became aware of the historical legacy of oppression of the West Australian Aboriginal people. His sympathy for the plight of Aboriginal workers in the Pilbara became known to *Marrngu* and, sometime in the 1940s, he was invited to a large ceremonial meeting at Skull Springs, west of Nullagine. This was a significant meeting for McLeod and he subsequently claimed that the widespread representation of Aboriginal people from various parts of Western Australia beyond the Pilbara gave him the right to be their spokesman on issues relating to their interaction with the non-Aboriginal domain. There seems no doubt that at this meeting McLeod was at least included in discussions about collective action on the Pilbara pastoral stations.

One of the main Aboriginal leaders involved in these discussions was a pastoral worker of mixed Aboriginal and European descent, Clancy McKenna. He had already been involved in some acts of resistance against the feudal power structures of the pastoral stations.[3] McKenna expressed an aspiration for *Marrngu* to acquire their own pastoral station, where they could have control over their own labour, develop economic independence, have a place for the old people to stay and run their own school for their children. There was also talk of a pastoral strike. McLeod claimed that he initially resisted the idea of a strike, wanting to focus on getting the new station. (At any rate, as he and McKenna argued, they should wait until World War II had been won.) In the meantime, McLeod made contact with sympathetic groups in Perth, such as the anti-Fascist League, to provide support in the struggle for improved conditions for Aboriginal pastoral workers.

In 1945, with the war over, *Marrngu* urged McLeod to join them in the strike, saying they would back him up. He agreed, and proposed May Day 1946, at the beginning of the shearing season, as the strike day. One of the leaders who emerged at this stage was a traditional lawman named Dooley Bin Bin. To ensure that the strike was coordinated across stations, Dooley Bin Bin travelled by train, truck and foot from station to station with a calendar to explain the proposed action, encouraging Aboriginal workers to stop work on 1 May. The strike on May Day was not a total success as it was quickly suppressed by the police and the local inspector of the Department of Native Affairs. It did, however, mark the beginning of overt political action.

A follow-up meeting was planned for 25 May. McKenna, Bin Bin and McLeod, however, were arrested, with McKenna and Bin Bin charged with 'enticing or persuading a native to leave any lawful service'. They received three-month prison sentences and McLeod received a fine for 'associating with natives'.

In July 1946, at the annual Port Hedland Races, *Marrngu* walked *en masse* to the Two-Mile Camp from the Four-Mile Camp, 5 kilometres outside Port Hedland, in defiance of a police order that they should not camp any closer to the town than Four-Mile. The group successfully used non-violent resistance when the police tried the next morning to get them to disperse. Confronted with mass action, and aware that through McLeod's contacts in Perth the usual police response would receive public criticism, the department and the police were at a loss as to how to handle the new defiance. One response was to deny the strikers access to the coupons that were required for the purchase of tea and sugar as part of the post-war rationing. These were available to Aboriginal people working on the stations but were denied to the strikers. On 2 August, a group of people from Two-Mile walked into the town to demand ration coupons. McLeod addressed the strikers and was arrested, but was released on bail pending a trial later in the month. The strikers had returned to Two-Mile and, unaware of his release, organised another protest in the town, marching four-abreast from Two-Mile to the police station, demanding Don McLeod's release. With the contacts McLeod had made with sympathetic groups in Perth some years earlier, the action was publicised and received national attention.

The collective action now had momentum. Many of the strikers decided not to return to the stations and, instead, established a camp at 'Twelve-Mile', 20 kilometres from Port Hedland, under Clancy McKenna's leadership. Others, including Dooley Bin Bin, moved to Moolyella near Marble Bar, where they started a tin-mining operation.

Over the following months, more *Marrngu* joined the strike camps at Twelve-Mile and Moolyella and, by the end of 1947, there were about 400 strikers. They came under sustained pressure from police, pastoralists and the Department of Native Affairs to return to station employment. According to Caroline Jula, who was one of the strikers, the police came 'every morning' to see Dooley, 'pressuring him to send workers back to the stations'. But the strikers continued to say no: 'We're not going any more. Strike, strike, we strike, in Moolyella. We got self, we got to work living self.'[4] The 'living self' that Caroline Jula proudly asserted in Aboriginal English is an indication of the sense of autonomy that was being achieved.

The strikers formed their own organisation, the North-west (Native) Workers Association. The strikers insisted that it be recognised and that the pastoralists apply to that organisation for labour. Many of the pastoralists responded to the strike with an increase in wages but wanted to maintain the old paternalistic and intimidating labour relations, and insisted that Aboriginal workers be employed on an individual basis. The Aboriginal organisation held its ground, and won. Commenting on the relationship between Pilbara pastoralists and the Aboriginal workers, Anne Scrimgeour suggests that, 'for pastoralists to concede the authority of an Aboriginal organisation by allowing it to intercede between themselves and Aboriginal workers did threaten to disrupt the system of controls that underpinned labour relations'.[5]

This was one of the first examples of the development of a government-registered Aboriginal organisation in Australia. Two decades later, there would be many more such Aboriginal organisations, with the emergence of what Tim Rowse has termed the 'Indigenous sector' (see chapter 8). Aboriginal community-controlled health organisations were to constitute a significant part of this sector. The *Marrngu* were one of the first groups of Aboriginal people to demonstrate the power of organising and collective action. They were also one of the first to realise that governments were not necessarily sympathetic or supportive of such organisations.

By the late 1940s, the strike had achieved improved conditions for Aboriginal labour, with many non-Aboriginal pastoralists negotiating with the North-west (Native) Workers Association to obtain workers. The Aboriginal movement continued with other economic initiatives, including mining operations using the yandy for winnowing and separation. In 1948 McLeod, who for the previous two years had been working on the Port Hedland waterfront without direct involvement with the strike, became more involved with the movement in its day-to-day activities. Prospecting and small-scale mining operations were initially successful and by the early 1950s, the group numbered about 700.

The government persisted in its efforts to undermine the activities of the strikers. As an example, around this time the West Australian government subsidised the establishment of a Roman Catholic mission at White Springs Station near Yandeyarra, with a school for children, in the hope that this would divert the Aboriginal people from their struggle for autonomy. However, *Marrngu* avoided it due partly to the belief that the mission would weaken traditional law, as appeared to be happening at Jigalong Mission, and partly due to suspicion of government intentions. There was an attempt in 1948 to have Twelve-Mile declared a prohibited area, perhaps to encourage a move to White Springs Mission. However, the Twelve-Mile residents threatened an escalation of the strike and the prohibition order was withdrawn. Due to a failure to attract Aboriginal people, the White Springs Mission soon closed.

With the growth in numbers of the strikers, a more centralised organisation was needed. A company was formed, called Northern Development and Mining Company and all profits were pooled for the benefit of the group, enabling greater expenditure on infrastructure. Yandeyarra Station was purchased with plans for a school, a home for the elderly, a clinic and sheep and cattle to provide meat. A school was built, but the Minister for Education refused to supply a teacher on the basis that it might entice people away from other stations, and that it would appear to be endorsing Don McLeod, who by now was anathema to many in authority in Perth.

When the company ran into financial difficulties in 1954, Yandeyarra Station was closed. In 1955 *Marrngu* and McLeod established a new company called Pindan and the group became known as the Pindan movement or the Pindan mob, with Ernie Mitchell, one of the original strikers, as leader. The Pindan mob had some initial successes but by 1959 differences in approaches to management of the company's resources emerged. These differences led to a major split in 1960 with Ernie Mitchell and Peter Coppin (also known as Kangkushot) as leaders of one group and McLeod and his supporters in the other group.

According to John Wilson, the people whose traditional country was the Pilbara coastal area tended to support Mitchell and Coppin while the people who had moved in from the desert supported McLeod. Originally the differences were over management issues but ultimately it came down to differences in kinship and ritual matters. Mitchell and Coppin established the Mugarinya Pastoral Company and re-acquired Yandeyarra Station. Jacob Oberdoo, with McLeod and other supporters, established a new company called the Nomads Pty Ltd. This group initially moved to Roebourne on the Pilbara coast to undertake mining activities. However, in 1971, the Nomads acquired Strelley Station, which soon became the base for their group as well as the name by which they became known: the Strelley mob. The increasing interest of large mining companies in mineral deposits in the Pilbara had made relatively small-scale mining ventures for a small company, particularly an Aboriginal company, increasingly difficult and, with the move to Strelley, the group again developed their pastoral activities. Through the 1970s, the Strelley mob acquired other pastoral properties.

The viability of the pastoral industry also declined throughout the 1970s. The large sheep stations had been converted to the raising of cattle and even this industry was not doing well. However, the Strelley mob retained their cattle-station activities. This was partly to ensure there were opportunities for training and employment for the next generation of young men, as it was recognised that cattle work was a source of not only income but also of self-esteem. There was also the hope that the industry might revive in future years. By the early eighties, the Strelley mob had six cattle stations: Strelley, Warralong, Coongan, Lalla Rookh, Carlindi and Callawa.

One of the aspirations at the time of the strike had been for Aboriginal people to run their own stations and to have a school for the children. The Mugarinya mob at Yandeyarra was more amenable than the Strelley mob to working with government and a state-run school was established at Yandeyarra. The Strelley mob, by contrast, wanted to run their own school and rejected a proposal for a school run by the West Australian education department. After several years of negotiations, funding was obtained from the Australian Government in 1975, as well as from charitable sources, to establish an independent community school, which started in 1976. Two teachers with experience in Aboriginal education, John and Gwen Bucknall, were recruited and under their guidance the Strelley Community School achieved a significant profile for its innovations in Aboriginal education. The education was bilingual, with an independent printing press producing material in Nyangumarta and Manyjilyjarra to support the bilingual program. Its success attracted teachers from various parts of Australia with an interest in Aboriginal education.

The Strelley mob had certain distinctive characteristics. They were fiercely independent and they were suspicious of government, which they attempted to keep at arm's length. They were also opposed to Christian proselytising as they had seen at Jigalong Mission and elsewhere its capacity to undermine traditional spirituality. They also recognised the destructive effect that alcohol can bring to families, communities and traditional law, and so they strongly maintained a ban on alcohol on their stations.

Martu country

While the *Marrngu* were collectively organising on the pastoral station country, many *Martu* continued to live a traditional lifestyle in the Great Sandy Desert. In the 1960s, Australia's Cold War activities, as we have seen, had an impact on other Aboriginal people from the Western Desert and this now also affected the *Martu*.[6]

In the 1950s, the UK developed plans for a long-range missile called the 'Blue Streak', designed to deliver nuclear warheads over a range of thousands of kilometres. Major trials of the Blue Streak were planned for the Woomera Rocket Range. Elaborate facilities were developed at Woomera itself, with a firing range as far as the Eighty-Mile Beach on the West Australian coast between the Pilbara and the Kimberley. The missiles were expected to land in the Great Sandy Desert. The Talgarno Prohibited Area—an area larger than France—had been declared in December 1958, most of it in the Great Sandy Desert.

After the Blue Streak tests were announced, there were plans for a township of Talgarno, which was to have over 1,000 workers on Anna Plains Station. However before the missile tests occurred, the British cabinet, due to financial pressures, and to the chagrin of the Australian Government, cancelled plans for the Blue Streak missile in February 1960.

At the same time however, the Cold War was taking another direction with the 'space race' between the US and the USSR. As it became clear that satellites had a significant communications and surveillance capability, Britain and other European countries also wanted to develop a space program. This resulted in the collaborative European Launcher Development Organisation, or ELDO.

In 1961 a conference in Strasbourg agreed that the collaboration would develop a three-stage rocket, the Europa, to launch satellites into orbit. This was an opportunity to revive the Blue Streak: the UK had responsibility for the first stage of the rocket and redesigned the Blue Streak for this purpose. France had responsibility for the second stage, West Germany for the third, Italy for the satellite carrier, Belgium for the tracking and guidance systems, Holland for the long-range telemetry system, and Australia was responsible for the range facilities. Ten trial firings from the Woomera Rocket Range were planned, to begin in 1963. The planned impact point was in the Percival Lakes area of the Great Sandy Desert—*Martu* country.

The West Australian Commissioner for Native Welfare advised the Weapons Research Establishment (WRE) that there were still Manyjilyjarra people living in the planned impact area. In early 1964, Walter MacDougall, the WRE native patrol officer, was called in with two native welfare officers from Port Hedland and an Aboriginal interpreter. They drove to the Lake Percival salt pan where, from their campsite on the edge of the salt pan, they could see fires but were unable to locate the *Martu* themselves, and they reluctantly gave up the search.

In the meantime, the first rocket firing into the area was postponed until 25 May 1964. MacDougall and a West Australian native patrol officer returned to Lake Percival, this time with the second WRE native patrol officer Bob Macaulay. Again they were unable to directly contact the *Martu* living in the area and concluded that they had moved south of Lake Percival clear of the expected impact zone.

As it turned out, the first rocket firing fell well short of the impact zone. The patrol officers returned to Giles but on the way found that the *Martu* had actually been camping near the expected impact zone. The second firing was planned for October 1964. MacDougall took two Aboriginal guides from Jigalong Mission to search the area. This time they located seven women, two adolescent girls, six boys and five girls. Another group of eight was located by Macaulay's group and both groups of *Martu* were taken to Jigalong. The second and third firings in 1965 were uneventful, landing near the expected impact site with no apparent effect on the *Martu*. Subsequent trials of the Europa rocket used a different firing line, heading north over Gove in the Northern Territory, across Papua New Guinea and into the Pacific. *Martu* in the Great Sandy Desert were no longer directly affected by the Cold War but, over the next few years, as the numbers decreased to below a critical mass that might have been required for ongoing ritual and other activities, the few remaining in the desert joined their relatives at Jigalong.

Jigalong, Strelley and the reoccupation of the Great Sandy Desert

The Strelley mob, with their ethos of self-determination and independence from government, saw themselves as different from their southern neighbours at Jigalong. The Apostolic Church that ran the Jigalong Mission saw traditional ritual life as pagan, which should be discarded and replaced by Christianity. Efforts to undermine traditional law were strongly resisted by the Jigalong mob. The mission closed in 1970 and the West Australian Native Welfare Department assumed control of Jigalong as an incorporated community with an Aboriginal Council. After the departure of the Mission regime, a new pastor and a Christian linguist introduced a less intrusive form of Christianity, which won some adherents. From the perspective of the Strelley mob, the Jigalong mob was too much under the control of government and also in danger of undermining the law by allowing a Christian influence to develop. In addition, with alcohol available in the mining town of Newman, a two-hour drive from Jigalong, the Strelley mob believed that the temptations of alcohol at Jigalong required an approach like their own strongly enforced alcohol ban.

On the other hand, *Martu* at Jigalong challenged the view that they were too influenced by government, mission and alcohol. By this stage they had a strong community council. Overt Christian proselytising no longer existed and they maintained their own ban on alcohol coming into the community. They also had concerns that the Strelley mob had made compromises with their traditional law, which had led to its weakening, and many declined periodic invitations from the Strelley mob to move away from Jigalong and join their collective approach to maintaining their autonomy. However, there were always intermarriages and cultural linkages and some *Martu*, particularly Manyjilyjarra people from further north in the desert, who had been the most recent arrivals into Jigalong, found an affinity with the Strelley mob.

In the 1970s, a significant number of these Manyjilyjarra people left Jigalong for Strelley. One motivating factor for this move was dissatisfaction with aspects of life at Jigalong: government control, Christianity and alcohol. More significant, perhaps, was the tension between the Manyjilyjarra and Kartujarra people, as the latter had generally lived at Jigalong for longer and tended to hold positions of influence. An even greater attraction for the Manyjilyjarra people to join with the Strelley mob, I believe, was that the Strelley mob had suggested that they would help them return to their homelands in the Great Sandy Desert. The fact that the Strelley mob supported bilingual and bicultural schooling for the children was also a factor.

In 1974 the anthropologist Robert Tonkinson, returning to Jigalong after undertaking his original ethnography there in the 1960s, noted that,

> some one hundred and ten out of about five hundred people identifying themselves as Jigalong Mob members are now living at Strelley, and some of these migrants now claim Strelley, not Jigalong, as their home. With the assistance of a few early converts from Jigalong, the northerners [i.e. the Strelley mob] have managed to divide the community along its line of weakest resistance: the basic tribal division between Manyjilyjarra and Kartutjara speakers. A majority of the once numerically dominant Manyjilyjarra group is currently at Strelley, leading some seventy of the number at Jigalong (out of a present population there of about 250).[7]

The Manyjilyjarra people who joined the Strelley mob in the 1970s were initially based on Strelley Station at what was called Middle Camp, under the leadership of Ditch Williams and Nyaparu (Billy) Gibbs. I would later come to know both men. They were both highly intelligent visionaries with an intense desire for their people to achieve autonomy and control of their country, to which they were determined to return.

In 1980 Ditch went on a reconnaissance expedition with Don McLeod and Brian Kelly and they identified a site north of Jigalong, known as Camp 61, located near a windmill on the rabbit-proof fence, as a potential base for an initial desert camp. Facilities were installed and in late 1981 a number of *Martu* from Middle Camp and Lalla Rookh moved there, soon to be joined by some *Martu* from Jigalong. In 1981 a branch of the Strelley Community School was established there with Janet Sharp as the first non-Aboriginal teacher, working with some *Martu* women in a bough-shelter school.

Camp 61 was always intended to be a stepping-stone back into the heart of Manyjilyjarra country, further north. A decision was made that the site where they would settle should be Dunn's Soak, near the north-west corner of a large dry saltpan named Lake Dora. In September 1981, an attempt to find a passable track from Camp 61 north along the Rudall River to Dunn's Soak failed due to the difficult terrain. Two months later, with the help of a bulldozer, a second expedition successfully reached Lake Dora and a camp was established at Rawa Soak (also known as Roha's Soak), 4 kilometres to the west of Dunn's Soak, and an airstrip was cleared to allow supplies to be flown in. The camp came to be known as Panaka Panaka, and a few years later the name of Panaka Panaka was changed to Punmu.[8]

Another road was subsequently constructed into Panaka Panaka, leaving the Great Northern Highway about 80 kilometres south of Sandfire Roadhouse (about half-way between Port Hedland and Broome), and heading east, utilising an oil exploration road called the Wapet Road. Although this route was longer, as it followed the direction of the sand-hills, it enabled easier access and became the main land route to Panaka Panaka.

Another desert community was established along this new road at a site named Paru or Spinifex although not as a result of the aspiration to reoccupy traditional homelands. Paru was established as a drying-out and rehabilitation camp. Concerned about their relatives who were destroying their health and dignity by drinking heavily in Port Hedland and other Pilbara towns, the Strelley mob arranged for regular pick-ups of people with alcohol problems from these towns, to be transported out to the desert community, away from the grog. The establishment of a small community at Paru also meant there was an overnight camp for *Martu* and *Marrngu* making the long drive out to Panaka Panaka.

Panaka Panaka was to become the base for the Manyjilyjarra *Martu*, but they had plans to reoccupy other sites, particularly Kunawarritji, or Well 33 on the Canning Stock Route, west from Panaka Panaka, and, to the south, Parnngurr, or Cotton Creek, in what was to become the Rudall River National Park.

These sites are in Manyjilyjarra country. East from Kunawarritji is a dry, stony desert plain and further east is Pintupi country. While the *Martu* were reoccupying their country, the Pintupi people were also reoccupying theirs, moving westward from Papunya and Haasts Bluff in the Northern Territory. As will be discussed in the next chapter, the Pintupi community of Kintore was established in August 1981, with plans to move further west into Pintupi country. *Martu* and the Pintupi have cultural and linguistic ties and a 'Desert Meeting' between the Strelley and Pintupi mobs was planned to be held at Kintore in May 1982, to discuss how they might work together to sustain the reoccupation, as well as the possibility of the Pintupi mob joining up with the Strelley mob.

Not long before the meeting was due, it emerged that a non-Aboriginal person at Kintore had invited some government officials. Don McLeod and the Strelley mob, with their tradition of going it alone without government interference, objected and called off the meeting. A short time later in July 1982, the meeting was re-convened, this time at Strelley with a group of Pintupi leaders and people from some other Western Desert communities present. However, nothing tangible seemed to come from the meeting apart from expressions of mutual support. The Pintupi, with their newfound autonomy at Kintore, firmly declined the offer to become part of the Strelley communal system.

The Strelley mob then convened a meeting at Jigalong, also in July, to suggest to the mob there that they should become more involved with the desert reoccupation and join up with the Strelley mob like the *Martu* who were now living at Panaka Panaka. Tensions still existed between the two groups and, as the planned day of the meeting approached, the Jigalong mob became apprehensive about the motives of the Strelley mob; there were rumours that the Strelley mob was intending to 'take over' Jigalong. The chairman of the Jigalong Community Council, Ned Gibbs, asked the community advisor, Peter Manning, to hide the key to the community safe to ensure that it would not be accessible to the Strelley mob if they tried to assume control. He also arranged for all the hunting rifles in the community to be collected and hidden away to avoid their use if a confrontation ensued.[9] The meeting proceeded without any major fracas and, although the Jigalong mob declined the suggestion that they should become part of the Strelley mob, the day ended with a ceremonial dance. Non-Aboriginal people living in Jigalong were asked to stay in their homes during the meeting, but were invited to the ceremony. To Robyn Withnell, who was present, the dancing—with the Strelley mob dancing towards the Jigalong mob, followed by the Jigalong mob dancing towards the Strelley mob as they retreated—appeared to symbolise the day's events. Despite the peaceful outcome, the *West Australian* newspaper, having been alerted to a possible fight, still managed to manufacture a front-page story on 27 July 1982 about a 'stand-off on the edge of the desert' in which it was claimed that the Strelley mob were 'threatening to use violence', requiring the Karratha police station to send in a 'peace-keeping force'.

The Strelley mob in the 1980s

From the early days, the Strelley mob operated as a co-operative, which meant that they pooled income, including welfare money. They put this money toward building equitable access to resources and services for all *Marrngu* constituting the mob. These services included the 'loading': food was purchased in bulk, and divided up into smaller bundles for each family unit, the amount depending on the size of the family. Adults received a small amount of disposable cash but most of the income was used for community services. In 1984, McLeod wrote:

> Our group known as the Nomads, who are the management committee of the Blackfellows of Western Australia, handle $1,000,000 a year. Some of this money comes from the Department of Aboriginal Affairs in Canberra, but most of it is received through Social Security payments.

> Even this small portion we received from the Department requires a massive input of bookwork to administer.[10]

This administration was managed at the Nomads office in the Perth suburb of South Guildford.

It is interesting to note that Don McLeod envisaged the Nomads as the 'management committee of the Blackfellows of Western Australia'. He believed that the co-operative system that had developed among the Strelley mob gave Aboriginal people genuine self-determination, and that the false promises of self-determination propounded at the time by the government did not really entail the government relinquishing control over the lives of Aboriginal people. McLeod, I think, genuinely believed that his actions were directed by Aboriginal people and that the co-operative system therefore represented real self-determination. He had a vision that ultimately all traditional Aboriginal people in Western Australia should join the movement, which he believed had been foreshadowed at the Skull Springs meeting some years earlier. This, in my view, was what Don hoped to achieve from the Desert Meetings with the Pintupi and the Jigalong mobs mentioned above.

I had also witnessed Don's efforts to develop a pan-desert movement at a Pitjantjatjara Council meeting in 1978 or 79, from memory, at Irrunytju. McLeod, with a couple of senior *Marrngu* men, arrived late on the day before the meeting. I was present at a meeting between them and a number of Ngaanyatjarra men and their advisors when McLeod proposed that the Ngaanyatjarra people join up with the *Martu* and *Marrngu*, effectively expanding the domain of the Strelley mob from the north-west coast of Western Australia to the borders with South Australia and the Northern Territory, with the Nomads company as the administration body. The Ngaanyatjarra people, at that time engaged in their struggle for land rights with the West Australian government and concerned about losing the momentum of their negotiations and potentially their autonomy within a wider group, decided to reject the proposal.

A year or two later, when I still was working with the Pitjantjatjara Homelands Health Service, I was contacted by someone from the Nomads office in Perth, asking whether I might be interested in coming to work with them as a doctor for the Strelley mob. My sister, Anne Scrimgeour, had started work as a teacher with the Strelley School in 1979, and they had heard about my work from her. I was not available at that time, but I said that I would be interested in working with them and, if in the future I became available, I would contact them.

In early 1981, after leaving the Pitjantjatjara homelands, I initially wanted some time to consider my career direction. I ended up travelling to India and, while there, thought more about my next moves. I decided that I had learnt a lot over the previous three years on the Pitjantjatjara homelands, both in terms of managing the medical conditions that occur in Aboriginal communities and also in terms of health-service development. I thought that I should build on this experience.

One aspect of the three years that I had found frustrating, however, was the constant negotiations with government departments over funding. From what I had understood about the structure of the Nomads company, I thought if I worked with them I might be able to concentrate more on healthcare without worrying so much about budgets, administration and bureaucracy.

Consequently, when I arrived back in Australia towards the end of 1981, I contacted the Nomads office and offered my services. I had arranged to return to the Pitjantjatjara homelands for six weeks over the summer as a locum medical officer while Howard Sadler, who had replaced me as the PHHS (now PHNS) GP, took annual leave. I suggested that I could be available to start work with the Strelley mob in February 1982. This was agreed and I was asked to come to Perth initially for some orientation, and then relocate to Strelley.

The Strelley Regional Aboriginal Medical Service

I had purchased a Holden Sandman panel-van on my return to Australia and drove from Adelaide to Kalka to work for six weeks. I had a few days in Alice Springs at the end of the locum work, and then intended to drive back through the Pitjantjatjara and Ngaanyatjarra homelands to Warburton, and then to Kalgoorlie and Perth. Soon after I left Alice Springs to commence the trip, heavy rains set in, making the roads impassable, so I diverted back to the Stuart Highway and drove south through Coober Pedy, across the Gawler Ranges and onto the Eyre Highway across the Nullarbor Plain to Perth. The trip took several days, longer than expected, as it turned out my second-hand Sandman was not the bargain I had thought it to be and I had a few breakdowns en route. Eventually, however, I drove into Perth.

I found the Nomads office in the suburb of South Guildford, and here I met the redoubtable Don McLeod, now in his early seventies. He was a fit-looking, wiry bushman with tanned and weathered skin, wearing a singlet and shorts. I was to get to know him better over the next couple of years. He was a complex and somewhat fractious character but the Strelley mob knew him well and they were fiercely loyal to him. Although based in Perth, Don visited Strelley from time to time, where he camped next to a campfire and, over time, I enjoyed some fascinating evenings around the campfire listening to Don's stories. Much of it was listening, rather than engaging in dialogue: Don did not show a lot of interest in other people's opinions. Like many visionaries, he had a firm idea of what was right and any divergence was, from his perspective, heretical and therefore to be expunged. As a result, he made many enemies over the course of his life but he also achieved a great deal. The sense of autonomy that was a hallmark of the Strelley mob is a testimony to his achievements.

The other two employees in the Nomads office were Jack Williams, the accountant, and Ray Butler, the manager. Both Jack and Ray had utmost trust in Don McLeod. The office managed all the finances and accounting for the Strelley mob, including all its cooperative ventures. It was a lean but efficient operation.

While I was at the Nomads office, we discussed how the proposed health service was to operate. Like all other services they ran, it was to be paid for from pooled resources. There was no specific government funding for a health service as such. It was agreed that I would 'bulk-bill' using Medibank, the Australian national-health insurance system that preceded Medicare.

Medibank had been introduced by the Whitlam Labor government and under the Fraser government had become less comprehensive. However, I was still able to use it for our service. The Medibank income went to a Nomads account and I was paid a salary. I was to be provided with a Toyota LandCruiser

Troop Carrier for the health service and when required I would have the use of a light aircraft that was based at Strelley and owned by the mob. Although it would be somewhat of a low-budget operation, I thought that the resources we had would be sufficient, and this turned out to be the case.

After a few days in Perth I drove north. Western Australia is a large state and I was on the road for three days before arriving in Strelley on a typical February day—fiercely hot. I was expected, and warmly welcomed. I had been told to contact John Bucknall, the school principal, who worked closely with community leaders, and had an associated role similar to the community advisor in other communities with which I was familiar. He had the trust of the community and, importantly, of Don McLeod. John introduced me to the community leaders who were based at Strelley such as Snowy Jittermarra, Jacob Oberdoo and Crow Yougala. These were proud and imposing men who had been involved in the strike thirty-five years earlier; they displayed a self-confidence that comes from a sense of autonomy and control over one's own life. They were impressive people.

I was provided with a house on the station, adjoining the house in which John and Gwen Bucknall lived. The population of Strelley itself was about 150 people; the Strelley mob itself numbered about 400. The only non-Aboriginal people living at Strelley were those employed by the community school that was based at Strelley with branches at other sites.

There were branches of the school at three other sites when I joined the Strelley mob: at Warralong (with three non-Aboriginal teachers), Lalla Rookh (with one teacher—my sister Anne) and Camp 61 (also one teacher). The other stations owned by the Strelley mob were all within a few hours' drive of Strelley. Warralong was the most populous with perhaps 100 people and a school, operating out of the old station homestead. Lalla Rookh had a small community of fifty or sixty people, with a small single-teacher school, also based in an old homestead. Coongan was a base for cattle-station activities. One of the two pastoral advisors, Ross Johnson, lived there with his wife Luana and their two children Clay and Messina. There were a few families living at Coongan and it was close enough to Warralong for any children there to attend the Warralong School. At Carlindi another pastoral advisor, Chris Wicks, lived with his wife Glenda and a few older *Marrngu*.

The desert communities were more distant. While they were accessible by road, it was a long two-day drive from Strelley to Panaka Panaka, and a similarly long drive in another direction to Camp 61. The use of a light aircraft was clearly advantageous so the Nomads had purchased a Cessna 207, and John Bucknall and Ross Johnson had both obtained their private pilot's licence.

The Cessna 207 was available for me to provide regular clinical visits to the desert communities. Initially, either John or Ross would pilot the aircraft to get me there, and although they usually had some work to do in the remote communities, it was obviously going to be more efficient if I obtained my own licence. I had actually started pilot training in the past, but had not completed it. I contacted a flying training school in Port Hedland and started intensive training. For a few months, I allocated every Thursday afternoon for flight training. Later, on many mornings when I was at Strelley, I would rise early, drive to Hedland airport, undergo an hour's training, then drive back to Strelley to start the day's work. In this way, I quickly progressed and before too long I was the proud owner of a private pilot's licence.

I developed a routine to ensure that I was able to provide continuity of healthcare to each of the communities constituting the Strelley mob. Every Monday, I would leave early from Strelley and drive to Warralong for a morning clinic. I would then drive across the riverbed to nearby Coongan where I would often lunch with Ross and Luana and attend to any medical issues there. In the afternoon, I would drive to Lalla Rookh Station, where there was a large permanent waterhole not far from the road called Jimakaninya, where I would usually stop and cool off with a swim. I would then continue on to Lalla Rookh for an evening clinic and dinner with my sister Anne, and then camp overnight in the homestead.

The next morning, I would consult again at Lalla Rookh and work with the Aboriginal health workers, before driving to Carlindi where I would hold a short clinic with the few old people who camped there before driving back to Strelley around lunchtime to work in the clinic throughout the afternoon.

My desert trips were scheduled over two days every fortnight. Every second Friday I would rise early, check the aircraft, fly eastward into the Great Sandy Desert, stopping initially at Paru to conduct a clinic. I would then fly on to Panaka Panaka where I would spend the afternoon, before camping overnight and undertaking any follow up the next morning. I would then fly south to Camp 61 for a clinic before heading back to Strelley on the Saturday afternoon.

Towards the end of 1982, a group of *Martu* moved from Panaka Panaka to Kunawarritji, near Well 33 on the Canning Stock Route. This then also became part of my fortnightly circuit. The track into Kunawarritji was widened for a short distance to allow a light aircraft to land and this became a rough bush airstrip. In January 1983, I was the first pilot to land an aircraft there.

There was also a more remote station called Callawa on the edge of the Pilbara pastoral country owned by the Strelley mob. There was periodically a small group of *Marrngu* living here, and given its distance, when necessary I would include a Callawa clinical visit in my fortnightly flight plan.

I suggested calling the new health service the Strelley Regional Aboriginal Medical Service. This was consistent with Aboriginal community-controlled health services that in recent years had been established in rural Western Australia—the Broome Regional Aboriginal Medical Service and the Geraldton Regional Aboriginal Medical Service. It also recognised the regional nature of the health service operations, involving all the sites occupied by people constituting the Strelley mob.

The Strelley Regional Aboriginal Medical Service worked well. The administration was handled efficiently by the Perth office. Primary healthcare delivery involved just the Aboriginal health workers and me. My experience in the PHHS stood me in good stead—I now had a better idea of how to manage common conditions and, with the Aboriginal health workers, we were generally able to meet the primary healthcare needs in each community.

Snowy Jittermarra was the *Marrngu* leader who had the health portfolio. He was the person to whom I went for advice on issues relating to health-service development. We did not have a health committee as such. There was an education committee that met regularly and if there were health issues that needed community discussion or ratification, this would be bought up at education committee meetings.

My clinical colleagues at each of the sites were the Aboriginal health workers: Puwarka, Neil Bidu, Nancy and Elsie at Strelley, Nabi Robinson and Mary Sambo at Warralong, Kathy Thomas at Lalla Rookh and Debra Lane at Panaka Panaka. Puwarka was also a *ngangkari*, or traditional healer. We worked well together, but when it came to his *ngangkari* work, he preferred to operate privately—a preference that I respected. As the only non-Aboriginal clinician for a dispersed population of around 400 people I was busy but not overworked and I found my life was less hectic than it had been when working for the PHHS.

Living at Strelley, I was not as distant from the trappings of civilisations as I had been while living and working with the Pitjantjatjara and Ngaanyatjarra homelands. We did, however, rely on radio for communications. A telephone line to Strelley was planned during 1982 and I think it may have been installed by the end of that year, enabling telephone communication with the outside world. Until then, telegrams could be received or sent via the Royal Flying Doctor Service radio base in Port Hedland.

The other stations were further away, and the desert camps were very remote. Communications with these sites was always by high frequency radio. I had a radio in my four-wheel-drive Toyota and I managed to set up a system where the transceiver was tuned to a particular frequency with a connection to an alarm. The radios in all the stations and desert camps had an emergency button; if the Aboriginal health workers wanted to contact me, they could press the button and the alarm in my Toyota would be activated. It was loud enough to wake me up but fortunately calls of this nature at night were rare. If there was a medical emergency, I could drive or fly to the scene; in the case of the desert camps, the Royal Flying Doctor Service based in Port Hedland could also be called to organise an evacuation when required.

As on the Pitjantjatjara homelands, we were mostly dealing with acute conditions, especially in children, but there were a number of people with chronic conditions. The referral hospital was Port Hedland, a few hours' drive from Strelley. There were no medical specialists residing there, however, and most of the specialist services at the hospital were provided by senior registrars, generally rotating up from teaching hospitals in Perth, and supported by occasional visiting specialists. A paediatric registrar did outreach visits to Strelley from time to time and I would arrange for any children from the other stations whom I wanted reviewed to come to Strelley on those occasions for the day.

The internal medicine registrars rotated up from the Royal Perth Hospital for three or six months at a time. One registrar I remember was Barry Marshall. I referred a patient to him for investigation of chest pain, so as to exclude a cardiac cause. I was in Port Hedland when the patient was ready for discharge and I caught up with Barry to discuss this and other cases. He said he was confident that there was no cardiac cause for the chest pain in this particular patient, and it was almost certainly due to reflux oesophagitis. He then said that I might like to try a course of antibiotics for the patient because, he said, he had been doing some research that seemed to show that there might be an infective cause for gastritis and oesophagitis. This was the first I had heard of this research, but a number of years later Barry Marshall and his colleague Robin Warren were awarded the Nobel Prize in medicine for this work identifying the role of the bacteria *Helicobacter pylori*.

In 1982 the only non-Aboriginal people living at Panaka Panaka were John and Trish Harold and their two young children. John, with long hair and a beard, came from an alternative lifestyle background and had been recruited by Don McLeod to provide administrative support to the *Martu* at Panaka Panaka. He also had plans for re-vegetation of the sand hills on the shore of the dry salt pan Lake Dora.

There was another non-Aboriginal person who supported the *Martu*. Brian Kelly was a Vietnam veteran who had fought with the SAS and had subsequently gravitated to the Australian outback. He was a rugged bushman with many practical skills that he was willing to put to use as required, for no pay, for the *Martu*. He would come and go, and sometimes on my visits to Kunawarritji he would be camped there with his partner Kate de Voy.

By 1983, most of the people living at Camp 61 had moved to Panaka Panaka and Kunawarritji or, in a few cases, back to Jigalong. Camp 61 continued to exist as an ephemeral place of residence, occasionally occupied, at least into the 1990s.

When I first started visiting Panaka Panaka in 1982, soon after its establishment, the *Martu* were very keen to have a school on-site. A bough-shelter school was built and a young woman, Cheryl Girgiba, was appointed as the *Martu* schoolteacher. The Strelley School, particularly its annex at Camp 61, provided some schooling support to Cheryl by two-way radio, but the *Martu* advocated for a full annex of the Strelley School with fully trained schoolteachers. At the beginning of 1983, a non-Aboriginal teacher was appointed to be based at the Panaka Panaka school. She was a young woman named Margaret Bridger, who had only just joined the Strelley School system that year. She was later to become my wife.

The split

The *Martu* at Panaka Panaka and Kunawarritji were back on their homelands and were determined to stay there. However, they became increasingly unhappy with their position in the Strelley mob. As with the rest of the mob, the *Martu* contributed their income to the general pool, but there was a view that they were not getting their share and were not being sufficiently included in the decision-making processes.

In 1983 there started to be talk of the *Martu* splitting away from the Strelley mob. John Harold, who was initially a strong supporter of Don McLeod, had been disillusioned with the way the community at Panaka Panaka was being treated and he agreed with the *Martu* that they were not being given the consideration they deserved. He let it be known that if they did decide to split he would stay with them and help manage their resources.

The issue came to a head in September 1983 with a big meeting at Strelley attended by large numbers of *Marrngu* and *Martu* as well as Don Mcleod, John Harold and John Sherwood, who was acting principal of the Strelley School while John Bucknall was on long-service leave. I was in Strelley at the time but not at the meeting. At the meeting, the *Martu* announced that they were cutting their ties with the Strelley mob. It was not an amicable parting; there was bitterness on both sides. Don McLeod blamed John Harold for fomenting the break, but I have no doubt that this was a decision made by the *Martu*—a sign of their intense desire for autonomy, which they believed they lacked. This was despite their gratitude to the Strelley mob for the key role they played in assisting them in returning to their homelands. They were now on their homelands, and they were going to make a go of it themselves.

Among the *Marrngu* the split in 1983 caused significant sadness, reminiscent as it was of the major split in 1960, when Ernie Mitchell and Peter Coppin had left to set up a different group based at Yandeyarra. One of the senior members of the Strelley mob, Monty Hale (Minyjun) remembered it thus:

> In 1983 people came from all the various camps for a meeting in the school building. The Panaka Panaka people said, 'We're going to split from you now and go out on our own. We're going out to Panaka Panaka.'
>
> We asked, 'What are you leaving us for? We are all living well together. Mirta [Don McLeod] told us long ago that we should stay together through good times and bad, with money and without money. That's how it was in the old days, and that's how it is now. We're not going to abandon Mirta. Mirta has always done the right thing by us; he did so before, when times were hard. It wasn't you who walked off the *walypila* [white-fella] stations. It was enough that in the old days they split from us at Warrlalkurra [Yandeyarra] and that Kangkushot [Peter Coppin] and Putungaja [Ernie Mitchell] took people away. The same thing is happening now; you are turning your back on us, and maybe it's because you don't like Mirta. It must be that, like them, you're resentful because you want to get more money. We're living well today. We know the different governments have said that Mirta is wrong. But he has always stuck by us. We're going to stay with him, he got the stations for us. Well, go if you must; we're going to stay here at Yurtingunya [Strelley]. He brought us *Marrngu* together and we going to stick with his word. You've rejected our way, so go on, you follow your own path.'
>
> And indeed they went east to Panaka Panaka, and we stayed at Yurtingunya.[11]

Monty Hale's lament demonstrates the strong loyalty the *Marrngu* had towards Don McLeod, as a result of their long association with him for about forty years, through good times and bad. The *Martu*, who had joined the mob only a decade earlier, did not have the same history. Their motivation for throwing in their lot with the Strelley mob was to facilitate the reoccupation of their homelands and this had now been achieved. The ostensible reason for the split revolved around concerns about alleged maladministration and unfair allocation of resources, but I believe the split was an inevitable product of the drive for autonomy. As with the previous major split in the Strelley mob in 1960, when the coastal and river-line people went with the Yandeyarra group and the desert people stuck with Don McLeod, the 1983 split was largely along kinship lines.

The split meant that the desert camps were no longer part of both the Strelley School system and the Strelley Regional Aboriginal Medical Service. One of the two teachers working at Panaka Panaka, Peter McGlew, was in Strelley at the time of the split and elected to remain employed by the Strelley School. Margaret Bridger, however, had developed strong links with the people of Panaka Panaka, and chose to stay there with them, even though it meant she was threatened with dismissal from her employment with the Strelley School. This allowed the education of the children of Panaka Panaka, or Punmu, to continue.

I might have had conflicting loyalties if I was continuing to work in the area. However, co-incidentally, I had resigned and was due to leave just after the split. I had worked with the Strelley Regional Aboriginal Medical Service for a little under two years. I had initially said I would come for a year to get the health service established and, after my first year, I was satisfied that I had helped to establish a functional health service, consistent with the aspirations of the Strelley mob. We started advertising for a replacement doctor early in 1983 and I agreed to stay until a replacement had been found. Eventually, a GP named Ken Bewley was appointed, and he commenced in October 1983. I decided to head back to Alice Springs.

I sadly said goodbye to the people with whom I had been privileged to live and work, and drove away. I drove my Sandman northeast to Broome and then across the Kimberley into the Northern Territory, staying at Katherine for a couple of days and then heading south back to Alice Springs.

Further developments of the Strelley mob

Meanwhile the Strelley Regional Aboriginal Medical Service was re-named the Nomads Health Service and continued to operate for a number of years with the Strelley mob, which was now reduced to the communities on the Pilbara pastoral stations. A movement back to country continued, but to the fringes of the settled Pilbara area rather than further out in the desert. In 1985 an outstation under the leadership of Pit Pit Thomas was established on Lochinvar Station, near the ruins of the station homestead that was called Mijijimaya, meaning 'the home of the Missus',[12] and the community came to be called Mijijimaya. In the same year a number of people moved from Warralong further east to Callawa. Another small community was established at Jirrpayirnya (Camel Camp) on the northern boundary of the rabbit-proof fence but this community was short-lived due to the failure of the water supply.

The movement to the fringes of the pastoral station country was partly due to a desire to be close to places where there were strong cultural links but it was also due to a desire to keep the culture strong by moving away, and keeping young people away, from the detrimental effects of town life.

But pressures persisted. The Strelley mob had always been wary of government, leading to tensions between government departments and the Strelley leaders. Public servants employed by DAA, and later ATSIC, wanted the Strelley communities to be absorbed into the bureaucratic system of grants that effectively gave the government greater control over their affairs. The public servants, no doubt, believed that the people were missing out on funding for which they were eligible.

The Strelley mob, on the other hand, valued their autonomy and the mob was prepared to forego some funding if the funding obligations reduced this autonomy. Over time, however, public servants were able to attract some of the younger adults away from the Strelley mob with promises of funding for projects, and as many of the original strikers grew old and died, their authority waned. Don McLeod's role with the Strelley mob also became a matter of debate among the younger generation and his death in 1999, at the age of ninety, was a significant milestone in the slow decline in the numbers of people in the Strelley mob. As the population decreased, the ability to maintain a medical service also decreased, and they stopped employing their own doctor sometime in the 1990s.

At the time of writing, the Strelley mob have left Strelley Station and consolidated the community at Warralong Station, where around 150 people live. The Nomads office in South Guildford still exists. Both Don McLeod and Jack Williams died some time ago, and the death of Ray Butler in 2018 meant the end of the old guard.

The Strelley story is a significant one. The strongly autonomous organisation existed for about fifty years. The famous strike that began in 1946 was partly about better working conditions, but more significantly for the *Marrngu*, I strongly believe, it was a struggle for autonomy. Hence Snowy Jittermarra asserted, in a documentary movie made about their story in 1987, 'We're still on the strike today, we're still on strike now.'[13] That struggle, however, was eventually undermined.

An unfortunate aspect of the story is that it did not get much attention from the activist Aboriginal leadership at a time when Strelley may have provided a model for emulation elsewhere. The great Aboriginal visionary and larrikin Tracker Tilmouth, who spent much of his life exploring options for economic sustainability in remote Aboriginal communities, and who was influenced by the time he spent as a young man on an Israeli kibbutz, said to his biographer Alexis Wright:

> The closest thing I can see to where we need to be is probably a kibbutz-type operation, where you get the whole family group doing certain things and looking after each other and kids are being looked after and going to school … people are working, you might not be earning so much money but at least you get a feed every day.[14]

Strelley was the place within Australia where Tracker's vision has come closest to realisation, but I am not sure that Tracker was aware of it. This can be attributed to Don McLeod's suspicion of the motives of educated Aboriginal people of mixed parentage who, he believed, had the same assimilationist ideas as the government. By keeping not just the government at arm's length, but also Aboriginal activists such as Tracker Tilmouth, as well as his increasing intractability as he grew older, it may be argued that he contributed to Strelley's isolation and eventual decline.[15]

Puntukurnu Aboriginal Medical Service

The *Martu*, having separated from the Strelley mob, did not have access to healthcare provided by the Strelley Regional Aboriginal Medical Service. The Royal Flying Doctor Service, from its base in Port Hedland, started fortnightly clinic flights into Panaka Panaka, re-named Punmu after the split. Other options for health-service delivery were explored.

About a year after the split, when I was working for the Pintupi Homelands Health Service to the east of Manyjilyjarra country, there were suggestions that the Pintupi Homelands Health Service could extend its operations to the west to include Kunawarritji and Punmu. This did not eventuate, and it was probably an impractical option, but there was a more informal mode of health support provided by the Pintupi mob. George Nyunmul Tjapaltjarri, known as 'Doctor George', a renowned *ngangkari* with whom I worked in the Pintupi Homelands Health Service, would frequently be asked to travel to Manyjilyjarra communities to attend to the sick. A vehicle would be driven from wherever he was needed to Kintore or Kiwirrkurra to collect him and Doctor George would travel long distances to provide his highly valued services.

The Western Desert Puntukurnuparna Aboriginal Corporation, or WDPAC, was formed in 1984 at a meeting in Kunawarritji. I happened to be there for the meeting as I was working at Kintore and had hired an aircraft with a couple of friends over an extended Easter break and was passing through Kunawarritji at the time of the meeting. WDPAC was set up as a land council to work towards land rights for communities in the northern part of the Western Desert but it became a more general resource agency particularly for the communities at Jigalong, Punmu and Kunawarritji and later at Parnngurr, near Cotton Creek in the Rudall River National Park, when people settled there in 1985.

In subsequent years, partly due to common interests as part of WDPAC, and also presumably for pragmatic reasons after the support from Strelley was withdrawn, a reconciliation between the *Martu* in the Manyjilyjarra desert communities and the *Martu* at Jigalong was achieved, all communities subsequently worked more closely together.

In 1993, ten years after I had left Strelley, I was living in Alice Springs with my young family, working with the Menzies School of Health Research. One day I received a call from Paul van Buynder, a former colleague who was now the public-health physician for the Pilbara region within the West Australian health department. He informed me that Jigalong, Parnngurr, Punmu and Kunawarritji, which by then were receiving health services from the department, had been having discussions about moving towards a community-controlled model of healthcare. He asked whether I would be interested in undertaking a consultancy to make recommendations. Consequently, I again found myself back in the Pilbara.

The Western Desert Puntukurnuparna Aboriginal Corporation (WDPAC), as the resource agency for the four communities, was the organisation managing the negotiations with the state health department over the possible transfer of health services to community control. The manager of WDPAC was Mark Chambers, whom I had met several years earlier when I worked with the Pitjantjatjara Homelands Health Service. After graduating from Mount Lawley Teachers' College, Mark had been appointed to the single-teacher school at Warakurna on the Ngaanyatjarra lands. He had become enamoured of the desert and Aboriginal culture and had given up teaching. He had married an Aboriginal woman from Warakurna, Judith Golding, who had been an Aboriginal health worker there when I worked in the area. He had developed an interest in early-contact history and, in between his historical researches, had worked in various support roles. He was now employed by WDPAC.

Mark met me when I flew into Port Hedland and we drove out to the communities. I had an opportunity to investigate the infrastructure for health-service delivery and I had meetings at each community to discuss the advantages and disadvantages of community control of their health services. The *Martu* were aware of the concept of community control of health services, particularly through their cultural links with Ngaanyatjarra and Pintupi communities and they saw the development as an important part of their aspirations for more autonomy and control over their own affairs.

I wrote a report for the health department outlining my findings and my support for the project, and included a plan for the transition to a community-controlled Aboriginal health service. The plan included employing a doctor to be based at Jigalong.

When I returned to Alice Springs, I discussed with my wife Margaret the possibility of applying for this position. We both thought that this was an opportunity to re-establish our links with the *Martu*. I took leave without pay from the Menzies School of Health Research in Alice Springs and in October 1993, with Margaret and our two young daughters Sophie and Laura, relocated to Jigalong, where we lived for the next two years in a house next to the clinic.

When I commenced work at Jigalong, I was employed by the West Australian health department. The plan was that, over the next few months, there would be a transition to community control and, when this happened as planned, I resigned from the health department to assume my role as the medical officer with the new health service. The *Martu* decided the health service would be called Puntukurnu Aboriginal Medical Service (PAMS); *puntukurnu* means 'belonging to the people'.

One of the aims of the health service was to ensure that *Martu* living on their homelands had access to healthcare. The health department's system of healthcare delivery, in general, worked better when close to larger centres. A greater distance from these centres generally meant less continuity of care. This was to some extent inevitable when healthcare is delivered out of a regional centre as there were always logistical obstacles to ensuring that small communities, remote from the centre, received the same level of care as was available closer to the centre. The Puntukurnu Aboriginal Medical Service, like the Pitjantjatjara Homelands Health Service, the Strelley Regional Aboriginal Medical Service and the Pintupi Homelands Health Service, was consciously designed to ensure, to the greatest possible extent, that people could live in small dispersed communities without compromising access to healthcare. Although I was based in Jigalong, there was a clear understanding that the Manyjilyjarra communities of Parnngurr, Punmu and Kunawarritji should have a similar level of primary healthcare as that available at Jigalong. In fact, when I started working for PAMS, I had proposed that consideration be given to our family relocating from Jigalong to Parnngurr, as Parnngurr was more central in the area covered by the health service. However, for various reasons, mainly of a logistical nature, the doctor's residence continued to be at Jigalong.

To contribute to effective primary healthcare in all four communities, we ensured that funding was available to employ a male and female Aboriginal health worker in each community. As it happened, some of these workers were already in place and we were able to ensure their employment was less precarious and more sustainable, and others were quickly selected by their communities and appointed.

Prior to the development of PAMS, non-Aboriginal health staff had not been based at the communities other than Jigalong. It was agreed that there would now be a registered nurse based at Punmu and Parrngurr, with the Punmu nurse doing outreach visits to Kunawarritji. We advertised these positions and flew shortlisted candidates to the communities to be interviewed by a community panel. I was a bit surprised when the Punmu community chose a young relatively inexperienced nurse over a more experienced one. It turned out however to be an excellent choice. Belinda Wozencroft was a very competent nurse who related well to the community and who intuitively understood what was needed for primary healthcare development. She stayed in Punmu for three years before studying medicine and becoming a GP.

The nurses and Aboriginal health workers had radio contact with me at Jigalong, where there was telephone contact with the wider world, but we continued to rely on radio communication for healthcare support between the communities. I arranged with the Royal Flying Doctor Service base at Port Hedland, which operated a high-frequency radio station, to have one particular frequency available for a half-hour session every lunchtime, allowing regular contact with the nurses and health workers

I visited Parrngurr, Punmu and Kunawarritji on a fortnightly basis. In the alternate weeks I drove to Parrngurr, a four-hour drive, and stayed overnight, but only on one occasion did I drive further north along the road from Parnngurr to Punmu and Kunawarritji along the Rudall River and around Lake Dora, as it was a long and difficult drive. Most of the time, we relied on travel by light aircraft for the fortnightly visits; an aircraft and pilot were hired to fly me around the communities for two or three days, usually staying at Punmu. My pilot's licence had lapsed and I decided not to renew it; at this stage in my career I was happy to rely on more experienced pilots.

It was decided that there should be a community health board to ensure community oversight over the transition from the health department to community control and as an ongoing mechanism to ensure accountability to the community. In order to ensure representation from each community, as well as equal gender representation, the constitution we developed stated that the board would consist of a man and a woman from each community.

As it happened, each community had a male and female Aboriginal health worker and all were mature and well respected. When a community meeting was held at which the board was to be elected, I was informed that the community had appointed the eight Aboriginal health workers to the health board. I suggested that this might not be appropriate; as employees of the health service, as well as members of the board of management, there may be potential conflicts of interest. I suggested that the community may wish to reconsider the choice, but after the next meeting I was informed that the community was clear that they saw these eight health workers as the most appropriate representatives and wanted them on the board of management. It eventuated that it was a very active and engaged board of management and when conflicts of interest arose we were able to manage them appropriately.

Reflecting the shift to a more sedentary lifestyle, chronic diseases in adults were more evident than they were a decade earlier; many people were on medications for hypertension, diabetes, high cholesterol or related problems. This necessitated regular reviews to assess the control of the problem as well as the potential development of complications and to ensure ongoing supplies of medication. A paper-based medical-record system was still in use and we had a system of cards to try to keep track of those who were due for medical review.

Electronic medical records were in their infancy but there were obvious benefits of a functional electronic system to provide reminders of when reviews were due. When the Australian Government offered grants to primary healthcare services to develop a system of electronic medical records, the PAMS board agreed that we should apply. After receiving the funding, I investigated whether there were any electronic systems available that would meet our needs. There did not seem to be anything available so we decided we should develop our own system. We found a Perth-based company willing to work with us in developing a system that concentrated on providing us with regular lists of people who were due for review or intervention. The principal of this company was Brian Dunstan, who later built on this experience of working with PAMS and other health services to develop an electronic health information system called Communicare that is now used by most Aboriginal community-controlled health organisations across Australia.

By the beginning of 1995, I was satisfied that the Puntukurnu Aboriginal Medical service was functioning well and started to make plans to find a replacement doctor and to return with my family (now with the addition of our son Callum, born in early 1995) to Alice Springs. In July I handed over to Ray Mackenzie, who had worked for many years with the Carnarvon Aboriginal Medical Service. He had agreed to work for a short time while awaiting the arrival of my friend and colleague Toby McLeay, who had worked for many years as the doctor with Urapuntja Health Service in Utopia and had since moved to the Adelaide Hills. He was ready for some more bush work and moved with his wife Lizzie and their three children to work with PAMS for two years.

The Puntukurnu Aboriginal Medical Service continues to provide healthcare to people living at Jigalong, Parnngurr, Punmu and Kunawarritji, as well as a *Martu* community in the mining town of Newman. Like many Aboriginal organisations it has had its ups and downs but is currently a well-functioning service, with Robby Chibawe as the CEO and Carol Williams as the chairperson of the board. Importantly, it continues to support the aspirations of *Martu* to continue to live autonomously on the homelands, which they reoccupied with the help of the Strelley mob in the early 1980s.

5

Pintupi country, Pintupi health

The magnificent MacDonnell Ranges extend east and west from Alice Springs. Westward, the ranges extend for about 300 kilometres from Alice Springs as far as Amunturrngu, or Mount Leibig, where the ranges peter out into flat desert country. Around 100 kilometres further west, there is a cluster of hills called the Ehrenberg Range, where a place known to the Pintupi people as Ilypili is one of the indications that Pintupi country has been reached. Another 100 kilometres or so further west, near the border between the Northern Territory and Western Australia, is another group of hills called the Kintore Range; its most dominant feature is Mount Leisler, or Yunytjunya. This area and further west across the West Australian border is the Gibson Desert, one of the most isolated areas of the world. The Pintupi people who occupied this remote region were among the last groups of Aboriginal people to have contact with settler-colonial Australia.

Early contact history

The reports of early explorers perhaps helped to keep the Pintupi people isolated from outside influences. In late 1872 when the explorer Ernest Giles reached the Ehrenberg Range he wrote: 'I can truly say it is dry, stony, scrubby and barren ... I saw few living creatures but it is occasionally visited by its native owners, to whom I do not grudge the possession of it.' Giles named the Gibson Desert (originally Gibson's Desert) after Alfred Gibson,

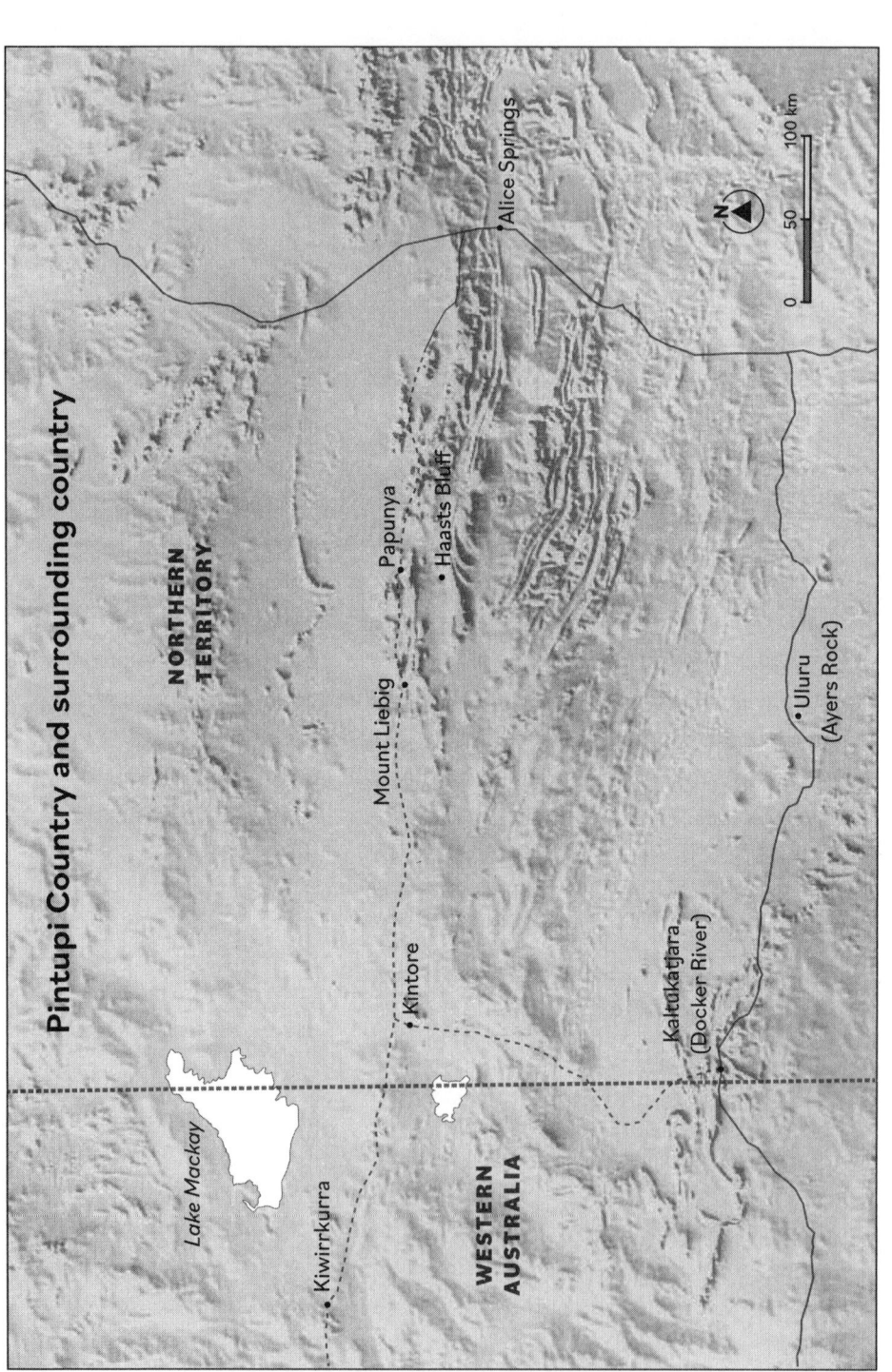

one of his party who, on another expedition leaving in 1874 from the Rawlinson Ranges to the south, became lost and perished in the harsh desert. Giles wrote that he 'called this terrible region … Gibson's Desert, after the first white victim to its horrors'.[1]

In 1889 William Harry Tietkens, who had been Ernest Giles' second-in-command, led the Central Australian Exploring and Prospecting Association Expedition into the area. Tietkens visited the Kintore Range and named its highest point Mount Leisler. He wrote that 'a strange wild panorama of desolation met our view: to the north round by west and the distant horizon was unrelieved by hill or range of any kind whatever. Spinifex plains extended as far as the eye could reach.' He also wrote that 'my wanderings through dreary and desolate regions to find the goal of my long cherished hopes in a still more desolate waste was a sad frustration that I had little anticipated'. He thought the country around the Kintore Range was absolutely waterless and that the spectre of Mount Leisler would fulfil a useful purpose by warning the future traveller to avoid its dry and waterless surroundings.[2]

Pintupi country is indeed harsh but it is, to my eyes, starkly beautiful. For Pintupi people it is the source of material and spiritual sustenance. They have lived in this country continuously for thousands of years (although, as we shall see, for a short period between the 1960s and 1981, the numbers living in Pintupi country were reduced to just one family group).

With the inexorable spread of European influence across the Australian continent during the nineteenth and twentieth centuries there was an inevitable, if rather late, encroachment on the Pintupi people. The Finke River Mission was established by the Lutheran church in Arrernte country at Hermannsburg (about 100 kilometres west of Alice Springs) in 1877 and in the first half of the twentieth century there was outreach work by missionaries into the country to the west of Hermannsburg. This outreach work made contact with some Pintupi people who for various reasons had travelled east from their country.

The cattle industry was also spreading throughout the area. In 1937 the area around a conspicuous breakaway mountain in the MacDonnell Ranges, 250 kilometres west-north-west of Alice Springs named Haasts Bluff, was earmarked to become a cattle station. In that year, Pastor Albrecht from the Finke River Mission and Dr Charles Duguid, founder of the Ernabella Mission on Yankunytjatjara country, as discussed in chapter 2, visited the area. Albrecht and Duguid convinced the Minister for Territories to revoke the grazing licence and instead to create an Aboriginal reserve in order to provide some protection for Aboriginal people in the wider area. Subsequently, after World War II, the Finke River Mission established the first permanent 'ration post' (a site for the distribution of food to itinerant Aboriginal people) at Haasts Bluff.

The Haasts Bluff ration depot was taken over by the Northern Territory administration in 1954 and five years later the welfare branch proclaimed the Pintupi Aboriginal Reserve to the west of the Haasts Bluff Reserve. Continuing immigration of people from further west led to a search by the Northern Territory administration for other sites for possible settlement. Better quantities of underground water were found 50 kilometres north of Haasts Bluff, leading to the sinking of bores and the beginning of the construction of Papunya settlement in 1956. By 1959 facilities had been established, enabling the transfer of significant groups of people to Papunya from Haasts Bluff. These facilities at Papunya included a school, a hospital staffed by two nurses (in a converted Nissen hut with three wards including a labour ward), and a kitchen/dining-room that provided three sit-down meals a day for all the settlement's residents.

The settlement of Papunya was officially opened by the Minister for Territories in 1960. A census in that year showed a population of 676 people living in the settlement as well as nearby outstations. The majority of these people were Pintupi speakers from the desert country to the west. Although they were away from their home country, Papunya was close to an important *tjala tjukurrpa* (honey-ant dreaming) site that linked to Ilypili in the Ehrenberg Range at the eastern edge of Pintupi country, meaning that there were cultural ties with the country for Pintupi people. Nonetheless, it was not their country.

The eastward movement of Pintupi people was part of a general movement of desert people speaking variations of the Western Desert language group into Arrernte country in the middle years of the twentieth century. This also included Pitjantjatjara people from the south. This led to the emergence of a lingua franca on the south-west of Arrernte country, which was a hybrid of Western Desert languages with some Arrernte influence. This language became known as Luritja, from a word meaning 'stranger' in Arrernte, and is the term used today for the people living at Papunya, Haasts Bluff and Mount Liebig.[3] This language continues to be used by some Pintupi today (the language spoken in Kintore today is sometimes called Pintupi-Luritja). The term 'Pintupi' was not originally used by the Pintupi people in reference to themselves. It was, I believe, a term applied by other Aboriginal groups to the Pintupi as a result of a long drawn-out exclamation of surprise—Pin-too-peee!—used exclusively by the people who came to be known as Pintupi and which I occasionally heard uttered by older people when I lived and worked with them.

In 1939 a German Pallottine Catholic mission called Balgo was established north of Pintupi country, on the south-eastern desert fringe of the Kimberley region of Western Australia. Some Pintupi people migrated into Balgo, along with Manyjilyjarra people who were able to travel north along the Canning Stock Route. The dominant language at Balgo is called Kukatja, which refers to the use of the word *kuka* for meat. The Kukatja language is a Western Desert language, very similar to Pintupi and it identifies the people from the country immediately north-east from Pintupi country.

Throughout the 1950s and into the 1960s, people continued to migrate into Haasts Bluff, Papunya and Balgo from Pintupi country. There were numerous pressures causing this migration. The severe drought in the late 1950s and early 1960s was one major cause. Even without the drought, the Pintupi people, like hunter-gatherers everywhere, were attracted by free food. The eastward migration was facilitated by Northern Territory patrols led by the anthropologist Jeremy Long, who was employed as an officer of the welfare branch. Long made nine patrols into Pintupi country from 1957 to 1964, returning with a number of people who would move into the settlements.

In 1960 a patrol found graded roads constructed to the south of the Kintore Range by Len Beadell's road-making team from the Weapons Research Establishment at Woomera, and of which they had not been aware. It appears that there was not much communication between the WRE and the welfare branch. In 1962 Long led a patrol to 'see what impact the new road was having on the people of this area'.⁴ He was joined on this patrol by the ubiquitous Walter MacDougall, the WRE patrol officer. On all his patrols, Long met a number of people, many of whom I would get to know two decades later in Kintore. For most of them, this was their first contact with non-Aboriginal people.

The degree to which the transportation of Pintupi people out of their country in the 1950s and 1960s was voluntary has been disputed, both at the time and later. A newspaper report in 1964 stated that the federal Labor politician Kim Beazley (father of the future Labor Party leader with the same name) claimed that tourism, oil and science had been the prime reason for shifting forty-two nomadic Aboriginal people to Papunya. In his response, the Territories minister Barnes denied that any force or false persuasion had been used to get them to leave their tribal land, and that they would be free to return when drought conditions ceased.⁵

Some retrospective accounts suggest that Pintupi people were unwilling to leave their country and were coerced into doing so. Other accounts give a more nuanced view. There were certainly reasons for government officials to encourage the migration; in particular the extant assimilation policy and the fact that Pintupi country lay within firing distance of the Woomera Rocket Range. However, pressures within Aboriginal society also contributed to the emigration from Pintupi country. These included the pressure from family members who had already migrated, the need to seek marriageable partners, the enticement of free and novel foods and concerns about *waramala* (bandits) and social breakdown as the remaining population thinned out. Christian evangelism also played a role, with Aboriginal evangelists moving back and forth from the Hermannsburg Mission. Marriage ties that developed allowed Pintupi people to live on country that was not their own.⁶

The accounts I have heard from Pintupi people suggest that there was little compulsion from government officials motivating their migration away from their country but most people did not envisage that the move would be permanent. Jeremy Long, who transported a number of people to Papunya, continues to be held in high regard among the Pintupi and he definitely recognised their strong attachment to their country. As early as 1957, in a report after his visit to the Kintore Range, he proposed that 'facilities such as are provided at the settlements should be provided to the Pintupi in their own country' as 'the adults do not like living at (Papunya) and are keen to return to their country if the Administration would assist them to live there and develop it'.[7] Kimber commented that this was 'totally unacceptable to the leading government officials' of the day, consistent with the policy of assimilation.

Whatever the reasons for being there, in Papunya and Haasts Bluff Pintupi people pined for their homeland. With exposure to unfamiliar infectious diseases and to alcohol, along with social and cultural breakdown associated with the move away from their country and the change in lifestyle, the mortality rate among the Pintupi was high. The linguists Ken and Leslie Hansen, who have had a long association with the Pintupi people, first went to Papunya in 1966. Fred Myers cites Leslie Hansen as saying: 'You'd hear crying and we'd say "Why are they crying?" and they'd say "All the Pintupi are going to die; they going to finish up."'[8]

During the 1960s Pintupi people continued to arrive in Papunya but there was simultaneous pressure from Pintupi within Papunya to move back towards their country at a time when official attitudes towards assimilation were softening. In 1967, recognising the problems faced by Pintupi people in Papunya, the Northern Territory welfare branch funded an outstation at a bore called Waruwiya, west of Papunya. However, problems with water quality led to its abandonment and the Pintupi returned to Papunya. In 1970 an outstation at Alumbara Bore, also west of Papunya, was established but an incident involving conflict with police led again to a return to Papunya. In 1973 a group of Pintupi people moved to Yayayi, further west towards Pintupi country, and within two or three years the population at Yayayi had reached around 300 people. After 1976, however, for various reasons the Yayayi community declined; some people moved further west to Yinyalingki, where a new bore had been drilled, and others moved back to Papunya. As Myers noted, 'Their difficulties in organising a group so much larger than any in their previous experience had never been resolved.'[9] There was also the fact that these outstations were on Luritja country; they were still not back in Pintupi country.

Reoccupying Pintupi country

Then, in 1981 the reoccupation of Pintupi country began with people moving back to the Kintore Range. The water supply was from a bore near a site called Walungurru and as people settled near the Kintore Range, they called themselves the Walungurru community. A few years later, when they were finally recognised by the Northern Territory government as a distinct community—rather than as an outstation of Papunya—and so eligible for direct funding, an incorporated body was formed, called Walungurru Community Incorporated. However, throughout the time I have been associated with the community, both local and external people usually refer to the settlement as Kintore, which I will also use in what follows.

The original move to Kintore was initiated by the Pintupi people themselves, with little government support or funding. One of the leaders, Jack Kunti Kunti, had access to a tractor and trailer, and he made a number of long, slow trips back and forth along the rough desert track from Papunya to Kintore (part of the network of roads made by Len Beadell and his team in the 1950s to facilitate access into the desert for the Woomera rocket-testing activities). He transported people with their blankets, dogs and other meagre belongings to their new residence.

They also had a non-Aboriginal man to act as a go-between with non-Aboriginal agencies. Paul Parker had worked in Papunya as schoolteacher and married his teacher's aide, a young Pintupi woman named Tilau. I had met Paul and Tilau in 1978 when they moved from Papunya to Irrunytju, when Paul became the community advisor after Tungku Tregenza had resigned to assume the role as administrator for the Pitjantjatjara Homelands Health Service. Paul and Tilau stayed there for several months but Tilau was homesick for her people and her country and they moved back to Papunya. When in 1981 the Pintupi people moved to Kintore, Paul moved with them and assisted with community management. Unfortunately, the following year, Paul fell out with the community. There was an angry response to a contravention of community expectations, which led to a confrontation in which Paul received a head injury. While the people were grateful for the work that Paul had done in helping to establish Kintore, they were adamant that he should permanently leave.

There were about 300 people in Kintore by 1982, which rose to about 500 by 1983. A governing body called the Western Desert Outstations Council was formed as the entity that could receive government funding, although this funding continued to be funnelled through the Papunya Council.

The people at Kintore, of course, needed health services and initially this was supplied by the Lyappa Medical Service, based at Papunya. Lyappa Medical Service (originally called Lyappa Congress) was the community-controlled service that had been operating in Papunya since 1978. It will be recalled that Trevor Cutter, in the 1976 Cutter Report, had recommended the establishment of a health service at Papunya. Funding became available in 1978, soon after funding had been released for the health services at Utopia (see chapter 1) and on the Pitjantjatjara and Ngaanyatjarra homelands (see chapter 3).

The health service started at Papunya in June 1978. Although the Cutter Report had recommended that the Haasts Bluff community should be included in the health service, this did not happen and Haasts Bluff continued to receive services from the Northern Territory health department. Also contrary to the recommendations of the report, the proposed governing Council of Ngangkaris was not established and the Papunya Council became the incorporated organisation that was funded for the health service. By 1981, Lyappa Medical Service employed a non-Aboriginal doctor, two nurses (one Aboriginal and one non-Aboriginal) and a number of local Aboriginal staff.

Not long after people had settled at Kintore, a meeting was held at Papunya to talk about health services. As there was tension between the Papunya Council and Pintupi people who had left Papunya, Yami Lester, a highly respected blind Yankuntjatjara man, was invited as an independent facilitator. It was agreed that Lyappa Medical Service would provide health service support to Kintore through a regular radio sked, supply of medications, employment of local Aboriginal health workers and regular visits by the doctor. The service had already provided health visits to outstations around the Papunya area including those in the west established by Pintupi people and now the Lyappa health staff provided regular health visits to Kintore. This increased the workload for the service and a second doctor was appointed.

Although the non-Aboriginal staff were very supportive of the Pintupi community at Kintore, the governing body of Lyappa Medical Service was still the Papunya Council, which consisted only of the Papunya people. Lyappa Medical Service was caught in the middle of the conflict between the Papunya Council and the Pintupi. Criticisms were made of staff that they were employed to provide a service to Papunya and that they should not be spending so much time with the Pintupi. In order to prevent staff travelling to Kintore, the council refused to provide diesel for the vehicles. However, the senior doctor at the time, Adrian Sleigh, purchased jerry cans that he would fill up in Alice Springs to allow regular visits to continue. The Papunya Council also changed the locks on the radio to prevent Adrian communicating with the people at Kintore.[10]

Some pressure was put on the Papunya Council by the DAA to ensure that the people at Kintore were not denied health services, and in January 1982, a registered nurse, Rob Amery, was appointed to work at Kintore. Rob spent most of his time at Kintore but found that his effectiveness was hampered by the lack of access to the Lyappa Medical Service doctor.

As Myers describes, Adrian Sleigh, as the senior Lyappa Medical Service doctor, had been an outspoken advocate of the health needs of the Aboriginal people in the area and in doing this had created tensions between himself and officials within both the DAA and the Northern Territory health department. In Myers' account, Adrian had a well-formed ideology of community control but this created tensions when there was contestation about which community exactly should have control. When tensions developed between the health staff and the Papunya Council, the staff found themselves isolated without support from their official governing body, the funding body, or the health department, and they were unable to mobilise support from the Papunya community.

Some sections of the health-service clientele probably would have had sympathy for the staff position, but some were themselves isolated (the Pintupi people being geographically removed and without significant power), whereas others in Papunya itself may not have been prepared to confront the council over the issue. In December 1982, the Papunya Council dismissed all their non-Aboriginal health staff and the Northern Territory health department, which had been in communication with the Papunya Council for some time, was ready to resume the provision of health services to Papunya and Kintore.

The Pintupi community at Kintore, however, were not party to this decision. They had good reason to be satisfied with the Lyappa Medical Service, and when they heard about the staff dismissals, spears were gathered and a contingent travelled to Papunya to argue with the council. The DAA and representatives from the health department flew in from Alice Springs to meet with the Pintupi people and assured them that health services would continue.

While the health department had said they would provide support, the people at Kintore were aware that, as they continued their reoccupation across the West Australian border, support from the Northern Territory health department would not necessarily follow over the border. They decided they should try to obtain funding to establish a community-controlled health service of their own. A government review of Kintore in early 1982 reported that Smithy Zimran, the president of the Western Desert Outstations Council and a trained Aboriginal health worker, had a definite view that the Outstations Council should form its own health service employing its own doctor and nursing sister. The review team thought that it was unnecessary for a resident doctor to be employed but that it was necessary for a nurse to be resident at Kintore, and the review team was ambivalent about who should provide the medical service suggesting it might be Lyappa Medical Service, the Northern Territory Department of Health, or an Aboriginal-owned health service.[11] Community leaders like Smithy Zimran were quite clear, however, that ultimately they wanted their own health service with a doctor resident in the community.

With the assistance of Congress and the National Aboriginal and Islander Health Organisation (NAIHO), Kintore lobbied the DAA for funding for a health service, including funding for a doctor's salary. Late in 1983 the Department of Aboriginal Affairs agreed to provide funding for the Pintupi Homelands Health Service to provide healthcare to the people of Kintore and surrounding outstations. During 1983, while awaiting news about whether their own health service would be funded, the people at Kintore received healthcare support from Congress in Alice Springs, which supplied some visiting services. The Northern Territory health department also ensured that services continued, with health staff flying out, particularly district medical officer Peter McCaul, on a regular basis.

When I left Strelley in September 1983 and returned to Alice Springs, I started working with the Pitjantjatjara Council to lay the groundwork for the development of Nganampa Health Council and the takeover of health services in the Pitjantjatjara and Yankunytjatjara lands in north-west South Australia. I considered applying for one of the medical-officer positions with the new Nganampa Health Council but when I heard that funding had become available to the Pintupi people at Kintore to employ their own doctor, I decided that this was my next challenge. I thought I should be able to contribute usefully after my experiences on the Pitjantjatjara and Ngaanyatjarra homelands and with the Strelley mob. It helped that I was still single (I had met my future wife Margaret while working with the Strelley mob, but it was not until a couple of years later that our relationship developed).

I applied and was shortlisted for an interview. The one other interviewee for the position was a strong candidate—my friend Peter Tait was a GP who had been working for the past three or four years at Congress in Alice Springs, and had been visiting Kintore regularly as part of Congress's contribution to supporting medical services there. I knew he was a very competent and caring GP and was known and liked by the Pintupi people. Peter and myself, and candidates for the two nursing and one administrator positions, were flown out to Kintore in a light aircraft in early December. The flight took us westward from Alice Springs along the MacDonnell Ranges and then west towards the Gibson Desert. Two hills gradually became visible on the western horizon towards which we were flying. This was the Kintore Range.

This was my first visit to Kintore and I liked the feel of it. To the south rose the angular features of Yunytjunya, a significant site in the network of *ngintaka tjukurrpa* (perentie lizard dreaming) tracks that has the appearance of a large perentie monitor lizard looking eastward. Yunytjunya was named Mount Leisler by the explorer Tietkens. Men's country, closed to women and non-initiates, lies at the foot of Yunytjunya. To the east of the settlement is women's country, which rises to a gentler mountain, Pulikutjara, with two soft rounded domes. This was named Mount Strickland by the explorers.

Having landed we were met by a number of Kintore residents and shown around the community and the clinic, a demountable construct with three small rooms and one entrance. On entering, one first encountered the general clinic area; the next room was an examination area, followed by a small office. It was small but obviously provided an important function within the community. We met Aboriginal health workers Benny Tjapaltjarri, his wife Kawayi Nampitjinpa, and Marlene Nampitjinpa.

The interviews were conducted under a shade shelter outside the clinic, with a significant proportion of the Kintore population sitting around and asking questions. When it was my turn, I responded to many of the questions in Pitjantjatjara, which is closely related to the Pintupi language. I hoped my limited facility in language might help my employment prospects. It may have helped, but I think opinion swung my way when I informed the interviewing group that I had a private pilot's licence. The homelands movement was still in process and, as on the Pitjantjatjara and Ngaanyatjarra lands and with the Strelley mob and the *Martu*, the use of a small aeroplane was seen as being an efficient way to provide services to dispersed small communities. Having a doctor with a pilot's licence would help their advocacy for an aeroplane.

Before leaving that afternoon, I was informed that I was the successful candidate. Peter Tait was understandably disappointed but accepted the result and continued to work with Congress. Some years later, in 1997, he returned to Kintore to work as the medical officer with the Pintupi Homelands Health Service with his wife Wendy and two young children.

Following interviews, the two nurses to be offered employment were Annie Dixon and Estrella Munoz, both experienced bush nurses. I took a liking to both of them and felt confident that we would work well together. A man was offered the health-services manager position but, after initially accepting, had to withdraw for family reasons. A young man named Nigel D'Sousa agreed to fill the position until a more permanent recruit could be found. D'Sousa had previously been employed by NAIHO on a temporary basis to help with the setting up of the health service and had organised our recruitment.

Pintupi Homelands Health Service: early days

On 1 February 1984, with a dog named Sid that I had acquired in Alice Springs, I returned to Kintore to live and work, joining Annie and Estrella, who had arrived a couple of days earlier. Our living conditions at Kintore were basic. There was one accommodation demountable for the health-service staff that did not have running water or a toilet. This was initially the accommodation for Annie, Estrella and me, and also Nigel when he was in the community. Estrella slept in the demountable while the rest of us camped in swags outside. We all shared the cooking, an activity at which Estrella excelled.

These basic living conditions were not limited to health-service staff. Kintore had two bores with windmills and two water-tanks. There were a number of taps throughout the community, and most people used these for both washing and obtaining water for cooking and drinking. Some people needed to walk up to 200 metres to access tap water. There were no toilets; for Aboriginal and non-Aboriginal people alike, defecation involved walking away from the community and discreetly squatting behind a bush.

The housing situation for PHHS staff improved as time went on. In April, I was able to move into a small caravan with hot water and a shower, and in November a pre-fabricated house was installed, which meant that I now had an indoor toilet with a septic tank.

It did not take long after my arrival to get to know the leaders in the community, both men and women. I remember men such as Smithy Zimran, Nosepeg Tjupurulla, Charlie Watama, Jack Kunti Kunti, Uta Uta Tjangala, Yala Yala Gibbs, Willy Tjungurrayi and Shorty Lungkata. They were generally unassuming people (despite some being well-known artists) but they were all visionary leaders who took pride in the fact that they had spearheaded the move back to Pintupi country. They were heroes and it was a privilege to know them. Sadly, most have now passed away.

When I arrived there were not many other non-Aboriginal people living in Kintore: the community advisor Ben Ryan, a building supervisor Steve Patman who lived in a caravan with his partner Kerrie, and the store manager Robert Novak. Rob had previously been the storekeeper at Papunya and had moved to Kintore to run their community store after Paul Parker left. Rob managed a goods store in a large tin shed with 'The Rob Shop' painted in large black letters on one external wall. Rob became a good friend. He was a very good chess player and during my time at Kintore many evening hours were spent hunched over the chessboard trying to beat Rob, usually unsuccessfully.

The Kintore School at that stage was still an outreach school from Papunya. Two schoolteachers were employed at the Papunya School, and they were paid a camping allowance to spend time at Kintore. One of the teachers, Barb Robinson, was Rob Novak's partner. They shared a caravan with Barb's son Danay, and Rob's dog Six-dollar. The other teacher, Jeff Holcombe, was more itinerant, but when he was in Kintore he camped in a swag.

The community-employed builder Steve Patman worked with local people to build a shed for each family group. While people lived in self-constructed *wiltjas*, these new sheds provided a waterproof area in which to store belongings and to sleep during rains. In an alcove next to the caravan that Steve shared with Kerrie, he had rigged up a shower with a wood-fired water heater. At the beginning of 1984 this was the only shower in the community, apart from a public shower near the clinic demountable that was little used. At the end of most days, we would line up to enjoy a shower at Steve's and Kerrie's place. By the end of 1984 Steve and his local team of builders had built eighteen shed-style houses, each with a shower facility.

There were a number of other non-Aboriginal people who were regular visitors to Kintore. The transport driver who brought supplies by road from Alice Springs every two weeks was a character named Jim Dooley. He was a staunch member of Alcoholics Anonymous and put a lot of effort into helping other people in Alice Springs kick their habit. Quite often when he drove out to Kintore he would bring a companion to help him resist temptation and remain abstinent. The Kintore community maintained a strong alcohol ban. I can recall one occasion when some people returned from Alice Springs in a car carrying alcohol and the car was burned as a punishment.

The Western Desert art movement, which had emerged in Papunya in the 1970s, was very strong at Kintore. The artists there had an association with the Papunya Tula artists cooperative. Daphne Williams, a middle-aged woman based in Alice Springs, was the manager of Papunya Tula, and she made regular visits to Kintore to ensure that artists had all the supplies they needed as well as an ongoing market for their products.

Another non-Aboriginal man who visited Kintore from time to time while I was there was Neil Murray. Neil was a musician who, while living at Papunya, had helped establish one of the early successful Aboriginal desert rock bands, the Warumpi Band. While living at Papunya, Neil had a relationship with a young Pintupi woman who had given birth to their daughter, Giselle. Giselle and her mother now lived at Kintore and Neil regularly visited to ensure that mother and baby were well and to provide ongoing support. Giselle still lives in Kintore, and, over thirty years later, we both sit on the board of directors of the Pintupi Homelands Health Service.

The new health service had been named the Pintupi Homelands Health Service, recognising that it was the health service for the Pintupi people as they continued the process of reoccupying their homelands. It also meant of course that once again I was working for an organisation with the acronym PHHS. By this time the other PHHS, the Pitjantjatjara Homelands Health Service, after having briefly changed its name to the Pitjantjatjara-Ngaanyatjarra Health Service had reverted to its original name. It by this point provided healthcare to the more restricted area around Pipalyatjara and Kalka in the north-west corner of South Australia. It would later be dissolved to be absorbed into Nganampa Health Council. The Pintupi Homelands Health Service, however, continues with the acronym PHHS to this day.

The move to Kintore was seen by the Pintupi as only the first stage in the reoccupation of their homelands. Within weeks of my arrival in 1984, hand-pumps for drawing water from bores had been installed at five sites around Kintore: at Pirnpirr, Ininti, Muyin, Tinki and Yuwalki. These sites were envisaged as small family-based residential places with services to be provided out of Kintore. There was also a significant proportion of people living in Kintore whose country was further west, deeper into the Gibson Desert. Initially I was told the plan was to establish a community at Jupiter Well, on the western edge of Pintupi country but a consensus soon formed that the Western Pintupi would settle at a site called Kiwirrkurra, near the Pollock Hills about 200 kilometres west of Kintore.

The new PHHS had funding for five Aboriginal health workers and when I started in February, there were already three employed—Benny, Kawayi and Marlene. This left two positions available, and it was left to the community to decide who might be nominated. A week or so later, Marlene informed me that the decision had been made and that Mantuwa Nangala and George Tjampu Tjapaltjarri would be joining the team. Marlene explained that they were both Western Pintupi and that they would move to Kiwirrkurra once it was established; this demonstrated recognition of the importance of having Aboriginal health workers there.

In the meantime, just meeting the needs of Kintore and the nearby outstations kept us busy. The main health problem we were dealing with was infantile diarrhoea, often complicated by chronic failure-to-thrive, sometimes with pneumonia. This was not dissimilar to the pattern I experienced when working in the Pitjantjatjara Homelands Health Service but the problem was possibly more overwhelming in Kintore. It was certainly more of a public health problem than I had found while working at Strelley, even in the relatively recently occupied desert communities of Panaka Panaka and Kunawarritji. The fairly primitive conditions at Kintore at the time, particularly regarding the water supply, no doubt contributed to the problem.

The small space we had in our clinic demountable was often quite crowded, especially when it opened in the mornings, mostly with mothers with young children. We decided it would be useful to create another space as a maternal and child-health centre, where we could attend to infants and support the (often quite young) mothers in improving infant nutrition and health.

Many babies were evacuated to Alice Springs Hospital. Diarrhoea was usually caused by viral gastroenteritis, which had no specific therapy and could cause death through dehydration. Treatment, then, took the form of rehydrating the child. In most cases this could be achieved with an oral rehydration mixture; severe cases would require parenteral rehydration, usually via intravenous drip. In many cases we were able to maintain hydration for several days, but sometimes the mother would report that the child was *uparinganyi* (becoming weak) and would sometimes have difficulty in lifting the head. This was usually a sign that potassium levels were dangerously low, and the child required urgent admission to hospital to correct the hydration and electrolyte imbalance.

I discussed these problems with my friend Bob Kass, who was senior paediatric registrar at Alice Springs Hospital. I decided it might be useful to spend a couple of weeks working there with Bob in the ward that was dedicated at that time to gastroenteritis in children, the 'gastro ward'.

I arranged to do an exchange with a hospital resident medical officer who agreed to relocate to Kintore for two weeks so as to enable me to spend the time in Alice Springs Hospital.

These two weeks were useful. I developed both knowledge and skills in managing the health problems of Aboriginal infants but also, with Bob's guidance, developed a strategy to prevent the problem of low-potassium levels in kids with gastroenteritis. The composition of the oral rehydration salts we were using had been developed based on clinical trials in developing countries, and we hypothesised that the formula had insufficient potassium for those in Central Australia. Consequently, I had a potassium mixture made up at the pharmacy attached to the hospital and, after I had returned to Kintore, I added 5 millilitres of this to each litre of oral-rehydration mixture used for treating cases of gastroenteritis. Although we did not have the resources to conduct a proper clinical trial this appeared to result in better management of infantile gastroenteritis, with fewer children needing evacuation.

Our patient information system in Kintore was based on hand-written notes in paper files. It became clear that these medical records were incomplete. All patients had medical records kept within the rural-health section of the Northern Territory health department. While I was working in the Alice Springs Hospital, I received permission to access these records for people living at Kintore and outstations so that I could then add this information to our records at Kintore. There was a 'Catch 22', however. I was told I could photocopy the notes but could not use the department's photocopier (the only photocopier in the building) or take the notes from the building. Such rules were indicative of the less-than-helpful attitude towards Aboriginal community-controlled health organisations that existed at some levels within the health department at the time. I laboriously went through the notes in the evenings transcribing relevant information by hand.

At Kintore, communication with the outside world was limited to short-wave radio and a weekly mail plane. The RFDS in Alice Springs managed the radio-communications network, which permitted the sending of telegrams or 'rad-phone' calls over the radio. Every weekday morning there was a 'sked' with the rural-health base so that all remote clinics could call in and receive updates on the progress of patients in hospital. There was also a lunchtime

'Congress sked' involving doctors and nurses from Congress, Urupantja Health Service at Utopia and Nganampa Health Council, which provided some mutual support and discussion of issues of common concern.

Estrella was a good and dedicated nurse. She wanted to find a community in which she felt comfortable and where she could contribute, and she had hoped that Kintore may be that community. Within a few weeks of her arrival, however, a combination of factors, including a couple of incidents of petty theft and intermittent outbreaks of violent behaviour, led to her decision to resign. We were sorry to see her go. She continues to live and work in the Northern Territory.

Another factor that frustrated Estrella was that the administration of the health service was not working as well as it might. As acting administrator, Nigel did his best but he was lacking in experience and spent most of his time in Alice Springs. He continued the attempt to find a permanent administrator and we were very pleased to hear in April that Gary Cartwright had been appointed. Gary had grown up in the Northern Territory and had lived as a child in Docker River, where his father was the first administrator. Gary's wife, Sally Ross, was a Kaytetj woman. They had met as high-school students in Alice Springs and now had two children. Gary and Sally decided to move to Kintore while the children boarded in Alice Springs to attend school.

Sally was a trained Aboriginal health worker. We had intended to recruit a nurse to take over Estrella's position, but when Gary and Sally moved to Kintore it was decided that with Sally on board, a second nurse wouldn't be necessary. This seemed to work well. Annie continued as the only nurse, with Sally, Benny, Kawayi, Marlene, Mantuwa and Tjampu as the health workers. We were, I felt, a great team.

All five of the local AHWs had been born into a hunter-gatherer lifestyle in Pintupi country and could remember their first encounters with non-Aboriginal people. Benny was the senior member of the team. An older man, he was a *ngangkari* as well as a respected lawman. He was also a natural comedian. On many occasions, when the clinic was quiet, he would regale us with stories, embellished with his acting, and would have us all laughing uncontrollably. Soon, however, Benny and Kawayi decided that, due to their age they wanted to spend time on their outstation Pirnpirr, and it was time to retire.

Their son, Victor Tjungurrayi, had initially been employed as the Aboriginal director of the organisation, working alongside Nigel, but he resigned early in 1984. Sometime later the community appointed his replacement, Riley Tjangala Major, who was a more senior man. He continued in this role for the remainder of my time with the organisation.

In 1984 a *ngangkari* joined the PHHS team. I had been greeted one day early in the year by a Pintupi man who had just relocated to Kintore from Warakurna. We recognised each other: George Nyunmul Tjapaltjarri, known as 'Doctor George', was a highly regarded *ngangkari* with whom I had worked on my visits to Warakurna a few years earlier, when I was with the Pitjantjatjara Homelands Health Service. Doctor George settled in Kintore in 1984, and was frequently sought out for his skills as a *ngangkari*. Inevitably, it was not unusual to find ourselves working together, and soon a partnership based on friendship and mutual respect developed. We became known as the 'two doctors'; when there was significant illness in the community, both doctors would often be asked to attend. After some time, at a community meeting, it was proposed that the partnership should be formalised and that Doctor George should become a salaried employee of the PHHS. This was arranged and he continued to be a valued employee of PHHS for many years after I had departed (often, as mentioned in the previous chapter, travelling far and wide to provide his healing arts). He passed away in 2017.

Kiwirrkurra and DLC

The aspiration to reoccupy homelands further west was evident when I arrived at Kintore and it remained strong thereafter. In May 1984, Charlie McMahon arrived to assist with the move to Kiwirrkurra. He was known as Charlie Hook as he had lost one of his hands in an accident while experimenting with rocketry as a teenager and had a prosthetic hook. He was an accomplished didgeridoo player and when he arrived in Kintore he had just returned from touring in the US with the famed Australian band Midnight Oil. He also had good bush skills and, through previous contact with the Pintupi while drilling boreholes, had agreed to work with them in supporting the next move west.

With Charlie's arrival, work started on getting the basic infrastructure installed—a bore with a windmill and tank, an airstrip and a store. The PHHS purchased a second-hand caravan that was transported to Kiwirrkurra for use as the Kiwirrkurra clinic. Initially people travelled back and forth between Kintore and Kiwirrkurra while the infrastructure was being developed but by August 1984 there was a permanent community; over the course of a few months it grew to around one hundred people. Most had come from Kintore but a considerable number had relocated from Balgo. Three of the PHHS Aboriginal health workers—Marlene, Tjampu and Mantuwa—had connections with the Western Pintupi and all spent time there. This meant there was usually at least one or two Aboriginal health workers in Kiwirrkurra. We ensured they had adequate supplies and radio contact with the health service staff at Kintore and we had a daily radio sked. Annie Dixon and I both visited regularly, making the three-hour journey by car and usually camping for one or two nights.

On one of my early trips out to Kiwirrkurra with Benny Tjapaltjarri, he pointed to the north and confidently told me there were still people living out there. He said there was an old man who had decided to continue the traditional Pintupi hunter-gatherer lifestyle and had stayed out there with his family after everybody else had moved to Papunya, Haasts Bluff or Balgo. I was intrigued by the story but tended towards scepticism—flights of imagination are not unheard of in the Western Desert. Benny, however, was right. In October 1984 contact was made with the family of nine people who were still living in Pintupi country north of Kiwirrkurra. The story of this contact is found in more detail in chapter 7.

With the movement of people further west, the PHHS had increased its advocacy to the DAA for the use of an aeroplane. The initial response was cool but, after the arrival of the newly contacted Pintupi in Kiwirrkurra, as well as the concern about ensuring access to timely healthcare as they were exposed to new diseases, the DAA agreed to provide funds for hire of an aeroplane, initially for two months and later extended to four months.

I had a particular aeroplane in mind. While working as medical advisor to help establish Nganampa Health Council in late 1983, my pilot's licence had proven useful to facilitate travel around the Pitjantjatjara communities.

I had access to a Cessna 207, a single-engine six seater with the call-sign DLC (Delta Lima Charlie), owned by a pilot friend who was employed in Alice Springs by the Missionary Aviation Fellowship. At that time, I had used DLC extensively. In April 1984 I had taken an extended Easter break and had hired DLC for a week or so to travel and to maintain my flying skills. With two friends I flew west from Alice to Kintore then to Punmu (Panaka Panaka) and on to Broome, and returned via Kunawarritji, where our arrival coincided with a big meeting of people from all over the northern part of the Western Desert. This meeting led to the formation of the land council called the Western Desert Puntukurnuparna Aboriginal Council which, some years later, would be my employing body at Jigalong.

When DAA agreed to provide funds for the hire of an aeroplane in October, DLC was still available. So, for the next four months it was based at Kintore and I flew regularly between Kintore and Kiwirrkurra.

The first time I flew DLC to Kiwirrkurra, not long after the arrival of the newly contacted Pintupi, I landed just before sundown and camped overnight. The next morning as my *ngangkari* colleague Doctor George and I were preparing breakfast on a campfire, we were joined by Warlimpirrnga and Piyirti, the two spokesmen for the group. They were both in their twenties and had already been recognised for their spiritual powers. They said they had both dreamt through the night that spirit-beings were going to pull wires from the plane and that they had sat up all night keeping the spirits away. They believed they had been successful but suggested I go to the airstrip and check the aeroplane and start the engine, which I did. I was a little apprehensive when I took off to fly back to Kintore later that day but I arrived without incident.

I also did a number of flights in various directions over Pintupi country. Many people living at Kintore and Kiwirrkurra wanted to see their country, which in many cases were not easily accessible with land vehicles. Consequently, people sometimes paid for the fuel and I was able to fly them out to do a few low circuits over important sites that they had not seen for many years. I was always impressed by the sense of wellbeing that followed these trips. People were happy to have seen their country and to have seen that it was in good condition.

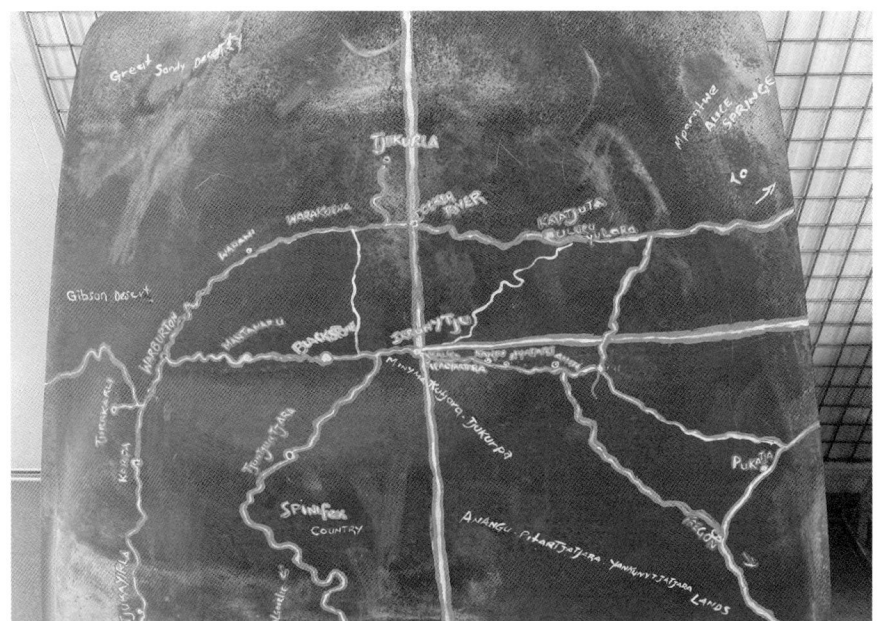

A mud map of the Pitjantjatjara and Ngaanyatjarra homelands, painted on an old Holden car bonnet by Ngaanyatjarra artist Diane Dawson (acrylic on metal), Minyma Kutjara Arts Centre Project, Irrunytju, 2020
David Scrimgeour

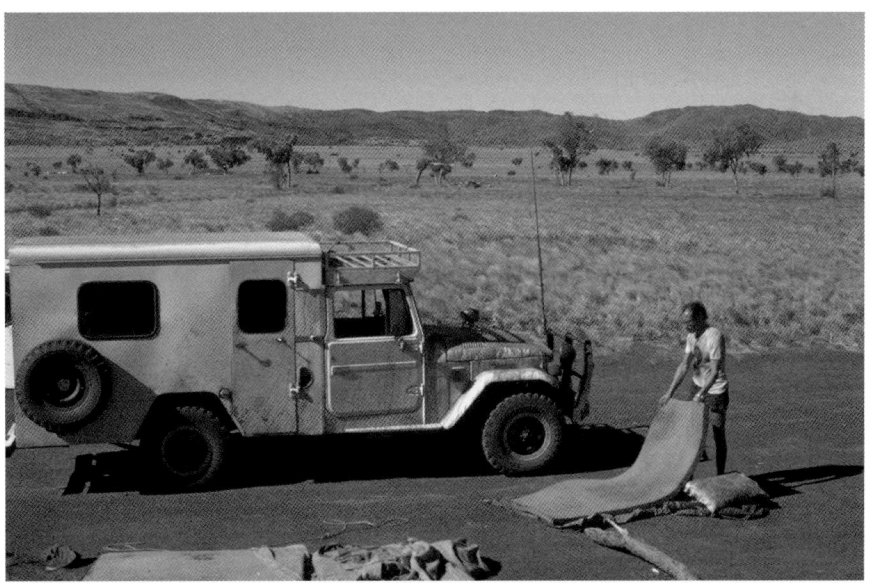

Unrolling the swag after a few days on the road, Kalka, 1978
Ara Irititja archive AI-0018451, Pitjantjatjara Council collection

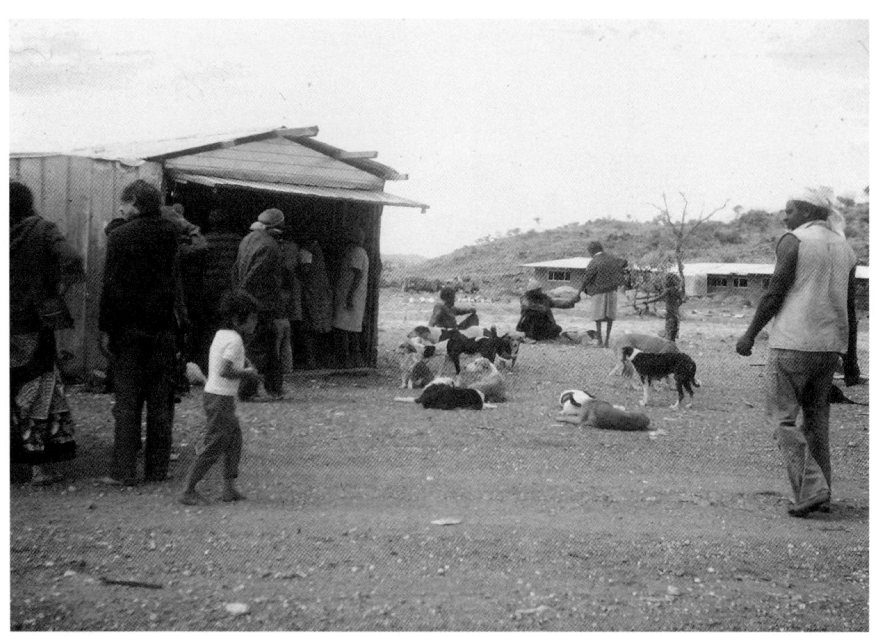

Outside the Piplayatjara Store, 1978
R.J. Scrimgeour

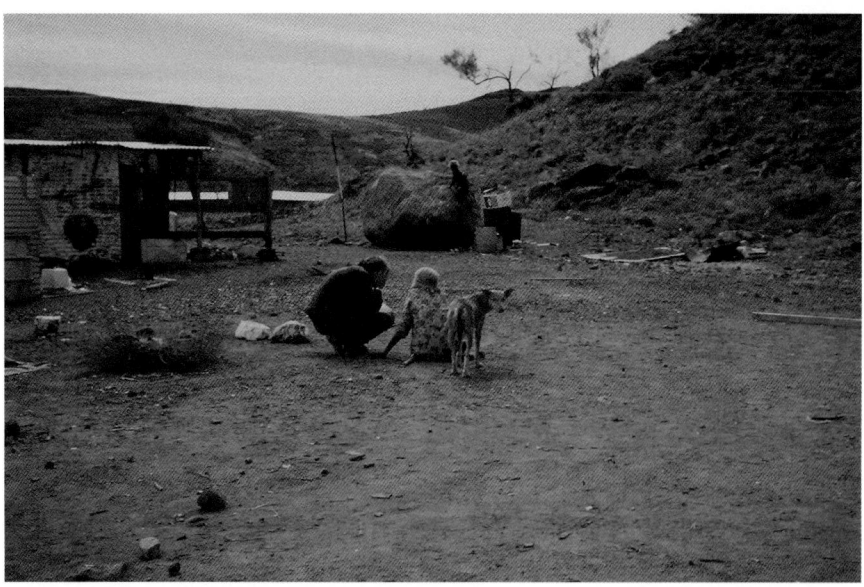

A medical consultation, Pipalyatjara, 1978
R.J. Scrimgeour

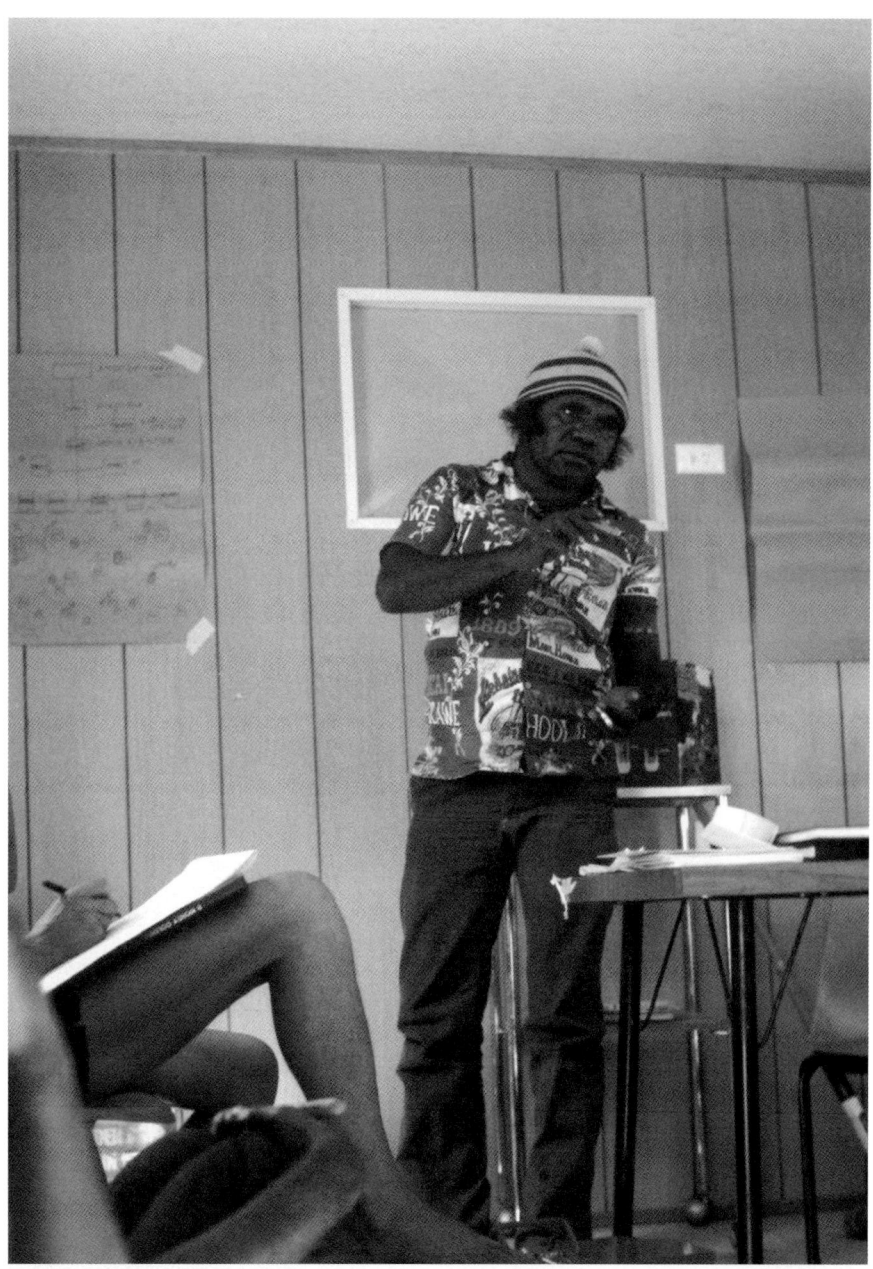

Ivan Baker (dec.) chairing a staff meeting of the Pitjantjatjara Homelands Health Service, Kalka, 1979
Ara Irititja archive AI-0018451, Mary Wighton collection

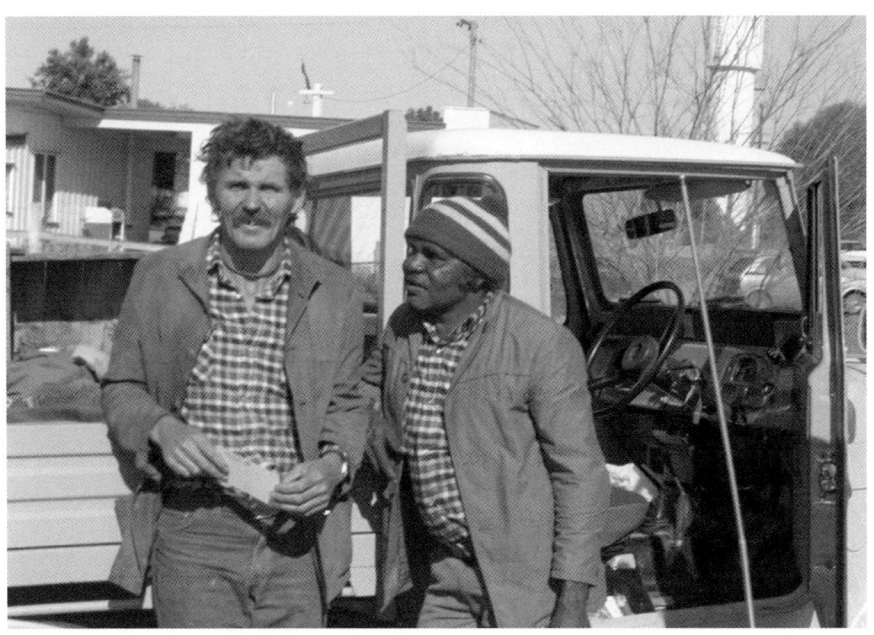

Friends from the Pitjantjatjara and Ngaanyatjarra homelands, Ushma Scales and Ivan Baker, on a road trip in 1982
Ara Irititja archive A1-0025554, Ushma Scales collection

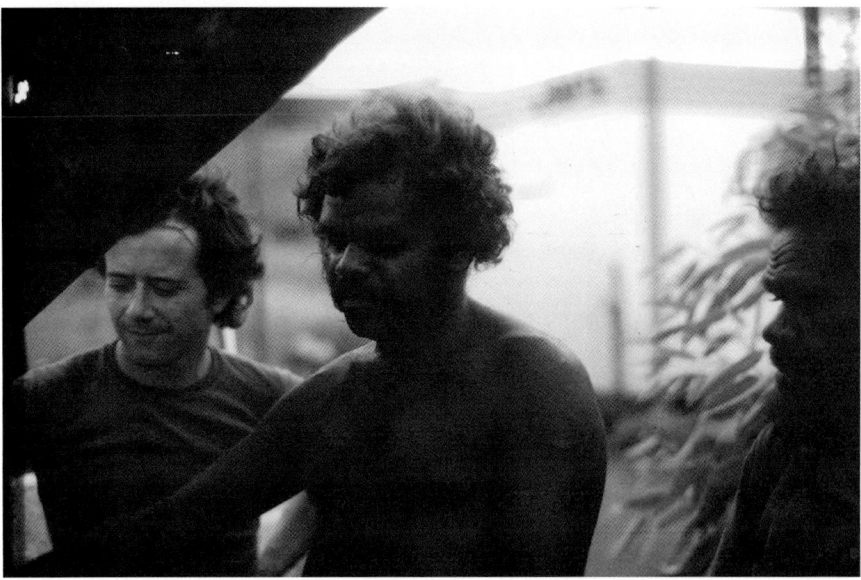

Aboriginal health worker and *malpa* Bobby Daniels (dec.) checking the oil and water in a Toyota before a bush trip, with Ian Baird looking on, Kalka, 1980
David Scrimgeour

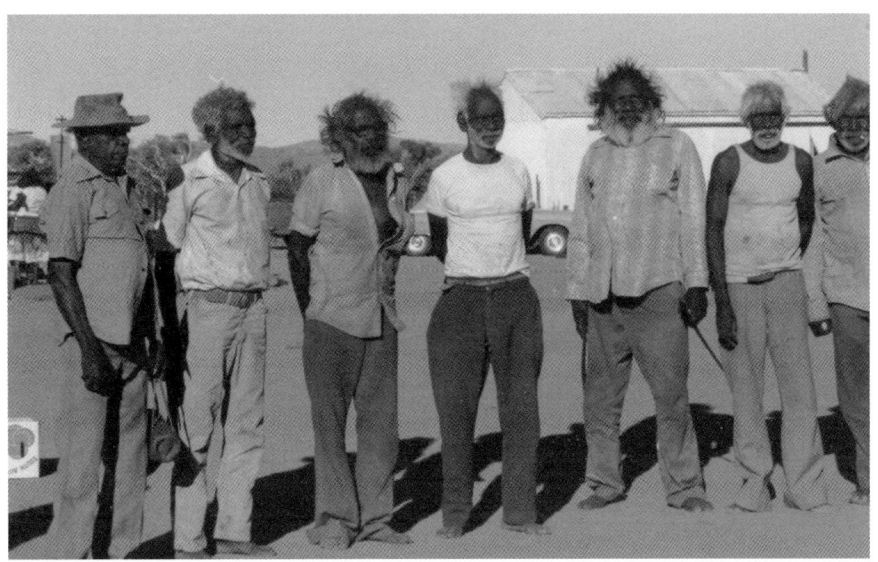

Strelley strikers: these men were community leaders who were all involved in the Pilbara Strike in 1946, Strelley, 1983
Anne Scrimgeour

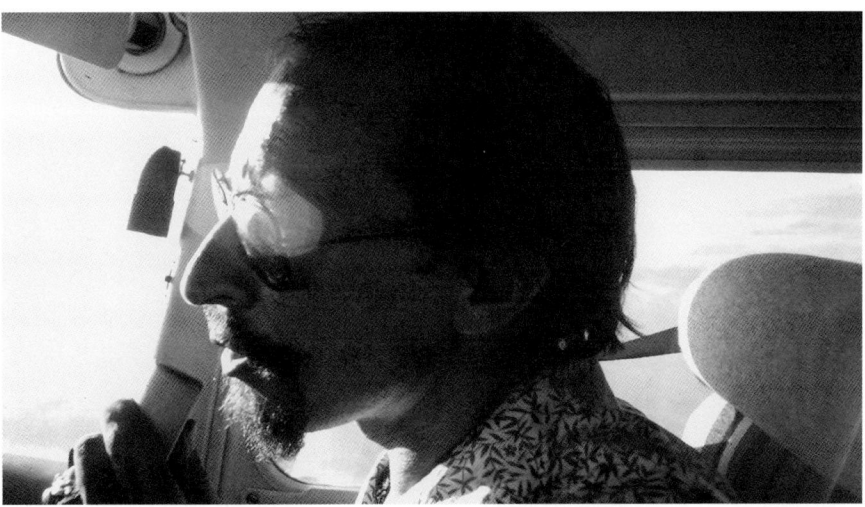

The author at the controls of Cessna 207 UGB, over the Great Sandy Desert, 1984
R.J. Scrimgeour

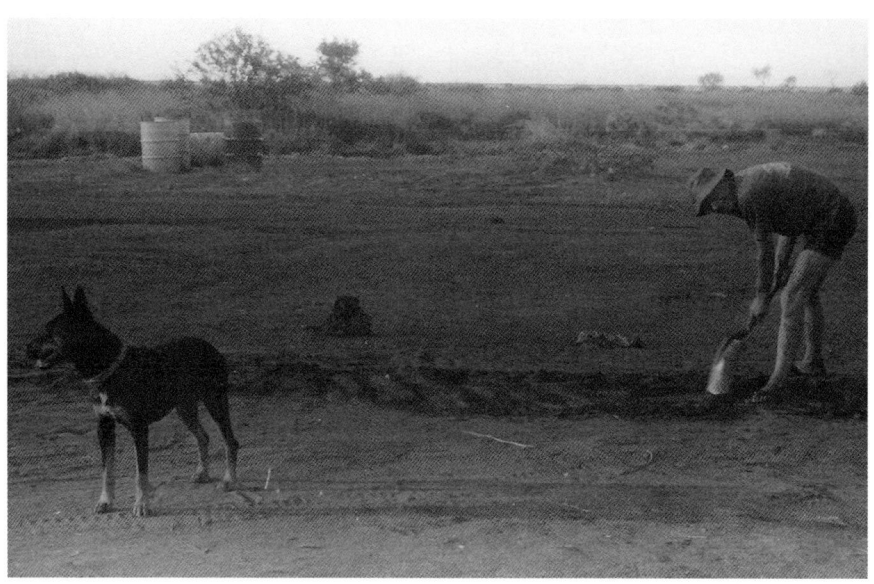

Digging a water channel to the original health service staff accommodation, Kintore, 1984
Annie Dixon

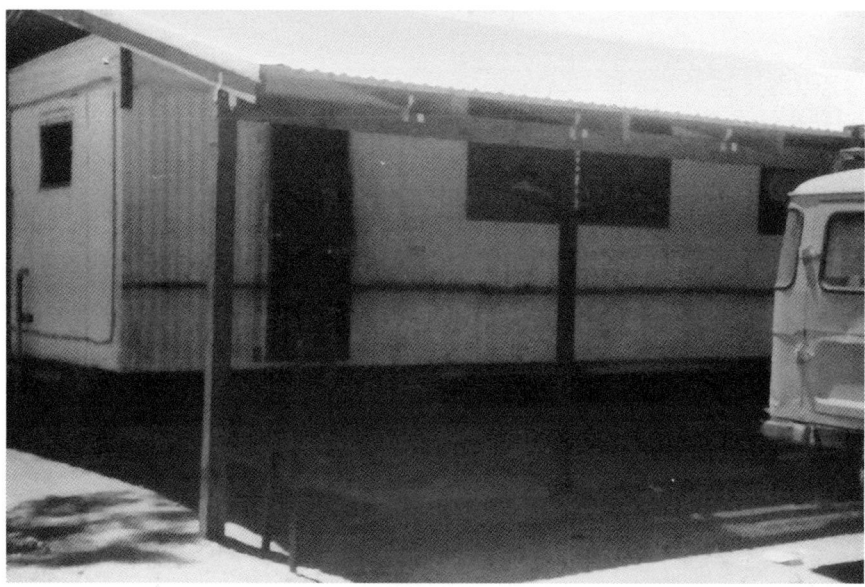

The original Pintupi Homelands Health Service clinic building, Kintore, 1984
Annie Dixon

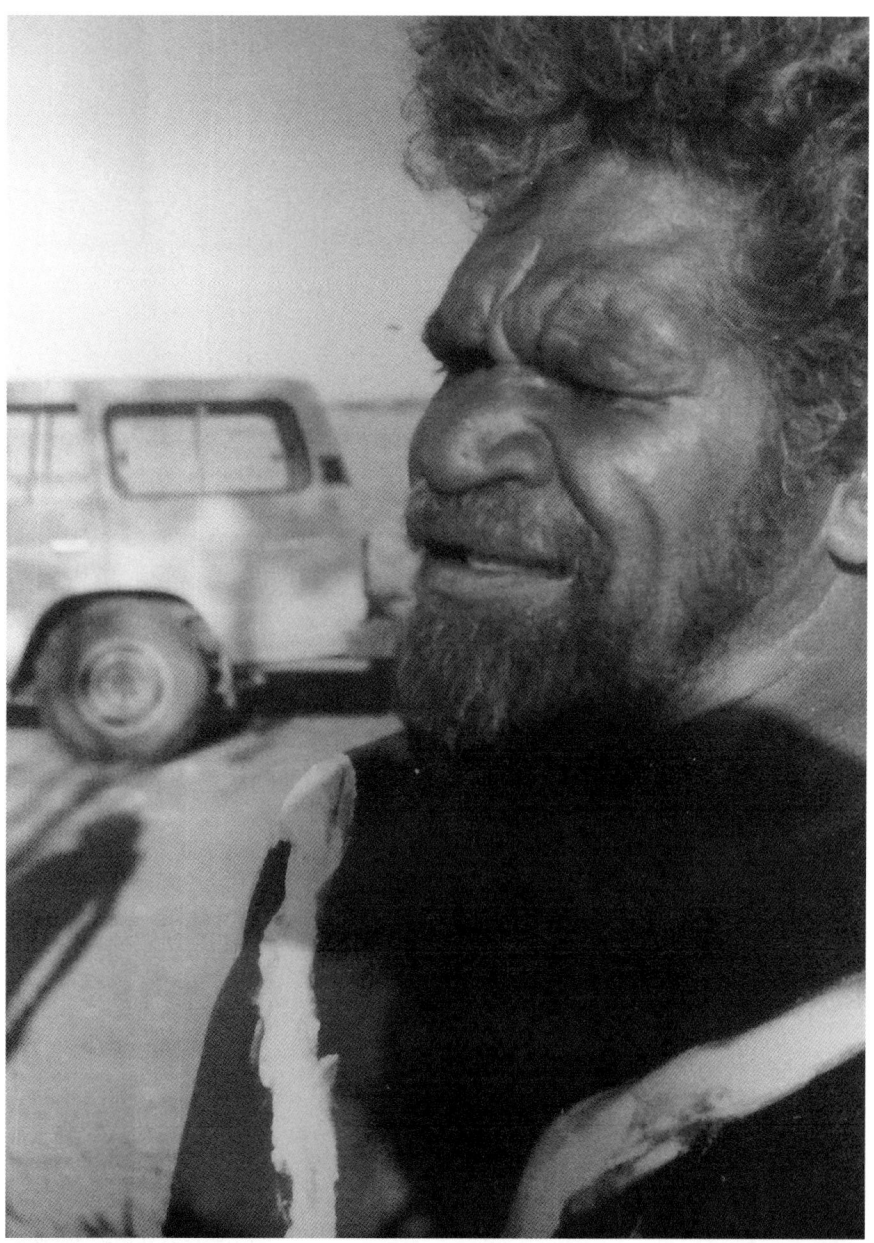

Ngangkari, friend and colleague 'Doctor George' Tjapaltjarri (dec.), Kintore, 1984
David Scrimgeour

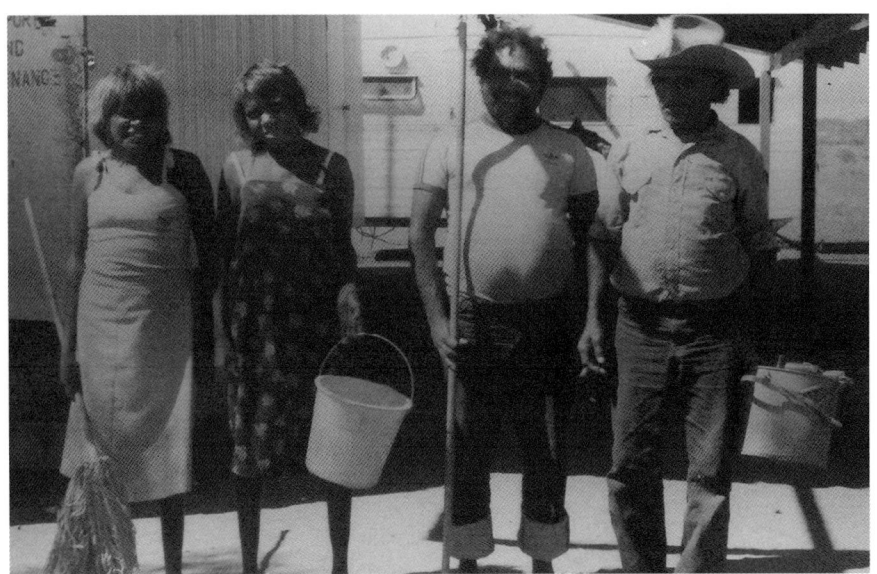

Pintupi Homelands Health Service Aboriginal health workers multi-tasking, after cleaning the clinic, Kintore, 1984. Left to right: Mantuwa Nangala, Marlene Nampitjinpa, George Tjampu Tjapaltjarri (dec.), Benny Tjapaltjarri (dec.)
David Scrimgeour

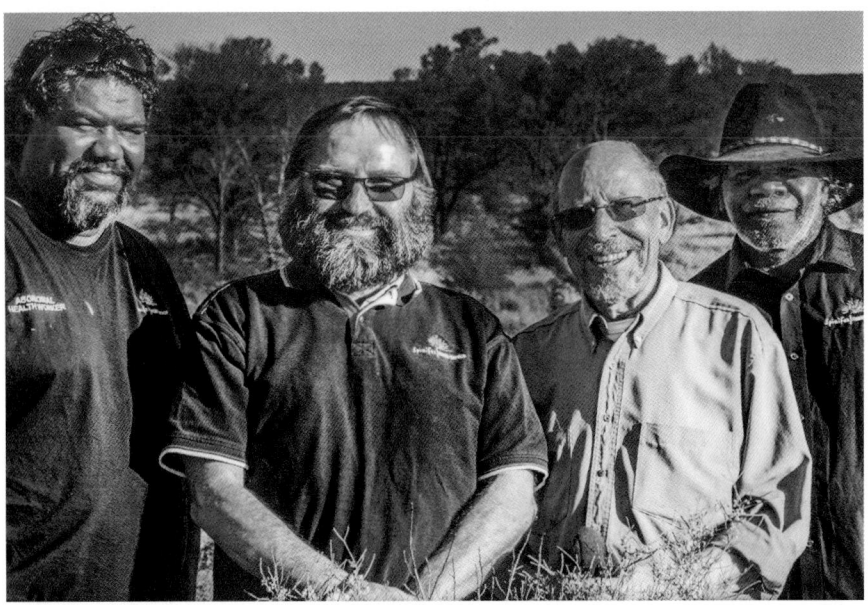

Spinifex Health Service colleagues, Tjuntjuntjara, 2017. Left to right: Aboriginal health practitioner Tyson Stevens; Remote Area Nurse Simon Gabrynowicz; author; Aboriginal health worker Winmati Roberts
Paul Bulley

On one occasion in December 1984, I was asked to fly out bush to retrieve a young man, Billy, who had been injured. Search parties, involving police and community members, had driven out into the bush hoping to find a missing man with an acquired brain injury alive. While monitoring their progress over the radio, I received a message one afternoon that one member of the search party had injured his leg and required urgent medical treatment. As it would take two or three days of driving to get him back to Kintore, I agreed to fly out to collect him. I was given a rough guide to the location and the search party lit a smoky fire to help me find them, as well as to determine the wind direction to show me in which direction to land. They also prepared a rough airstrip by driving repeatedly up and down over an area of spinifex to flatten it. I landed there in the late afternoon and quickly took off again with Billy; under the limitations of my licence, I was required to land back at Kintore by last light. When I arrived back at Kintore I found the rough bush airstrip landing had caused the nose-wheel strut to collapse.

I thought I would have to get DLC into Alice Springs for repairs. However, the next day I spoke to an aircraft mechanic over the 'rad-phone' and he explained how to rig up an old radiator-hose to cushion the wheel and make it functional. It was a 'bush job', with the hose tied on to the nose-wheel strut with fencing wire, but it worked until I was next able to fly DLC into Alice Springs.

Health problems

Annie was an experienced bush nurse and midwife. We had a good working relationship throughout the year we worked together. As a midwife, she was happy to encourage women with uncomplicated pregnancies to stay in Kintore to deliver their babies with the support of Annie and some of the older women. In my first year at Kintore we had seventeen births, of which five occurred in Kintore itself. Unfortunately one of these involved a premature labour at thirty-six weeks; there was a breech delivery and the baby did not survive. I was not in Kintore at the time and I am not sure whether my presence would have made a difference. It was, however, a factor in my decision to get more obstetric training. It should be noted that, as this event occurred at thirty-six weeks gestation and women who were planning to deliver in Alice Springs usually went there at thirty-seven weeks, this probably would have happened at Kintore regardless of the intended place of delivery. The other four deliveries at Kintore were uneventful from an obstetric point of view and were always happy occasions. There was also one case of intrauterine death at eighteen weeks due to syphilis.

During my time at Kintore there was one infant death from pneumonia at age two months and one death of a child from a motor-vehicle accident close to Kintore. The only other death that occurred while I was there was a rather sad story. There was a young middle-aged man who had limited mental capacity due to an acquired brain injury early in life. He was prone to violent outbursts and frequently ended up in trouble with the law. He had spent a considerable amount of time in gaol, and also sometimes in mental-health units, but neither of these institutions addressed his needs. He arrived back in Kintore not long after my arrival, having been released from gaol. He was related to Marlene and she and her extended family took responsibility for caring for him, although there were others in the community who did not want him there.

One of my first encounters with this man ended badly. Somewhat ineptly, I tried to convince him to take a tablet to help calm him down when he was mildly agitated but with an iron bar in his hand. This led to a blow with the iron bar on my foot. This was the only occasion in all my years of working in remote communities where I had been the victim of any violence.

Sometime later, the same man walked out of the community and was missing for several days. Despite his cognitive deficit, he knew how to live off the land and a few days later he walked into Muyin, about 30 kilometres to the west, in a physically healthy condition. His next solo venture into the bush, however, ended tragically. This was in December when the weather was much hotter. When he did not return after a week or so, a search party involving police and the community was mounted. Eventually, his dead body was found.

After I had been living and working in Kintore for a year, I wrote a report on progress and problems of the PHHS. It covered various operational issues and also included some comments on the common health problems encountered, such as statistics on birth and deaths, evacuations and transfers, immunisations, infant anthropometry, and a range of infectious diseases including infant diarrhoea, chronic ear disease, trachoma, hepatitis B, leprosy and sexually transmitted diseases.

Hepatitis B was a recently identified condition. It is a blood-borne virus that was first identified in the blood of an Australian Aboriginal person in 1969, leading to its nomination as the Australia Antigen. Subsequently it was recognised as a virus that caused hepatitis (liver inflammation) and was named hepatitis B to distinguish it from hepatitis A, a virus transmitted through the faecal-oral route. In 1984 little was known about the epidemiology of hepatitis B but it had been noted that there appeared to be a significant prevalence in Aboriginal people. That year, I tested eighty-two adults in Kintore for hepatitis B serological markers and found that twenty-two of them (26 per cent) had chronic hepatitis B. This was possibly the first epidemiological survey of hepatitis B in Central Australia and it showed that it was a significant problem—people with chronic hepatitis B may develop liver cirrhosis, liver failure or liver cancer. Although there was no evidence of morbidity from hepatitis B while I was working in Kintore, at least one of the people I identified with chronic hepatitis B went on to die from liver cancer some years later. At that time, there was little that we could do to treat complications arising from chronic hepatitis. More than three decades later, however, there are good treatments available and a preventative vaccine so with good healthcare, hepatitis B and its sequelae in Aboriginal communities should become much less of a problem. It continues to be an interest of mine; at the time of writing I manage a hepatitis B control program for the Ngaanyatjarra Health Service.

It is interesting to note that there was no mention in my first annual report of adult chronic diseases such as diabetes and kidney disease, which are now recognised as a major cause of morbidity and mortality in remote Aboriginal communities. There were a few people on medications for diabetes and there were probably a number of undiagnosed cases. Our treatment options were limited. A now frequently used medication, metformin, had recently come under a cloud as there was evidence that it caused potentially fatal lactic acidosis. (It can, but the incidence of lactic acidosis due to this medication is much less than was thought at that time.) The only other oral medication was a class of medicines called sulphonylureas and the evidence for the efficacy of these medications at that time was limited. Insulin was available but problems with storage as well as difficulty in ensuring that people received regular injection limited its use. The consensus among most of my colleagues in Central Australia at the time was that we should concentrate on improving nutrition, both as a preventative and a therapeutic intervention, rather than on medical solutions.

At the time, there were no treatments available for kidney disease. If, as occasionally happened, a patient went into kidney failure, they died. There was no dialysis available in Alice Springs, and certainly not in Kintore.

At the time of writing, thirty-five years later, the situation with chronic diseases has changed significantly. The prevalence is much higher but there are also more treatment options available. Currently in the PHHS, as in other remote health centres, managing adult chronic diseases is a major activity. I will discuss the response of the Pintupi people to the increasing prevalence of renal disease below.

Leaving Kintore

After my first year with the Pintupi Homelands Health Service I felt satisfied with the contribution I had made to help the Pintupi people reoccupy their homelands. I believed that by this stage I had a much greater understanding of what was required to develop an effective health service in remote communities. As my experience had grown, I believed I was becoming more effective than I had been in my earlier positions. With the Pintupi Homelands Health Service, I felt more confident that I had a reasonably systematic and proactive approach to working within a community health service. I was also comfortable that the Pintupi people had a sense of ownership and control over their primary healthcare service.

I was happy to continue living at Kintore and doing this kind of work. However, though I now had a good understanding of health service development, I was less confident about whether I had all the clinical skills that were required. Although I was part of a team, when it came to clinical decision-making, the buck stopped with me. When I had relocated to Alice Springs in 1977 to work at Congress, I had been in the fledgling Family Medicine Program but I had never completed formal training as a GP. One particular area of clinical expertise that I wanted to develop was in obstetrics and neonatal paediatrics. As mentioned above, Annie had supported women who wanted to give birth in Kintore. As it was 'women's business', I had usually stayed in the background to allow Annie and other women to manage the delivery. However, I was ready to be called in if there was a complication. I was very aware that I would be more useful if I could update the skills required to manage an obstetric or neonatal paediatric emergency.

I decided it was time to return to hospital for some up-skilling, with the idea that I would then return to Kintore. I explored a number of options, and when I was accepted for a six-month term in obstetrics and neonatal paediatrics at King Edward Memorial Hospital in Perth, starting in July 1985, I decided to accept this position. This would allow me time to continue working at Kintore until the end of March and then fit in a break with some overseas travel. I had an English friend, John Holliday, who was a GP with an interest in Aboriginal health and the politics of Aboriginal affairs. He had visited Strelley when I was working there and I thought he might be interested in applying to take over my role with the PHHS. He applied, and was accepted.

Other changes were happening with PHHS staff. Gary Cartwright and Sally Ross resigned for family reasons in October 1984—they wanted to be closer to their children in Alice Springs. Sally sadly died in a motor-vehicle accident a few years later and Gary became a member of the Northern Territory parliament. Gary was replaced as the health-service administrator by John Keane, an arts curator who had a close connection with Pintupi artists. In Sally's place, we decided to look for a second nurse rather than another health worker. When Annie indicated that she planned to resign in January 1985, we advertised both nursing positions and two capable nurses, Joan Adams and Rosalie Jones, commenced work with the PHHS when Annie left.

In mid-March 1985, I flew DLC to Alice Springs to meet John Holliday and his partner Claire, who had arrived from London. We spent a week or two in Alice Springs, Kintore and Kiwirrkurra to allow time for orientation and a handover. Then it was time to leave Kintore. I was sad to leave but I knew I would be back—though my return would be sooner than anticipated.

I took off in DLC early on a Monday morning, but about ten minutes after departure the engine started to splutter. I did not like the sound of it, and returned to Kintore. When I contacted an aircraft mechanic over the radphone, he agreed to fly out and have a look. He arrived at around 3 p.m. and after he had tuned up the engine I took off again, with the mechanic waiting to see how it went. There was still a splutter, so I again returned to Kintore. The mechanic worked on it some more and assured me that it seemed fixed. To make sure, we went on a check flight and all seemed well. He returned to Alice but the requirements of my licence to only fly in daylight hours meant that I had to wait until the following morning.

The next morning I took off again but before long the splutter recommenced. Once again I returned to Kintore and this time decided to leave DLC there until it could be properly repaired. Perhaps the spirit-beings that Walumpirr and Piyirti had fought off some months earlier had finally got to the aircraft. Or perhaps something was drawing me back to Kintore. In any case, the store truck had arrived that morning, so I hitched a ride into Alice Springs sitting in the cabin alongside the driver Jim Dooley.

I had thought that after up-skilling I would return to work at Kintore, but after finishing my time at King Edward Memorial Hospital, I was offered a position working in a refugee camp in Sudan, which I decided to accept. I did however return early in 1986 for a few weeks, while John and Claire had a holiday. After that I had intermittent contact with the Pintupi over a number of years, which gradually became less frequent until my connection was revived in 2011, as I describe below.

Later developments

Health services to Kiwirrkurra continued to be supplied by PHHS after I left. At times, staff were subject to criticisms from Kintore people for spending too much time at Kiwirrkurra (somewhat ironically, given the history of Lyappa Medical Service). There was also a body of opinion at Kiwirrkurra that in the provision of services, including healthcare, Kiwirrkurra was perceived as a mere outstation of Kintore rather than as a community in its own right. (This was a struggle that Kintore itself had undergone earlier in its efforts to be seen as separate from Papunya.)

In the late 1980s, Kiwirrkurra started negotiating with the Ngaanyatjarra Council, the resource agency for Ngaanyatjarra communities to the south. It eventually decided to join the Ngaanyatjarra Council. The possibility of joining the Ngaanyatjarra Health Service was also raised and, as the Ngaanyatjarra Health Service offered to place a nurse at Kiwirrkurra, this option was chosen. In 1989 Kiwirrkurra left the Pintupi Homelands Health Service to become part of Ngaanyatjarra Health Service. The health centre at Kiwirrkurra is named after my late colleague George Tjampu Tjapaltjarri, who started work with the PHHS in 1984 and subsequently became an Aboriginal health worker at Kiwirrkurra.

In the 1990s the prevalence of adult chronic diseases had risen and an increasing number of Pintupi people were developing end-stage kidney disease, requiring dialysis. Dialysis had become available in Alice Springs and a number of older Pintupi people had to relocate there to access it. This caused significant distress; many of the people in dialysis were those who had led the movement back to Pintupi country and who were now not able to live there.

There were calls for a dialysis unit to be established at Kintore but the response from funding bodies was that it was too complex and expensive. The Pintupi were not deterred. They had a marketable resource—their art. An exhibition of Pintupi art was organised and held in Sydney in 2000; over a million dollars was raised from the sale of paintings. Paul Rivalland, a GP who had worked for a while as the PHHS doctor following John Holliday, was hired to undertake a feasibility study, and an organisation called the Western Desert Nganampa Walytja Palyantjaku Aboriginal Corporation (known as the 'Purple House') was formed. By 2004, under the capable management of an ex-nurse, Sarah Brown, a base had been established in Alice Springs and a dialysis unit at Kintore, enabling Pintupi people on dialysis to spend time back on country. The Purple House has since extended this service to a number of other remote communities.

In 2011 while living in Adelaide I received an invitation to an event in Kintore, celebrating the thirtieth anniversary of the reoccupation of Pintupi country. I travelled back to Kintore for what was a happy event, demonstrating that the movement of people out of Papunya to Kintore in 1981 was still remembered with pride. It also allowed me the opportunity to reconnect with Pintupi friends as well as a number of non-Aboriginal people from earlier days, including my friend and colleague Annie Dixon. Not all the Pintupi people I remembered from 1984 and 1985 were there. Political tensions still existed between Kintore and Kiwirrkurra and a number of people from Kiwirrkurra did not attend. Also, sadly, many had died. Annie and I had a poignant walk around the cemetery, reading names on gravestones of people we had known who had now passed away.

I met the current health team at PHHS, including Simon Madin, who had been working there for a number of years as the doctor, and Leon Chapman, the administrator. I gave Leon my card and said to contact me if I could help at any time in the future. A year or so later he did and in the following years I did a number of short-term locums working as the PHHS doctor. I was happy to find the PHHS was a reasonably well-resourced and well-functioning health service, and I was happy to be making a contribution again.

Kintore had changed in a number of ways. There were more buildings and infrastructure and it had become a well-established Aboriginal community. There was, however, a sense that in many ways the people did not have as much control over their lives as they had previously when they had taken matters into their own hands to establish the community, or to demand dialysis facilities in their own country. In particular, there was no longer a governing council for Kintore itself; the Northern Territory government had abolished community councils and amalgamated them into larger 'shires', later called 'regional councils'. The MacDonnell Regional Council, to which Kintore belongs, is based in Alice Springs. As one woman said to me, 'we are an outstation again'. Currently, the only community-controlled organisations based in Kintore are the PHHS and the community store.

At the present time the PHHS continues as the health service for the Kintore community. Kiwirrkurra continues to receive health services from the Ngaanyatjarra Health Service, although I believe healthcare in Kiwirrkurra could improve if the people there decided to re-join the PHHS. The small outstations that existed around Kintore when I was there in 1984 and 1985, such as Pirnpirr, Ininti, Muyin, Tinki and Yuwalki, are no longer inhabited. There are a number of reasons for this, which I discuss in chapter 8.

In its early days, the PHHS had an informal governing structure with management decisions made at community meetings. Over the years the governance structure was formalised and a board of directors, consisting of elected community members, was established. PHHS is incorporated with the Office of the Registrar of Aboriginal Corporations (ORIC). The registrar encourages Aboriginal organisations to consider inviting skills-based directors onto the board and, while many Aboriginal organisations continue to prefer to restrict board membership to community members, others, including PHHS, decided that it would be useful to have external input. Consequently, in 2015 I was invited by the PHHS board of directors to join as a non-voting independent director; my role is to provide expertise in primary healthcare. Another independent non-voting director was appointed at the same time— Graham Dowling, an Alice Springs-based Aboriginal man with expertise in management.

At the time of writing I continue to sit on the board as an independent director. Board meetings are held about six times a year and, on most occasions, I am able to get to Kintore to attend (although most meetings for 2020 and 2021 were conducted online, due to the pandemic). It pleases me that over thirty years since I helped develop the PHHS, I am still able to provide support and that, from time to time, I can be out in Pintupi country with the Pintupi people. It is a source of satisfaction that the Pintupi people's struggle to live autonomously on their own country and to have control of their health services has been maintained.

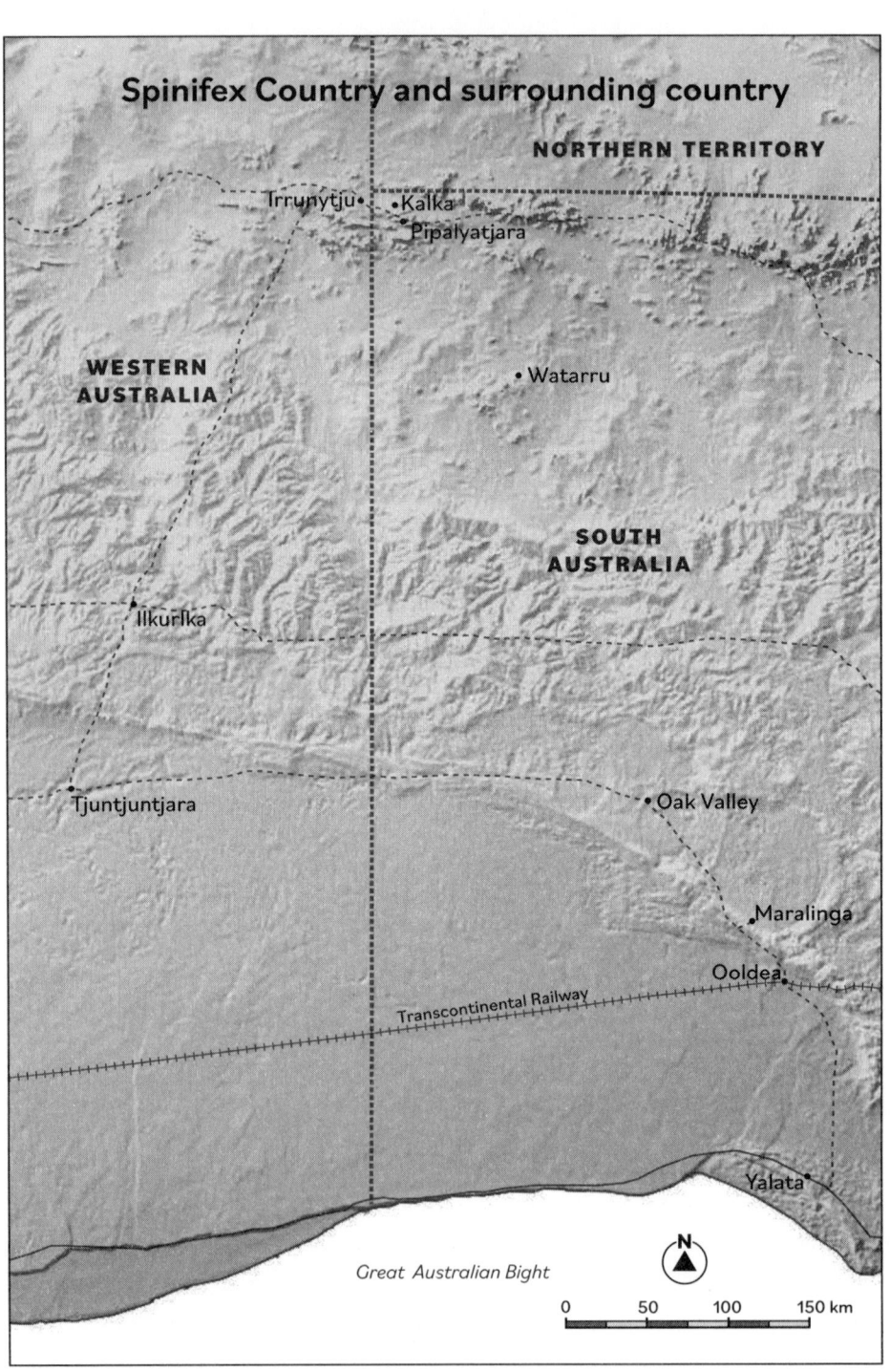

6

The Spinifex people

The Spinifex people hail from the sandhill and spinifex country in the Great Victoria Desert in Western Australia.[1] Like the Pintupi and the *Martu*, they have made the transition from a traditional nomadic lifestyle to a more modern Australian lifestyle in living memory. This has entailed a move away from their country to more settled regions, followed by a return to reoccupy the homelands.

The Spinifex people differ from other Western Desert peoples in being referred to, not by the particular Western Desert language they speak (such as Pitjantjatjara, Ngaanyatjarra, Manyjilyjarra and Pintupi), but by the nature of their country. They are, in fact, southern Pitjantjatjara speakers, along with the people living at Oak Valley and Yalata in the south-eastern portion of the Great Victoria Desert across the border in South Australia. Their language is very similar to the language I learnt when living on the Pitjantjatjara homelands forty years ago, with occasional vocabulary variations and, I am told by native Pitjantjatjara speakers, with a slightly different accent, although this is too subtle for my linguistic ear. As the term Pitjantjatjara is usually associated with the APY Lands of South Australia to the north-west of the country of the Spinifex people, it seems that the Spinifex people are comfortable to have that denotation. In Pitjantjatjara, they refer to themselves as *pila nguru* (meaning 'from the spinifex valleys between sand-dunes').

Their country, often called Spinifex country or just Spinifex, is in the Great Victoria Desert, in the south-east of Western Australia bordering with South Australia; in spinifex, mulga and sandhill country north of the

Nullarbor Plain, the Transcontinental Railway Line and the Great Australian Bight; and south of the ranges where the Ngaanyatjarra and Pitjantjatjara communities of Papulangkatja and Irrunytju are situated.

Early contact history

The Great Victoria Desert was named by the explorer Ernest Giles, who travelled through the area in 1875, leaving from Port Augusta, stopping at Ooldea Soak in South Australia and then at a small waterhole named Boundary Dam near the West Australian border. As he travelled west for the next 500 kilometres, passing through the southern edge of Spinifex country, Giles found no water until his team reached a permanent soak that he named Queen Victoria Springs. By now he was beyond Spinifex country, but Queen Victoria Springs was not far north of a place that would later be called Cundeelee and would have a significant role in the story of the Spinifex people.[2] The discovery of gold in the Kalgoorlie area in the late nineteenth century led to an influx of prospectors and pastoralists to the east and north of Spinifex country. However, the Great Victoria Desert, with its paucity of water and difficult terrain, was deemed unsuitable for mining and pastoral development and the Spinifex people were left alone.

The construction of the Trans-Australian Railway Line between 1909 and 1917, connecting the east coast of Australia with the west coast and running along the southern fringe of Spinifex country, had an impact on the Spinifex people. Ooldea Soak, on the South Australian side of the Great Victoria Desert, was identified as a source of water to supply workers during the construction of the line and more importantly for the steam locomotives after the construction. The soak was bored for water and it supplied up to 320,000 litres per week. Ooldea had been an important ceremonial and trading place, and a permanent water source in times of drought for Spinifex people as well as Aboriginal groups from both coastal and desert areas. The construction of the railway line led to a more established Aboriginal presence. In 1919 the self-taught anthropologist Daisy Bates moved to Ooldea and stayed there for sixteen years, providing food and medicine as required to *Anangu* in the area.

Bates lived in a tent and received little support from the railway or from the government for the care she provided to the Aboriginal people.

In 1933 the United Aborigines Mission established a mission at Ooldea. The South Australian Aborigines' Protection Board provided the first missionary, Annie Locke, with rations and basic medicines for distribution to the local Aboriginal people. Bates had opposed the establishment of a mission, which she believed would encroach upon her work. Relations between Bates and Locke were strained and, two years after the establishment of the mission, Bates left the area and the mission continued. In 1936 Harrie Green had taken over from Annie Lock as superintendent of Ooldea Mission. In the early days of the mission there were usually around a hundred people living at Ooldea but this number was fluid as most people alternated their periods of residence at Ooldea with time spent back on their homelands. By the 1940s there were houses, a church, a school and other buildings.

The anthropologist Norman Tindale wrote in his field notes at Ooldea in November 1934 that 'the "Spinifex Natives" were at Ooldea for the first time'. The anthropologist A.P. Elkin, visiting Ooldea in the 1930s, referred to people from the 'far west or Spinifex tribes'. In 1941 Ronald and Catherine Berndt undertook fieldwork at Ooldea Mission, which by this time had a ration depot, a school and a dormitory for the schoolchildren. The Berndts refer to 'a group known as the Spinifex people' from the area to the north and north-west of Ooldea, which they refer to as 'the great comparatively unknown desert, the Spinifex country'. On their map, showing the country of the various tribal groups they heard about at Ooldea, the desert country north-west of Ooldea has the label 'The *Pila* or Spinifex people'. The Berndts referred to a distinction between *pila* (the spinifex valleys between sand-dunes), the people occupying Spinifex country and *yapu* (stony country) and those from the Pitjantjatjara and Ngaanyatjarra homelands among the rocky ranges further to the north and west. Similarly, Bill Edwards made a distinction between the *apu* (or *yapu*) *murputja*, the hill people, and *pilatja*, the plains or Spinifex people. Tom Gara has suggested that by the 1930s a springtime visit to Ooldea had become part of the Spinifex people's annual migration, partly for ceremonial reasons.[3] When the Berndts arrived in 1942 there were about 200 people living at the main camp at Ooldea, but 'when the water-holes were filled at the beginning of what turned out to be a rainy season, they went out north and north-west into the Spinifex', leaving about eighty people at Ooldea. Some months later they returned and for a while the numbers swelled to about 500 due to ceremonial activities.

The Transcontinental Railway Line attracted Aboriginal people from Spinifex country to trade artefacts and dingo scalps in return for food at other railway sidings on the West Australian side of the border with South Australia. From 1935, the West Australian government established a number of native reserves and ration depots east of Kalgoorlie in an attempt to control the movement of Aboriginal people. In 1937 a ration depot was established at Karonie, on the railway line 90 kilometres east of Kalgoorlie. A 'tea-and-sugar train' dropped off basic foodstuffs at Karonie for railway workers, as well as for Aboriginal people camped along the railway line.

Anthony Carlisle was the West Australian Department of Native Affairs 'Protector and Ration Superintendent' in the area from 1933 to 1949; he did not have a high opinion of Aboriginal people. In a 1933 report to the Commissioner for Native Affairs R.O. Neville, he stated that,

> the trouble with the poor creatures is, I am convinced, that being feeble-minded, or intellectually weak, they are consequently vulnerable and pliant tools in the hands of despoilers ... I am now able to give you a much better report of their behaviour.[4]

Later that year he reported that

> the natives around the area are wholly undisciplined and possessing as they have the means of transporting themselves anywhere at any time, they do and will not recognise the authority of any superintendent of a reserve and simply make their own plans at all times, leave the reserve without consulting me, and at one time (they are getting a little more submissive now!) would treat with contempt any instructions I gave them.

In 1937 159 people were listed as Karonie ration recipients. The Department of Native Affairs put pressure on Carlisle to stem the movement of people from Spinifex country. There were cost concerns but also there was a sense that dependence on rations was possibly detrimental to *Anangu*. Consequently, the department decided in 1939 to move the ration depot north-east, to a place named Cundeelee, which was officially gazetted as a ration depot and native reserve. Carlisle, however, found it difficult to convince the Aboriginal people at Karonie to move and, in 1941, Karonie was declared a prohibited area, meaning that Aboriginal people, unless gainfully employed, could not camp within a 5-mile radius of the former depot. With the help of police from Kalgoorlie, Carlisle dispersed the Karonie mob and Cundeelee became the source of rations for the Spinifex people who had been based around Karonie.

In 1948 S.G. Middleton became Commissioner of Native Affairs, signalling a change from the more paternalistic approach of the previous commissioner towards a more welfare-oriented approach of assimilation and institutionalisation. Middleton's policy was to encourage Christian missions to administer Aboriginal affairs in the more remote areas. In 1949 the Australian Aborigines' Evangelical Mission (AAEM), with affiliation to Protestant churches in North America, submitted a proposal to establish a mission at Madura Station, south of Spinifex country. When, for various reasons, this proved difficult, it was proposed that Cundeelee rather than Madura should be the site of the mission. The missionary Albert Sofer moved to Cundeelee in 1949, to be joined a year later by an American missionary Bob Stewart and later the same year by another American, Bob Anderson. Establishing the facilities at Cundeelee proved difficult but, with missionary zeal, the three AAEM missionaries and their families persisted. The number of people at the mission was initially quite small but the influx of Spinifex people into Cundeelee in 1952, following the closure of Ooldea, helped to boost the numbers.

At Ooldea the population had become less transient, and more people had arrived from Spinifex country. However, the soak was running out of water and in 1948, the South Australian Aborigines' Protection Board declared Ooldea unsuitable as a mission site. It identified Yalata, a pastoral property further south, as the new site for a mission. Rivalry developed between the UAM and Lutheran missionaries (who ran a mission at Koonibba, near the town of Ceduna 200 kilometres east of Yalata) over who should manage the new mission. Conflict within the UAM, which resulted in Harrie Green resigning from the UAM, weakened their position, and the Lutherans were asked by the Aborigines' Protection Board to establish Yalata Mission.

In 1952 Lutherans from Koonibba arrived at Ooldea to transport people to Yalata. They took sixty-seven people, mainly Kokatha. Harrie Green, apparently offended that he had been overlooked to run the new mission, may have spread rumours that the move to Yalata might lead to a loss of autonomy.[5] Consequently, the Spinifex people at Ooldea with relatives at Cundeelee Mission waited for a train to take them west to Cundeelee, leading to the boost in the population there. Another significant group who had been based on Ooldea decided to move north to Ernabella. However, the native patrol officer employed by the Woomera Weapons Research Establishment, Walter MacDougall, found them and, perhaps with concerns about the impending atomic tests in the area, arranged transport south for that group to Yalata.

While the decision to establish a nuclear testing site at Maralinga came after the decision to relocate the mission from Ooldea to Yalata, the nuclear tests meant that the people now living at Yalata were not able to return to their country to the north. Walter MacDougall now had the task of attempting to ensure that no Aboriginal people entered the Maralinga Prohibited Area. During the preparations, MacDougall had decided that there were no Aboriginal people in Spinifex country west of Maralinga at risk from the nuclear tests—despite having been told by some Aboriginal informants that the area was inhabited. Consequently, there were no patrols into Spinifex country until after the major trials had been completed.[6]

The patrols, attempting to locate Aboriginal people and keep them away from the prohibited area, were concentrated in the north (where people might travel south from Pitjantjatjara and Yankunytjatjara lands) and south (to prevent people who had been removed to Yalata trying to move back to the area around Ooldea). Even so, the task was hopeless. In November 1957 a family of four, the Milpuddies, was found camping alongside a crater created by the only Maralinga bomb detonated at ground level seven months earlier. It was classified as a contaminated area. The family had walked south from the Everard Ranges along an established trail of water-holes, heading for Ooldea, which unbeknownst to them had closed five years earlier. The family were showered and transported to Yalata. The woman, who was pregnant, subsequently miscarried. The four dogs traveling with the family were shot on the direct order of the Minister for Supply, Howard Beale.[7]

The Spinifex country to the west of Maralinga was ignored by MacDougall but, in 1955, he visited Cundeelee and was told that eighty people had recently walked in from the Shell Lakes in Spinifex country. He travelled to this area, and found a group of twenty adults and some children. He thought they were not at risk as they were sufficiently distant from the Maralinga Prohibited Area, so he allowed them to stay. He was told that some of the group had walked north to the hill country to replenish their stocks of *mingkulpa* (native tobacco). Two years later, MacDougall and his newly recruited fellow patrol officer Robert Macaulay were at Watarru (Mount Lindsay), south of Pipalyatjara, which was being considered as a site for underground nuclear testing. They were with the anthropologist Norman Tindale and some Pitjantjatjara guides when they came across footprints of 'strangers', who MacDougall thought must have been the Spinifex people who had travelled north to collect *mingkulpa*. I assume this site at Watarru was the place that I was shown twenty years later, where MacDougall had apparently established a base (see chapter 2).

In 1959, after the major trials had been completed, Macaulay visited Cundeelee and was told that the missionaries, concerned about the impact of the tests on Spinifex people, had conducted a number of 'rescue missions' into Spinifex country in the preceding five years, and had brought about eighty *Anangu* to Cundeelee. The missionaries informed Macaulay that there were people still living there, so he travelled to the Shell Lakes, where he found a camp of about thirty *Anangu*. Through interpreters, he discovered that they and other Spinifex people travelled over a wide area. It now became clear that possibly over one hundred *Anangu* were living in Spinifex country during the major nuclear tests, sometimes entering into the Maralinga Prohibited Area. Consequently, Commonwealth police patrols into the western side of the Prohibited Area were commenced in late 1959.

Over the following few years, these patrols, as well as MacDougall and Macaulay, found frequent signs of the Spinifex people, but the decision was made that this information should be kept secret from the Australian public. When people were located, they were encouraged to travel west to Cundeelee.

When Macaulay and two police officers found a family near the state border, they were told to walk west to Cundeelee and follow the roads constructed by Len Beadell. The roads had not been constructed with any knowledge about the location of water or food supplies, and as a result three members of this family died of thirst at Neale Junction, 400 kilometres west of where they had been located. The surviving members of this family reached Cundeelee; one of these survivors lived in Tjuntjuntjara until she died in 2022.

Through the fifties and early sixties, despite the nuclear tests, many family groups continued to walk the long distance between their country and Cundeelee Mission, and back. However, by the time the survivors of the last family arrived in 1963, most of the Spinifex people were settled at Cundeelee. There was, as we shall see in the next chapter, one family who continued to live on country, having returned from Warburton Mission around the same time that the last group left for Cundeelee.

From Cundeelee to Coonana to Tjuntjuntjara

The Cundeelee Mission was seen as a safe place, particularly in comparison with Karonie. Cundeelee was also a *minyma tjuta tjukurrpa* (Seven Sisters dreaming) site, with connection to Spinifex country, which added to its appeal. Another factor that gave comfort to the Spinifex people was the fact that parts of the Cundeelee landscape were reminiscent of Spinifex country, with spinifex, mulga and sand-plains. On the other hand, the imperative to retain connection to their country remained. In addition, water supplies were unreliable at Cundeelee and facilities were limited. A government report in 1973 commented on the poor conditions at the mission and the poor health of the people.

In the early 1980s, when there were about 250 *Anangu* living at Cundeelee, the government told them that, due to the inadequate water supplies, they should relocate to Coonana Station. There was some resistance to this, as the Spinifex people would have preferred to move back to their country to maintain their traditional ties. Coonana has no spiritual significance for the Spinifex people, was further away from their homeland and, in fact, had worse water supplies than Cundeelee. The government forced the issue, nonetheless, and a settlement at Coonana was established, to which most of the people from Cundeelee relocated. As the anthropologist Scott Cane has observed, the Spinifex people were probably the only desert people forced to move further from their homelands in the 1980s, a time when the homelands movement in most of the Western Desert was at its peak.[8]

The majority of the Spinifex people, still aspiring to return to their country, after a year or so at Coonana established a camp at Double Pump on the Nullarbor Plain, closer to their country. Local pastoralists were not happy about this camp, and to allay these concerns the local federal member of parliament obtained an Australian Government grant to drill a bore at a place called Yakatunya, closer again to Spinifex country, 100 kilometres north of the railway line. Later, a 99-year lease was obtained for 16,000 hectares around Yakatunya. This became a base for people to live while they continued to work towards reoccupying their country. While south of the actual Spinifex country, Yakatunya, immediately north of the treeless Nullabor Plain, is a place of mythological significance for the Spinifex people.

A key figure in helping with the reoccupation was my friend Ian Baird, with whom I had worked some years previously at Kalka. Ian had become inspired to work in Aboriginal communities in 1979 when he had enrolled in a course in Aboriginal Studies in Adelaide. His lecturer was Tungku Tregenza, who had moved to Adelaide from Kalka but had retained his links with the Pitjantjatjara people and the Pitjantjatjara Homelands Health Service. Through Tungku, Ian obtained some relief work at Kalka, which is where I first met him. After leaving Kalka, Ian had been employed as culture and recreation officer at Cundeelee. He learnt to speak the Pitjantjatjara language, became absorbed in the culture and ultimately married a woman from Cundeelee, Debbie Hansen. Ian and Debbie moved to Yakatunya with the *Anangu*, where they were joined by Jon Lark, a friend of Ian who had also been influenced by Tungku Tregenza's lectures in 1979. Both Ian and Jon helped to maintain the community in its remote location and support its further development and onward movement.

From the base at Yakatunya, the Spinifex people wanted to make a road to improve access into their country with the aim of ultimately settling back there. Across the border in South Australia, *Anangu* living at Yalata also aspired to move north to their homelands in the Maralinga area which, despite the fact the tests had ceased twenty years earlier, was still closed to the public and potentially contaminated with radioactive material. There was also increasing concern expressed in the media, supported by public campaigns, about the effects of the tests on the health of Australian and British personnel involved in the trials, as well as that of local Aboriginal people. In 1984 the federal government, led by Labor's Bob Hawke, established the Royal Commission into British Nuclear Tests in Australia, which produced its report in 1985. The report's recommendations led to a clean-up of the test sites and the restitution of the Maralinga lands to the Aboriginal owners. In 1987 *Anangu* from Yalata established a community at Oak Valley, 200 kilometres away from the old Maralinga township. Yalata had had a community-controlled health service since 1984 and, when the Oak Valley community was developed, the Yalata Health Service changed its name to Yalata Maralinga Health Service, which provided healthcare to both Yalata and Oak Valley residents. Some years later, the Yalata Maralinga Health Service split into two health services, one at Yalata and one at Oak Valley.

The royal commission also awarded compensation to the Spinifex people, allowing them the resources needed to work on the road construction from Yakatunya north into Spinifex country and from there east across the border to facilitate contact with their relatives re-establishing themselves at Oak Valley. In 1986, while the road was being made and the Spinifex people were re-connecting with their country, they re-established contact with a family that had continued to live in Spinifex country. The story of that family, the last group of hunter-gatherers to come out of the desert in Australia, is related in chapter 7.

The Spinifex people continued their efforts to reoccupy their country. The intention had been to establish the community at a place called Ilkurlka, in the heart of Spinifex country. Ultimately, however, the initial settlement was established on the southern edge of Spinifex country at Tjuntjuntjara, or the place of the *tjuntjun*, the small brown bush babbler (*Pomatostomus superciliosis*). People moved to Tjuntjuntjara from Yakatunya in 1989 and Tjuntjuntjara became a small but thriving community. At Tjuntjuntjara a community council was formed called Paupiyala Tjarutja Aboriginal

Corporation (PTAC). Paupiya is an important site in the heart of Spinifex country, associated with the *kipara tjukurrpa* (bush turkey dreaming), about 70 kilometres north of Tjuntjuntjara. Paupiyala Tjarutja effectively means 'radiating outward from Paupiya'.

From Tjuntjuntjara, there were aspirations to continue the movement and establish another base at Ilkurlka, as well as smaller outstations at Tawun, Tjintirrkara and Miramirratjara—all places of significance for the Spinifex people. In 1994, when Scott Cane worked with the community on a development plan, this was still a definite aspiration.[9] However, the main effort went into establishing the required facilities at Tjuntjuntjara and, with declining government support for the homelands movement as time went on, the Spinifex people accepted that Tjuntjuntjara would remain their residential base allowing access to their country. Some facilities were developed at Ilkurlka, including a roadhouse that services tourists travelling east–west along the remote Anne Beadell Highway and *Anangu* travelling north–south along a track connecting Tjuntjuntjara with the Pitjantatjara and Ngaanyatjarra lands. It also provides a base for cultural activities for Spinifex people within the heart of Spinifex country.

Healthcare at Tjuntjuntjara

Once established back in their homelands, a priority for the Spinifex people was to ensure they had access to healthcare. At Coonana, the West Australian health department ran a nursing post where two registered nurses were employed. The department was reluctant to commit resources for health services at Yakatunya, and later at Tjuntjuntjara, but support was available from Bega Garnbirringu, the Aboriginal community-controlled health service in Kalgoorlie. In the early years of Tjuntjuntjara, Bega health staff, particularly doctors David Dunn and Anne Stevens, provided regular monthly visits to the developing community. Bega funded a monthly charter-flight to enable the visits and eventually funded a position for a nurse to live in the community.

In Scott Cane's report on the community plan in 1994, he stated that four options were being considered by the community regarding health services. These were: to continue with Bega Garnbirringu Aboriginal Health

Service; to operate as an annex of the state health service from Coonana; to join the Yalata Maralinga Health Service; or to use funding from the Aboriginal and Torres Strait Islander Commission to employ a nurse. Cane stated that the community seemed to favour the last option but a firm decision had not yet been made.[10]

The community ultimately chose a combination of the second and fourth options. There was sufficient money available from ATSIC to employ a nurse but not for relief when the nurse was on leave away from the community. An arrangement was reached with the West Australian health department for PTAC to use their own funding to employ one nurse, bringing the combined number of nurses at Coonana and Tjuntjuntjara to three, and these nurses provided on-site care at Tjuntjuntjara on rotation. A demountable was supplied to accommodate the nurse at Tjuntjuntjara and another demountable was used as a clinic. In 1995 an actual clinic building was constructed. At around the same time, the provision of visiting GPs by Bega Garnbirringu ceased and the Royal Flying Doctor Service began to provide a visiting GP service, generally fortnightly.

In 1998 the Commonwealth funding (now coming from the Office of Aboriginal and Torres Strait Islander Health (OATSIH) within the health department rather than from ATSIC) was increased to allow the employment of two nurses, both to be based at Tjuntjuntjara. This gave more independence for the local health service, and the rotational arrangement with Coonana ceased. In the context of a small remote community, however, this independence led to some difficulties. The health service was administered by the community council, PTAC, which was a well-managed organisation but lacking somewhat in health service management expertise, so that these management decisions were often guided by the nurses. There was a relatively high turnover of nursing staff and, as new nurses arrived, they sometimes had different ideas about how things should be done or what needed to be purchased, which sometimes conflicted with advice from other nurses.

This management difficulty led to my first visit to Tjuntjuntjara in 2009. At that time I was living in Adelaide and working as Public Health Medical Officer with the Aboriginal Health Council of South Australia. One day I received a visit from Ian Baird and Jon Lark, who told me about the developments at Tjuntjuntjara and, particularly, about its Aboriginal community-controlled health service. They told me about the management difficulties and were concerned that the health service was not as effective as it might be. They had funding for a review and asked whether I would be interested in conducting it. I happily agreed.

In August 2009 I drove from Adelaide to Tjuntjuntjara—a two-day journey, with an overnight stay in Ceduna, a coastal town in the far west of South Australia, and then through the Aboriginal communities of Yalata and Oak Valley before crossing the border into Western Australia towards Tjuntjuntjara. I had not visited Tjuntjuntjara before but I was familiar with Yalata and Oak Valley.

Control of Yalata had been handed over from the Lutheran Mission to Yalata Community Council in 1974. It was now a community of about 300 people, mostly Pitjantjatjara-speaking, situated 200 kilometres west of Ceduna. I had had a connection with Yalata since 2000, when I was approached by the then manager of Tullawon Health Service, David Kilgarriff. Tullawon Health Service was the name given to the Aboriginal community-controlled health organisations in Yalata, following the split in the Yalata-Maralinga Health Service the previous year. Tullawon Health Service at that time employed two nurses and a number of Aboriginal health workers, while the RFDS base in Port Augusta flew in a doctor once a week to conduct a clinic.

David's concern was that he and the board often needed medical advice, and he asked whether I might be available to provide it. In particular, he said, when new nurses started, they often had different ideas on policies and procedures in the clinic. This, of course, was similar to the problem I was now being asked to address in Tjuntjuntjara. In 2000 it was the Tullawon Health Service board seeking expert independent advice to ensure that there was consistency in clinic policies. I had agreed to provide this support and, for the next few years, I was employed part-time as Medical Director of THS, spending three days every two months at Yalata working with the staff and meeting with the Board.

In 2007, when I commenced full-time work as Public Health Medical Officer with the Aboriginal Health Council of South Australia, Jill Benson, a GP who had recently started providing some clinical services to Tullawon, took over as medical director. However, in my role at AHCSA, as the peak body for all Aboriginal community-controlled health services in South Australia, including Tullawon Health Service and Oak Valley Maralinga Health Service, I had ongoing contact with both health services.

I have digressed from the account of my road trip to Tjuntjuntjara. From Yalata and Oak Valley, I drove to Tjuntjuntjara where I spent several days investigating how the health service was operating and talking to local people. I wrote a report based on my findings, with a number of recommendations. The following is an extract from the executive summary of my 2009 report:

> Tjuntjuntjara is a small, very remote Aboriginal community in the south-east of WA, with a usual population of around 150 people. Its remoteness is one of its strengths: it is a relatively healthy community. Being a long way from alcohol outlets, it is largely free from many of the problems which beset many remote Aboriginal communities. It is noticeable that the demographic structure of Tjuntjuntjara differs from many other Aboriginal communities in that it has a relatively high proportion of older people, with almost one in five people seen at the clinic being over the age of fifty years. However, it is not exclusively an old people's community; the demographic structure is fairly even throughout all age groups, and 28% are under the age of fifteen.
>
> The fact that it is a healthy, happy community means that Tjuntjuntjara is worthy of support if Australian governments are committed to 'closing the gap'. This support includes ensuring that the people living at Tjuntjuntjara have access to good quality comprehensive primary healthcare, as there are still significant health risks and issues existing in the community.
>
> The health service at Tjuntjuntjara is community-controlled, under the direction of PTAC. Funding to PTAC for health services comes from the Office of Aboriginal and Torres Strait Islander Health (OATSIH) in the Commonwealth Department of Health and Ageing (DoHA). The service employs two nurses and two Aboriginal health workers (AHWs). At the time of my visit, both nurses were short-term agency nurses, and one of the AHWs was away for training. All four health providers were women.

The fact that the two nurses were providing short-term agency relief meant that they did not have the more comprehensive knowledge about the service and its issues that could be expected with longer-term staff. However, both had been in the community for four months, which was sufficient to allow a number of issues about the quality of healthcare services to emerge. This, combined with discussions with other community staff and residents produced a reasonably comprehensive picture of the strengths and deficits of the health service.

Credit should be given to community administrative staff for the efforts in managing and maintaining a health service with little health knowledge and while attending to many other pressing problems. Credit should also be given to the health staff who work hard to provide healthcare in a difficult environment.

However, all readily conceded that the current level of healthcare provided is very basic, and in general is limited to reacting to issues that present to the clinic. It is widely recognized that to improve health outcomes, people living in Aboriginal communities should have access to good-quality comprehensive primary healthcare, and Tjuntjuntjara is no exception to this. There are examples in other parts of remote Australia where such healthcare is provided, but in these situations there are better support systems in place than currently exist in Tjuntjuntjara.

The challenge for Tjuntjuntjara is to build on what currently exists in the health service to ensure that sustainable support systems are in place to ensure good-quality, appropriate, comprehensive primary healthcare is available. This should be achievable, if current problems are addressed.

In my report, I made a number of recommendations as to how these problems might be addressed. The OATSIH was situated in the Commonweath Department of Health. Having provided funds for the review of the health service, it was willing to invest some resources to help implement my recommendations, including employing some key staff. Graham Townley, an anthropologist with a good knowledge of the Tjuntjuntjara community, played a crucial role. He was employed initially as a consultant but later worked in a salaried position as health service manager, a position paid by an OATSIH grant. A clinic manager was also appointed. Katie Pennington was originally employed as a remote-area nurse in 2010, and subsequently went on to become clinic manager, which contributed significantly to the improved provision of comprehensive primary healthcare. Both Graham and Katie, although they did not always see eye to eye, made a major contribution to the development of the health service.

The Kakarrara Wilurrara Health Alliance

My 2009 report made two other recommendations which, thanks to an alignment of the planets, were achieved when a particular funding stream became available just at the right time. One of these recommendations related to the need for a medical director, similar to the role I had previously held within Tullawon Health Service. I stated in my report:

> There is a definite need to include within the structure of the health service a role for one or more persons with clinical skills who can provide ongoing leadership, supervision, advice and support for health service development. This need not be a full-time person: in fact, a person based away from the community, but visiting regularly, is probably the only way to ensure the long-term sustainability that is required. Other health services in remote Aboriginal communities have found having a person in this role beneficial. The title of the role is often 'Medical Director' although this can be misleading as the function is not just 'medical' but also has an important function of developing public or population health programs and activities. However, for the purposes of this report the title of Medical Director will be retained.
>
> The role of the Medical Director would include: providing advice to the Health subcommittee of the PTAC Board, and the Board itself when necessary, on public health issues; providing supervision and leadership to members of the primary healthcare team; supervising the development of public health and medical policies and programs; providing some clinical care while in Tjuntjuntjara as required; supervising chronic disease management and management plans; etc.

The related recommendation was on the need to develop linkages with neighbouring health services. I suggested that, given the small size of the service at Tjuntjuntjara, developing some formal linkages with other health services for mutual support and resource-sharing may be beneficial. Bega Garnbirringu in Kalgoorlie to the west, and Ngaanyatjarra Health Service to the north were both considered. However the consensus of opinion within Tjuntjuntjara appeared to be that the strongest cultural connections were with Oak Valley and Yalata to the east across the border with South Australia. I stated:

> It is with the remote communities of Oak Valley and Yalata in SA that Tjuntjuntjara has the closest links, and the greatest movement of people is between these communities. (At the time of my visit to Tjuntjuntjara, most of the usual residents of both Oak Valley and Tjuntjuntjara were in Yalata for a funeral.) Oak Valley is a very remote community of about 80 people, with its own health service, which like Tjuntjuntjara Aboriginal Health Service struggles with inadequate support systems. Yalata has a well-established health service, Tullawon Health Service, which benefits from the engagement of a Medical Director.
>
> There are potential benefits from exploring the development of closer ties between these three health services, which could be to the advantage of all three communities but particularly Oak Valley and Tjuntjuntjara. It is possible to develop linkages and a regional approach to certain activities, without each community losing their autonomy or becoming just an outreach service from a larger community. This would need careful negotiation and the support and co-operation of each health service and their communities. As an initial step, a workshop involving each health service could be held, to explore possibilities for working together.

There was support from the Spinifex people as well as from the Tullawon Health Service and Oak Valley Maralinga Health Service for developing these linkages across the border. The Commonwealth Department of Health, which had recently been encouraging regionalisation of health services, also supported the idea and agreed to fund a meeting between the three health services. Some of the buildings at the old Maralinga Village that had housed workers during the Maralinga nuclear tests had been maintained and were looked after by a couple of caretakers. Catering and basic accommodation were available here and as it was on the homelands and convenient for all three health services, it was chosen as the venue for the meeting.

Board members and management staff from the three health services attended a two-day meeting at the Maralinga Village in 2011. Due to my previous involvement, I was also invited. There was unanimous agreement at the meeting that an alliance should be formed which, as I had recommended in my report, should maintain the autonomy of each health service but facilitate resource-sharing and mutual support. The *Anangu* present proposed the name of Kakarrara Wilurrara Health Alliance (KWHA) meaning the East–West Health Alliance. The original ATSIC Regional Council, which had covered both sides of the border, had been called the Kakarrara Wilurrara Regional Council. When, without consultation, the John Howard–led Coalition government reduced the number of ATSIC Regional Councils and changed the areas covered by councils, the Kakarrara Wilurrara Regional Council was abolished, and Tjuntjuntjara became part of a regional council entirely in Western Australia (until the Howard government subsequently abolished the whole ATSIC structure). The revival of this title appeared to be recognition by *Anangu* of the links across the border and they were glad to again have the opportunity to re-establish formal connections.

It was agreed that the KWHA should have an overall medical director to provide clinical and public-health advice. Jill Benson, who had taken over the role of medical director of Tullawon Health Service from me in 2007, was at the Maralinga meeting and agreed to expand her role to be the medical director of KWHA as well. Given Jill's dedication and dynamism, this was a fortuitous choice.

One of the potential roles for the KWHA was to help develop a program of visiting health professionals to the three health services. Serendipitously, a Commonwealth-funded program was available with the potential to support such a program. The Medical Specialists Outreach Assistance Program— Indigenous Chronic Disease (MSOAP-ICD)[11] provided funds for general practitioners, specialists and allied health practitioners to support chronic disease management for Indigenous people in rural and remote communities. The funding went to non-Indigenous organisations in each state and territory, as had become the practice of the Commonwealth health department (see chapter 10). In Western Australia the fund-holder for this program was Rural Health West (RHW), and in South Australia the Rural Doctors Workforce Agency (RDWA). This complicated the process of getting funding directed to KWHA, which operated on both sides of the border, but Jill Benson negotiated with both RHW and the RDWA to allow an amount of money to be pooled so as to provide outreach services to all three health services.

The financial support provided was sufficient to fund a monthly charter-flight from Adelaide to take a GP and two or three other health professionals to each community for two days each month. This monthly charter flight became, and continues to be, the main activity of the KWHA. By providing regular visits from various health professionals it has added significant value to the primary healthcare provided in each community. Perhaps the most valuable component was the monthly visit by a GP. Each health service had a regular GP identified to provide clinical and public health support to the nurses and Aboriginal health workers resident in the community.

Growing Spinifex Health Service

Spinifex Health Service was in need of a GP. Once again, the planets were aligned. David Johnson was an experienced GP who had recently entered the training program to become a public-health physician and, as part of the training, had started a six-month rotation working at the Aboriginal Health Council of South Australia, with me as his supervisor. I suggested to him that he might like to become the GP for Spinifex Health Service and work on a project in health-service development as a contribution to his public health training. David accepted the challenge. Recognising that his role went beyond just the provision of clinical services, he was given the title of medical director of Spinifex Health Service, as I had recommended in my review.

David spent at least two days in Tjuntjuntjara every month. However he recognised that he needed to spend more time there and, on several occasions, arranged to stay for one or two weeks. At an early stage, senior men took David on a trip into Spinifex country to show him important sites and to provide an orientation to their culture and priorities. David was the first doctor employed by the Spinifex people's own health service and this gesture by senior people within the community is an indication of the importance they placed on the position.

Another development was an improvement in access to dental care—an important but often neglected component of comprehensive primary healthcare. When I had been medical director of Tullawon Health Service at Yalata, I had been able to negotiate an arrangement with the South Australian Government Dental Services for a regular visiting dentist to Yalata. I was able to recruit a very experienced remote-area dentist named Colin Endean, whom I had met many years before on the Pitjantjatjara lands. Another achievement of KWHA was to consolidate dental-care funding for the three health services. It has been a number of years now that Colin and his partner Roxanne Gallegos have provided a regular high-quality dental service to the three communities. (This is unfortunately not typical; many remote Aboriginal communities do not get anything approaching adequate dental care.)

Spinifex Health Service continued to develop. In 2011 I was invited back to review the program since my original review two years previously. The results were impressive. Most of my recommendations had been implemented and there had been an effective transition from a basic nursing post to a comprehensive primary healthcare service. In my original review I had listed the components of comprehensive primary healthcare that people living in Tjuntjuntjara should expect. In my report two years later I was able to comment on whether or not these separate components were now available. As the list in my original review gives an overview of what, by this stage of my professional development, I envisaged as significant components of comprehensive primary healthcare in a remote Aboriginal community, I will quote it in full:

> People living at Tjuntjuntjara should be able to access the following components of comprehensive primary healthcare:

All people should have access to appropriate information about health issues, including how to prevent health problems.

Pregnant women should have culturally safe, appropriate antenatal care, with check-ups commencing early in pregnancy and continuing at frequent intervals throughout the pregnancy.

Childbirth should occur in a safe environment with adequate social support.

Infants should be monitored regularly, initially weekly and then monthly until two years of age, with appropriate support and intervention if weight-faltering or other problems occur.

All children should be offered immunization according to national guidelines at the appropriate times.

All children under 15 years of age should have their ears checked monthly, and all children found to have ear disease should be appropriately treated and monitored closely until the disease has resolved.

All children should have audiometric screening annually, and appropriate action taken for children with hearing loss.

All children aged 5–9 should be screened for trachoma annually, with appropriate follow-up according to national guidelines.

All adults aged 15 years and over should be offered an annual health check-up, with appropriate follow-up to manage any abnormality identified.

All women should have access to regular cervical screening, and mammographic screening if aged over 40 years.

Pneumococcal vaccination and annual influenza vaccination should be offered at the appropriate times to all people for whom it is recommended.

All teenagers and adults should have access to appropriate education about sexual health matters, and should have freely available access to condoms, and to other appropriate contraception methods when desired.

All people should have early access to appropriate and confidential advice about, and diagnosis and management of, sexually transmitted infections.

All people with addiction issues (including tobacco, alcohol, marijuana and other drugs) should have ready access to advice and support to assist in dealing with the addiction.

All people with mental health problems should have access to appropriate ongoing management and care.

All people should have access to regular dental checks, and appropriate and timely management of dental problems.

All people with chronic diseases should be reviewed at least six-monthly, with appropriate action to facilitate optimal control and the prevention of complications.

All people with diabetes should have access to a podiatrist and a nutritionist at least annually.

All people with renal disease should be reviewed three-monthly, with adequate preparation for dialysis if this becomes necessary.

All people with terminal disease should have access to appropriate palliative care to allow them to die with dignity in the place of their choice.

All people with disabilities should be regularly reviewed and have access to appropriate care, including specialist and allied healthcare when appropriate.

All people requiring specialist care should have timely access to the appropriate specialist.

All people requiring elective surgery (e.g. cataracts, trichiasis, perforated eardrums) should have the opportunity to have surgery within a year of diagnosis.

All people with acute medical problems or injuries should have access to timely diagnosis and management.

All people should have access to appropriate medications required for their medical conditions, without encountering financial hardship.

By mid-2011, much of this was happening. This was an impressive achievement, demonstrating that SHS had developed significantly in two years. There was still work to be done and services continued to improve.

David Johnson continued as GP, a position all the more essential as in 2012 the Royal Flying Doctor Service ceased its provision of a visiting GP service out of Kalgoorlie to Tjuntjuntjara for cost-saving reasons. By late 2014, David wanted to reduce his time away from home and I expressed an interest in taking over his role as medical director. The health service agreed and, early in 2015, I resigned from the Aboriginal Health Council of South Australia to assume my new position. It was clear that two days a month on the ground in Tjuntjuntjara was not sufficient, so I arranged to spend at least a week there every month. Generally this involved flying from Adelaide (where I live) to Perth, with a connecting flight to Kalgoorlie, and then a mail plane the following morning out to Tjuntjuntjara. After eight or nine days in Tjuntjuntjara I usually returned with the KWHA charter-flight, taking a more direct route back to Adelaide.

In between my visits I maintained communication with the health staff in Tjuntjuntjara. We had a weekly teleconference to discuss patient management and other issues and I was available by phone or email at other times as required. I had remote access to the Health Information System on my laptop, so I could review pathology and radiology results and discharge summaries as they became available, and review patient notes. With a good primary healthcare team in the community (four Aboriginal health workers and three nurses) this system worked well. Early in 2019, having decided it was time to take a break, I happily handed over the role to Janelle Trees, a general practitioner of Aboriginal descent who had some previous experience working with the Spinifex people.

Since I wrote my report two years after the initial review, visiting services had been extended and consolidated. Spinifex Health Service now receives regular visits from a number of regular specialists. An eminent renal physician who also has an interest in diabetes management, a general and respiratory physician, an ear, nose and throat surgeon, an ophthalmologist and a paediatrician each visit two times a year. The renal physician, Mark Thomas, also provides extra case conferences over the telephone four times a year. A podiatrist, a physiotherapist, a dietician, an audiologist and a diabetes educator all visit two times a year. The ophthalmologist and the ENT surgeon facilitate access to surgery, so waiting lists for these problems are kept to a minimum.

The value of these visits is optimised by having good primary-healthcare systems in place. At each visit, a list of people who need to be reviewed is generated from the electronic health information system and, with the assistance of the Aboriginal health workers, the people on the list are notified and usually attend for the review. It is also important that the type of specialist or allied-health practitioner is determined by the needs of the service, largely because the KWHA has had control of the funding. In this way, the specialists and allied health practitioners provide support to the ongoing primary healthcare rather than, as sometimes happens elsewhere, being essentially a parallel service.

Spinifex Health Service is a branch of the Tjuntjuntjara Community Council, Paupiyala Tjarutja Aboriginal Corporation (PTAC). Given the relatively small size of the community, this currently seems to be the most appropriate structure, although sometimes there are discussions about the health service incorporating separately. For the moment, the board of directors of PTAC has a health subcommittee that usually meets every couple of months to discuss issues relating to the management and future directions of the health service.

The Spinifex people continue to live in Spinifex country. The old people, who grew up in their country and spearheaded the return, still live in Tjuntjuntjara. Tjuntjuntjara has a thriving art centre, called Spinifex Arts, under the guidance of Amanda Dent and Brian Hallett. This provides an opportunity for the older people to express themselves creatively, enjoy the sociality of their peers and to contribute to the economic development of their community.

Another vibrant activity operating from Tjuntjuntjara is the Spinifex Ranger Program, which falls under the rubric of the Pila Nguru Aboriginal Corporation (PNAC), the native-title landholding organisation based in Tjuntjuntjara. Ian Baird continues to be the coordinator of PNAC, which includes the Spinifex Ranger Program. A number of young and middle-aged adults work as rangers, involved in a variety of land-care activities, providing employment and maintaining their links with the land, as well as contributing to environmental sustainability. In 2018 the Spinifex rangers won the Indigenous National Land-care Award. I will discuss further the importance of activities such as this in chapter 8.

Like many other remote Aboriginal communities, Tjuntjuntjara has its problems. I have no doubt, however, that living on their country benefits the health and wellbeing of the Spinifex people, which is a testament to their struggle for autonomy.

7

First contact, last contact

The demise of hunter-gatherers

The settler colonisation of the Australian mainland may be envisaged as occurring in three waves. In the late eighteenth century, European settlement of the south-east coast began. In the first half of the nineteenth century settlements spread to some other coastal areas and to the Murray Darling Basin. Finally, in the second half of the nineteenth century, settlements spread into other parts of Australia. European settlement remained predominantly in the east and around the coast, and there were some areas in the interior where permanent non-Aboriginal settlement was never established. In particular, the large Western Desert region in the central-western interior—which appeared inhospitable to the encroaching non-Aboriginal settlers, resistant to agriculture, and distant from markets—remained largely untouched by the tide until well into the twentieth century. In the Western Desert, Aboriginal people maintained a traditional hunter-gatherer lifestyle until relatively recently. Eventually, however, the settler-colonial frontier advanced inexorably towards these people.

This advancing frontier was not just the frontier between the non-Aboriginal settlement of Australia and the lands of the remaining traditional Aboriginal people. On a larger timescale, and a broader spatial scale, it can be seen as one of the last phases of a global process that has been happening for around ten millennia—the remorseless takeover of land occupied by hunter-gatherers by agriculturalists and pastoralists, a process that began with the

Agricultural Revolution. For about 99 per cent of the history of *Homo sapiens*, people have lived as hunter-gatherers. Of the 150 billion people who have lived on earth, more than 60 per cent were hunter-gatherers. Around 35 per cent were agriculturalists, and only a few per cent have lived in industrial societies. It is, however, this recent development of industrial society that has created the unstable ecological environment in which we now all live.

Hunter-gatherers are often associated with marginal lands but, prior to the Agricultural Revolution, hunting and gathering was the lifestyle of humans wherever they lived, which presumably would have been mostly in the more fertile regions where game and other foods were plentiful. In the past, the accepted wisdom was that the Agricultural Revolution was a major step forward in the development of humankind in that it was an advance from a precarious struggle for subsistence to a more sustainable and comfortable mode of living. Over the past fifty years this assumption has been challenged. A conference called 'Man the Hunter' held in Chicago in 1966 was the occasion for a number of papers suggesting that the hunter-gatherer lifestyle was not necessarily a Hobbesian state of nature where life was nasty, brutish and short. It was at this conference that the economic anthropologist Marshall Sahlins, speaking of hunter-gatherers, coined the term 'the original affluent society'. His evidence-backed research showed that hunter-gatherers lived well, requiring only a few hours of effort each day to maintain their subsistence, which allowed a significant amount of leisure time for other activities including socialising and spiritual performances. Sahlins suggested that affluence was due partly to the ability to extract a living from nature, but also from having few and finite material needs.

Another often-noted feature of hunter-gatherer societies cited by Sahlins was a tendency to resolve conflict by fission. When arguments arise, those involved part company rather than allowing the dispute to accelerate into violent conflict. We have seen how, in the Western Desert, this tendency to fission has led to the homelands movement itself and to particular developments within it.

Sahlins' notion of the original affluent society has been challenged,[1] but it is now generally accepted that the transition from a hunter-gatherer to an agriculturalist lifestyle was not necessarily one that led to an improved life.

Agriculture is thought to have started in the Near East around ten- to fifteen-thousand years ago. It also happened independently in other parts of the world, transitioning in fits and starts over millennia to a new lifestyle, involving growing crops and domesticating herds of animals for food. This is not to say that hunter-gatherers did not practise a form of agriculture. David Graeber and David Wingrow suggest that hunter-gatherer modes of production varied immensely, with frequent experimental forays into differing techniques of food production and harvesting. This is consistent with the evidence that the Australian landscape was modified by land-management practices that Aboriginal people had developed to harvest flora and fauna for their consumption.[2] In recent work with *Martu* at Punmu, Parngurr and Kunawarritji, Doug Bird and Rebecca Bligh Bird have demonstrated that mosaic burning enhanced the efficiency of hunting burrowed prey.

I have also experienced evidence of similar practices. I remember on one of my first trips from Kintore to Kiwirrkurra, when people were just starting to move back to Kiwirrkurra, I was travelling in a vehicle with George Tjampu Tjapaltjarri, munching on *pura*, or bush tomato (*Solanum diversiflorum*) that had been collected near Kintore, as we went. I asked whether *pura* could be found around Kiwirrkurra. Tjampu replied in the negative. 'We have not been there for a long time, so the country has not been burnt,' he said. 'But now we are going back, and will start burning properly again, and *pura* will grow there again.'

While hunter-gatherers, including Australian Aboriginal people, often had sophisticated modes of production and land-management techniques, the so-called Agricultural Revolution over time led to a qualitative change in lifestyle resulting in a more settled mode of living and ultimately led to the development of cities and city-states. Some have suggested that the first step was permanent settlements, perhaps for defensive purposes, and that this was the impetus for developing agriculture.[3] Whichever came first, the expansion of intensive agriculture in the ensuing millennia resulted in the decline of hunting and gathering in steadily increasing parts of the world. This may have been due in some cases to a gradual adoption of agriculture by people who had been hunter-gatherers, but it is likely that, in most cases, it was through conquest of land by agriculturalists and pastoralists and eradication of the hunter-gatherers who depended on the land for a living. Hunter-gatherers do not readily give up their lifestyle but, where there has been conflict over land, they have always been vulnerable to the hierarchical and militarised organisation of agriculturalists and their political formations.

The anthropologist Hugh Brody makes the point that the accepted notion of hunter-gatherers as 'nomads' and agriculturalists as 'settled' is understandable and appropriate when thinking in the short-term, but in the longer term the reverse is true. Farming and sedentarisation leads to higher fertility rates and population pressures and, consequently, to the inevitable desire for more land for crops, pasture and for the natural resources required for other activities in settled communities. In the longer term, hunter-gatherers continue to live and move around their homelands, while farmers migrate. Over generations, the land occupied by hunter-gatherers is remorselessly taken over by agriculturalists and pastoralists. The Industrial Revolution, in more recent history, merely accelerated the process.

The Agricultural Revolution also led to an increase in the risk of infectious diseases. As Hugh Brody has stated,

> The spread of farming through the world has meant the occupation and eventual destruction of most of the world's hunter-gatherer societies. Yet there is a characteristic of farming peoples that has caused more death to others that even their genius for warfare. They have created and spread diseases.[4]

In farming settlements, people generally had large families and lived in crowded buildings, in close contact with domestic animals and in situations that encourage the breeding of vermin such as rats, lice and mosquitoes. This close contact with animals facilitated the crossing of species-barriers by organisms causing infectious diseases. Many epidemic diseases in humans began in domestic animals; for example measles, tuberculosis and smallpox are derived from diseases found in cattle; influenza is from viruses in pigs and chickens. Large families living in close contact facilitated the easy spread of these diseases between people. It also allowed the development of natural immunity in those who survived exposure to infectious diseases.

Hunter-gatherers were less likely to be exposed to these diseases, at least until they had contact with expanding farming societies. Without the opportunity to develop immunity to these infectious diseases, the historical record shows that there were often high mortality rates among the newly exposed hunter-gatherers in the initial contact period. This was just one of the catastrophic impacts of the spread of farming societies into hunter-gatherers' lands, but it was a particularly significant one. In many parts of the world a high proportion of hunter-gatherers were killed by infectious diseases that came with the expansion into their lands of farming societies. Australian Aboriginal people were no exception.

In a review of disease among Aboriginal people in 1932, Basedow stated that 'at the rate that havoc is at present being wrought by civilisation among the pure-blooded sections of the Aboriginal community, it will not be many years before the last of them have shared the unenviable lot of their Tasmanian brothers'.[5] There have been a number of recorded epidemics of infectious diseases that devastated Aboriginal communities. A highly contagious epidemic (previously thought to be smallpox, but quite possibly chickenpox) caused a high mortality among Aboriginal people in the Sydney area within a year of the arrival of the First Fleet. Between 1829 and 1845 and again in 1869, there were similar epidemics, leading to many Aboriginal deaths in other parts of Australia. Typhoid fever epidemics were recorded in Aboriginal communities in Queensland and South Australia in the early twentieth century. A measles epidemic in Western Australia in 1867 was estimated to have halved the Aboriginal population there. Spanish Influenza in 1918 also had a devastating effect; in some areas it was estimated there was an up to 50 per cent mortality rate among Aboriginal communities.[6] When the Pintupi people moved west into Papunya in the 1960s, there was a high death rate from infectious diseases. Dick Kimber noted that the main causes of death were 'the infections, largely pneumonia or viral (measles) that destroyed more than half the population'.[7]

One hundred years ago, there were still large areas of Australia where the hunter-gatherer lifestyle persisted. This was the case in spite of the remorseless global advance of the farming-society frontiers into Australia, with its associated violence and devastating diseases, and the take-over of the more fertile parts of the continent. Forty years ago, when I started work in the Western Desert, the process was still occurring. Almost all hunter-gatherers had to some extent adapted their lifestyle to a more sedentary life. But not quite all of them.

There were two families still living in the Western Desert as hunter-gatherers: one in Pintupi country and one in Spinifex country. Contact was made with both these families in the 1980s. These contacts were different from most previous episodes. In both these cases, the contact was not between Aboriginal hunter-gatherers and non-Aboriginal settler-colonialists. These contacts were between the hunter-gatherer families and their own relatives returning to their country. I happened to be involved with both these episodes.

The last hunter-gatherers in the Gibson Desert

To the west of Lake Mackay in Western Australia near its eastern border, north of the track between the Kintore Range (where the Kintore community was established in 1981) and the Pollock Hills (where the Kiwirrkurra community was established in 1984), ten people were living: an older man with the skin-name Tjungurrayi, his two wives (both Nangalas) and seven younger people, Tjapaltjarris and Napaltjarris. Tjungurrayi had been known to his peers as a wise man. In the 1960s when Jeremy Long and others were intruding into the Gibson Desert and transporting people into Papunya, Tjungurrayi understood, probably more than others, the implications of succumbing to the attractions of settlement life. He chose, it seems, to stay with his family on their country.

Tjungurrayi died around the time that the reoccupation of the Pintupi country was occurring. In 1984 the nine remaining family members became aware of human activity in the region of Kiwirrkurra. They ventured nearby, remaining hidden, and by observing footprints in the sand realised that the people settling at Kiwirrkurra were relatives they had not seen for twenty years or more. They did not make immediate contact. They were aware of Tjungurrayi's aversion to abandoning their lifestyle, but now there were relatives living back on their country and, with the young people reaching adulthood, the question of marriageable partners was becoming an issue.

In October 1984 two of the Tjapaltjarri brothers made the first approach. An older Pintupi man, Pinta Pinta Tjapananka, and his son Mathew were camping near their newly installed hand pump at Winparku, about 50 kilometres east of Kiwirrkurra when, late in the afternoon, they heard a call. They were approached by the two naked young men and a conversation ensued with Pinta Pinta. The men explained that they belonged to a family group and that the rest of their family were camped further north. Pinta Pinta's son, however, panicked and fired a rifle into the air. The two young men immediately ran off into the desert.

The reaction of Pinta Pinta and Mathew was panic. They drove back to Kiwirrkurra in their car without stopping to fix flat tyres, arriving on the tyre-hubs. They alerted the rest of the community to the fact that the contact had been made. A community meeting was called where it was debated whether or not they should follow the young men to find the family and, by the next morning, the decision had been made. Two Toyotas left Kiwirrkurra and for two days followed, with difficulty, the tracks of the two young men. Eventually the family was found hiding in a hollow between two sandhills.

The reunion between the long-lost relatives was a happy one, but there was still ambivalence about whether the family should leave their desert lifestyle to live in Kiwirrkurra with the other Pintupi people. Eventually, consensus was achieved and the return journey was made into Kiwirrkurra with the newly contacted family. The family consisted of two old women, two young men and a young woman, two teenage girls and two teenage boys.

I met the newly contacted group the day after their arrival in Kiwirrkurra. The good health of the nine people was evident. They were all of slim build, without excess fat, and obviously fit. Before meeting them, I had asked my Aboriginal health worker colleague Tjampu Tjapaltjarri Martin whether it would be appropriate for me to conduct a basic physical examination. He chuckled and said, 'No—they might spear you!' Instead I was introduced to them, and a number of men and women explained my role. Thus I was accepted by them and at the appropriate time I was able to examine them. Within a week, consent was given for blood samples to be taken. When required, we were able to treat their illnesses and provide immunisations.

Based on their own experience of their first exposure to settlement at Haasts Bluff and Papunya not long previously, the Pintupi were aware of the health risks faced by the newcomers. They recognised that staying at Kiwirrkurra allowed some degree of quarantining from the wider world and decided they should limit the number of visitors. The news, however, leaked out about the contact, and a journalist flew in and out and published a story in the print media. The Pintupi people then placed a ban on further media intrusions. There was significant interest from various medical personnel, many of whom wanted to visit, but the Pintupi were quite clear that they wanted their own health team, the Pintupi Homelands Health Service, to take responsibility for their healthcare. I was aware of the high mortality rate of the Pintupi people who had arrived at Papunya twenty years earlier, and of data from the records of newly contacted tribal populations in other parts of the world demonstrating a high mortality rate in the immediate post-contact period, so I was conscious of the fact that this entailed a significant responsibility.

Pressure persisted on the Pintupi to allow both media and external medical teams to visit. The community did agree to allow the Commonwealth Minister for Aboriginal Affairs, Clyde Holding, and the Permanent Secretary of his department, Charlie Perkins, to fly to Kiwirrkurra to meet their newly arrived relatives and to discuss how they were caring for them. Perkins tried to convince the community they should at least allow an Aboriginal media organisation to visit, but the Pintupi were adamant that they would look after their relatives without external intrusion. Perkins also advocated for the government health officials to be allowed to visit, but the community strongly asserted that they employed their own health staff and insisted that the ban on outsiders included people from government health departments. This was a prime example of the importance placed by the Pintupi people on the re-assertion of their autonomy associated with the reoccupation of their country.

One medico who particularly wanted to meet the new arrivals was a respected physician based in Darwin, John Hargraves, who had been involved in an expedition into the Gibson Desert some decades earlier. John had done much good work in Aboriginal health over a long period of time, but his views had not changed from a time when Aboriginal voices were unheeded.

He believed his previous expedition involvement entitled him to return, and that the expressed wish of the Pintupi people to decide for themselves who should provide healthcare was evidence of 'political manipulation'. He used his influence to commandeer a Royal Flying Doctor Service aircraft to fly him from Alice Springs to Kiwirrkurra via Kintore. I was in Kintore when the plane stopped en route; I spoke to John and reiterated to him that the Kiwirrkurra people had said he should not visit, but he said he was going anyway.

On arrival at Kiwirrkurra, John tried to examine the new arrivals but the local community strongly insisted that he was not welcome and forced him back on the aircraft to return to Alice Springs. John subsequently sent a telex to Canberra stating that the nomads were 'mixing in the extremely unhealthy environment of other infected Pintupi at Kiwirrkurra'. This caused concern. Charlie Perkins stated that 'nine people could die within the next two months. So the blood of these people is going to be on the hands of who? It's going to be on the hands of the Minister for Health and the Minister for Aboriginal Affairs and the Central Land Council ... and the so-called independent Kintore health service.' (The 'so-called independent Kintore health service' was in fact that Pintupi Homelands Health Service, funded by his own department.) He went on to say that the new arrivals should be

> protected from their own kinfolks [who] were giving them diseases and deciding what sort of health they should have. It's an infringement of civil liberties. How dare they decide that you can't have a doctor because we don't like government doctors so they just die. They die. That's literally what's going to happen.[8]

Perkins' concerns were genuine, based on advice he was receiving. But the advice was coloured by an implicit belief that uneducated 'traditional' Aboriginal people were not capable of making decisions about the lives of their kinfolk. The Pintupi cared for their relatives and recognised the importance of quarantine, as well as having trust in their own health service. The events demonstrated actual self-determination and autonomous decision-making in practice, but the actions of John Hargraves and the words of Charlie Perkins (both good men who achieved a great deal in Aboriginal affairs) showed that support for genuine self-determination for Aboriginal people in remote parts of Australia was tenuous.

When the suggestion was made that there might be a role for anthropologists, the Pintupi said they would only agree if they could choose the anthropologists. They insisted that the only acceptable anthropologists were Fred Myers and Bette Clarke, both of whom had a long association with the Pintupi. A deal was negotiated between the Central Land Council and the Department of Aboriginal Affairs for Fred and Bette to be flown in from the US to spend some time in Kiwirrkurra and report to government on the implications of the situation.

As I have discussed in chapter 5, we were able to convince the local Alice Springs office of the DAA to provide funds for the short-term hire of a light aircraft to facilitate my travel between Kintore and Kiwirrkurra. Support was also available from the medical staff of the Central Australian Aboriginal Congress, particularly my old friend Trevor Cutter, and advice from the communicable-disease control sections of the Northern Territory and Commonwealth health departments. In this way, informed healthcare was provided by people who everybody at Kiwirrkurra knew and trusted. This healthcare and the health outcomes will be described further below.

The last hunter-gatherers in the Great Victoria Desert

While these events were unfolding in Kiwirrkurra, further south, close to Western Australia's eastern border, another family continued to live as hunter-gatherers. This was in Spinifex country in the Great Victoria Desert.

Sometime in the 1960s a man from Spinifex country walked into Warburton Mission. The mission was on Ngaanyatjarra country, and some tension arose between him and some Ngaanyatjarra men. A violent argument ensued and, fearing retribution, he left with his wife and a young girl for whom they were caring. For the next twenty years they lived as hunter-gatherers in Spinifex country. Three boys were born to the older woman and, when the young girl grew up, she bore a son to the older man. This family occasionally saw evidence of the reoccupation of the Ngaanyatjarra lands, at Papulangkatja and Irrunytju, on the northern fringe of the country on which they lived, but chose to continue to avoid contact. In these communities, there were occasional reports of evidence that there was a family in this area. In 1979 I had been on an expedition into country south-west from Pipalyatjara with some *Anangu*, and we came across what appeared to be a recently used campfire. From time to time, other such reports emerged.

In the 1980s, their relatives from Spinifex country, having moved from Cundeelee to Coonana and to Yakatunya (as explained in chapter 6), were eager to re-establish their traditions on their homelands and had begun to make exploratory trips back into their country. This involved travelling on roads made by Len Beadell during the time of the Maralinga tests—the Anne Beadell Highway and the Connie Sue Highway—and then travelling around and over sandhills to locate significant sites. One particular site associated with the *kipara tjukurrpa* (bush turkey dreaming) proved hard to locate. In September 1986, a group of people travelling in three Toyotas made the journey from Yakatunya into Spinifex country, specifically to locate this site. They travelled along the Anne Beadell Highway, and camped at Ilkurlka. From here the Toyotas drove towards Wyarra Rockhole, hoping to locate the site.

Ian Baird was the only non-Aboriginal person on the trip. He remembers a sudden call of 'Stop! Stop!' Some of the group had noticed signs of recent digging for *maku* (witchetty grubs). The site was examined and an older man, Ian's father-in-law, found some footprints and (with the amazing skills desert Aboriginal people use to identify people from their footprints) announced who had made the prints. It was the man who had left Warburton Mission many years previously. A series of footprints were then found leading north over the sandhills.

Discussion ensued. Should they follow the group to reconnect with them, or should they leave them to their self-imposed exile? Eventually it was decided that one vehicle should follow the tracks and find the family so as to talk, while the rest of the group returned to Ilkurlka. By this stage food and water were running low and had to be rationed. However, there was a sense of wellbeing from being back on their country and potentially reconnecting with long-lost family. In the evening the men went out from the camp to sing the songs of the surrounding country.

In the night the Toyota returned with the long-lost relatives; agreement had been reached between them that re-connection should be established. The next morning, everybody was introduced. The newly arrived group consisted of seven people. The man and wife who had briefly stayed at Warburton twenty years earlier had subsequently had three sons, who were now adolescents. The young girl who had been with the older couple when they left Warburton was now in her twenties, and she had borne a son—fathered by the older man—who was now aged about four years old. Ian recalls how slim and healthy they appeared when he met them that morning, just as I had been struck by the healthy appearance of the newly contacted Pintupi two years previously.

There was a debate about whether they should return to Yakatunya or Coonana and the decision was made that Coonana was preferable, at least initially, as medical help was available there if needed. As in Kiwirrkurra, there was recognition from prior experience that contact could lead to health problems, and it was thought that as soon as possible they should move from Coonana to Yakatunya, where they would be more isolated.

On the drive back to Coonana, the old man of the family learnt about the passing away of a number of relatives since he last had contact with the rest of the Spinifex people. Aggrieved, his response was to spear his informant and then to run away from the group back into the bush. The rest of the group returned to Coonana to allow the newcomers to settle in, while Ian Baird and the middle brother (who adopted the same first name and became Ian Richter)[9] travelled along the Connie Sue Highway to track down the old man. His tracks were found and followed until he was located. Following negotiations the old man agreed to accompany them back to Coonana.

I had just returned from working in a refugee camp in Sudan and was staying in Perth when I read a short item in the *West Australian* newspaper stating that contact had been made with a previously uncontacted group of Aboriginal people in the Great Victoria Desert. I was intrigued, particularly given my experience at Kiwirrkurra two years previously but, this time, I thought, it was not my business.

However, the next day I had a phone call from an officer of the Department of Aboriginal Affairs, who had somehow tracked me down and who asked whether I would be available, given my previous experience in Kiwirrkurra, to travel to Coonana and Yakatunya to prepare a report to help plan for the healthcare of the newly contacted group. I was, of course, interested but sought, and obtained, reassurance that the Spinifex people had given informed consent for my involvement. The next day I was flown to Kalgoorlie from Perth and was met there by Ian Baird, who drove me to Coonana, where I spent a day or so. I then joined a group of Spinifex people and the new arrivals on a drive to Yakatunya, where it was planned that the new family would stay. I camped at Yakatunya for several days. As with the Pintupi family, I was impressed with how fit and healthy the newly contacted Spinifex people appeared. Again, I allowed time after I was introduced to them to develop a rapport before carrying out physical examination and taking blood samples, and to develop a plan for their ongoing healthcare.

Aware of the pressure put on the Pintupi at Kiwirrkurra two years earlier, the Spinifex people were keen to avoid publicity about these events, and the Department of Aboriginal Affairs respected this. This lack of publicity facilitated the reincorporation of the new arrivals with their kin, and also meant that there was less public awareness of the events. The nine people who walked into Kiwirrkurra in 1984 are often referred to as the 'last of the nomads', but in fact they were not quite the last.

Health and healthcare

In the case of both the Pintupi family and the Spinifex family, clinical examination confirmed their good health. Their skin and teeth were in excellent condition. Cardiovascular and respiratory examinations were normal. Blood pressures were low, with systolic pressures between 80 and 100 millimetres of mercury and diastolic pressures between 50 and 70 millimetres of mercury. This was consistent with findings in other hunter-gatherer societies such as Kalahari Bushman. Total cholesterol levels were very low, with total cholesterol levels between 2 and 3.0 mmol per litre. This was even lower than had been found in Kalahari Bushmen, where the average total cholesterol level was 3.1 mmol per litre.[10]

As expected for people living in a small isolated group, antibodies to acute infections such as measles, mumps, rubella, influenza, respiratory syncytial virus, polio and hepatitis A were absent. There were cases of positive hepatitis B serology, and two of these had chronic hepatitis B (hepatitis B surface antigen positive, surface antibody IgM and IgG negative). There is evidence that hepatitis B has been endemic in Australian Aboriginal people since the first arrival around 60,000 years ago.[11] The finding of positive hepatitis B serology in the new arrivals appears to support this.

There were also some cases of positive treponemal serology (positive RPR and TPHA), which is usually an indicator of syphilis infection. In these cases, positive serology was very likely due to yaws, a treponemal infection unrelated to syphilis, which is spread by direct contact rather than sexual contact. It was known to be endemic in Aboriginal societies in the early contact period, and probably preceded European contact.

In 1964 a combined West Australian health department and Native Welfare expedition had travelled through the Gibson Desert and examined a number of Pintupi people from this region. They found that twenty-seven out of thirty-four people tested had positive Wasserman reactions (an earlier treponemal serology test). Seven of these cases had signs attributable to yaws and there was no clinical evidence of syphilis.[12] In the new arrivals in 1984 and 1986 there was no clinical evidence of either syphilis or yaws. While I attributed the positive serology to yaws, as both syphilis and yaws are susceptible to penicillin, the treatment given would have been effective for both.

The finding of hepatitis B and yaws in these groups suggests that (in contrast to most diseases prevalent in Aboriginal communities today) these were chronic diseases that existed in Aboriginal society prior to European contact. The impact of settler colonialism cannot be totally ruled out, however. The older members of the Spinifex family had had brief contact with the people living at Warburton Mission, and while the Pintupi family had not left their country, there had been some travel by foot of Pintupi people back and forth into their country in the early contact days. It is conceivable, but unlikely, that these infectious diseases could have been transmitted on these occasions.

There were some positive chlamydia serology results, probably due to the causative organism of trachoma. There were two cases of slight scarring of the upper eyelids that would probably be attributable to previous trachoma infection, but there was no evidence of the repeated intense infections that in previous years had led to blindness in Aboriginal people living in more crowded conditions.

There was serological evidence of past exposure to some other infections including cytomegalovirus, herpes virus, and Australian encephalitis (a mosquito-borne virus) but these appeared to have no clinical significance. All subjects had negative Mantoux tests, showing that none were infected with tuberculosis.

About one week after contact, exposure to the pool of infection existing in the community led to many of the new arrivals developing muco-purulent conjunctivitis, which responded to tetracycline eye-drops. A few days later, most developed a cough with a mild fever and signs of an upper respiratory tract infection. On the advice of an infectious disease specialist, all were placed on a course of a broad-spectrum antibiotic, co-trimoxazole, for five days. They were then placed on 250 mg of prophylactic penicillin orally twice daily for one month (unless substituted by a course of co-trimoxazole for intercurrent infection). After a month or so, all patients were given an intramuscular course of long acting benzathine penicillin as treatment for the treponemal infection, as well as prophylactic antibiotic cover. They continued to have chronic upper respiratory infections, with thick nasal discharge and coughs, but no clinical evidence of lower respiratory infections. Three patients had episodes of acute otitis media with inflamed bulging eardrums, which responded to co-trimoxazole.

Immunisation was provided against polio with Sabin oral vaccine, measles and mumps and pneumococcus. All subjects were given an intramuscular injection of human immunoglobulin. In my notes, I have no record of administering influenza vaccine, but it was available for purchase in the mid-1980s and I assume it was given.

In both cases the healthcare plan appeared to be successful in that none of the newly contacted people succumbed to serious infections. Over time, they settled into life in their remote Aboriginal communities. Their experience differed from their relatives around twenty years earlier, when many Pintupi and Spinifex people died following contact. There are a few reasons for the better outcomes.

Kiwirrkurra was different from what Papunya had been like when people had migrated there from Pintupi country twenty or thirty years earlier. Similarly, Yakatunya was different from Cundeelee in the 1950s and 60s. The newly arrived families had been 'found' by their own relatives, and they arrived to a relatively small community of their own people; this remoteness provided a form of quarantine. Moreover, they were still on or close to their own country so did not suffer from the spiritual malaise that had occurred when Aboriginal people had been removed from their land. On the contrary, there was a degree of spiritual reinvigoration. After re-establishing contact there was an exchange of spiritual law and experience that reinforced rather than denigrated their cultural heritage. The Richter family at Yakatunya were found when their relatives were searching for the elusive *kipara tjukurrpa* site and the search was abandoned when contact with the family was made. However, on the next trip into Spinifex country from Yalatunya, the old Mr Richter was able to take his countrymen directly to the site.

In the case of the Pintupi people, they had their own health service, including medical staff who lived with the people and who had some knowledge of the language. This meant that medical care was readily available in an acceptable form. The Aboriginal health workers at Kiwirrkurra had known the five older subjects when they were children before white contact. This meant that they were an indispensable part of the medical team, overseeing the provision of medications, providing daily reports and ensuring rapid management of illness. Doctor George, the *ngangkari*, also worked with the medical team and provided a bridge between the two systems of healthcare.

The healthcare was not just a one-way process. In particular, the two men aged in their twenties in the Pintupi family were themselves credited with having highly developed spiritual healing powers and they were regularly sought out for treatment of illness. All members of the group had a warm friendliness, a sense of humour and a social cohesiveness that had made getting to know them an enriching experience for both their relatives and the non-Aboriginal medical staff.

The new arrivals from Pintupi country and Spinifex country were also fortunate to have made contact at a time when there was government support for self-determination—even if, as I have suggested, this could be tenuous. It was communities asserting their autonomy that led to contact being made among their own people; the steps taken by the communities to protect them were good examples of self-determination in action.

Unfortunately, as we shall see in the following chapters, support for self-determination was not to last. As such, what follows will differ in presentation from the previous chapters. We will now look at government responses to the social movements I have been describing through my experiences in the Western Desert: the homelands movement and the Aboriginal community-controlled health movement.

8

The reoccupation of the Western Desert and the counter-attack

Homelands or outstations?

The Western Desert was one of the last areas within Australia to be affected by the steady advance of settler colonialism and, on a longer time-scale and globally, by the destructive impact of the Agricultural and Industrial revolutions on hunter-gatherer lifestyles. By the 1950s and 60s, however, colonialism had caught up with people in the Western Desert. By then, various pressures on most desert dwellers resulted in them living in missions, settlements or pastoral properties, generally leading to a more sedentary existence compared to their previous lifestyle. In 1974 the anthropologist Robert Tonkinson reported that

> Today almost all Western Desert Aborigines are congregated in fringe settlements or even further afield in small towns. Although physically separated from their desert homelands, most maintain close spiritual ties with their birthplace and earlier life.

Indeed, the connection with country was never completely extinguished and most of those in the fringe settlements probably did not consider that the separation from the homelands was permanent. Within two decades of Tonkinson's report many parts of the Western Desert had been reoccupied. We have seen in earlier chapters how the Pitjantjatjara and Ngaanyatjarra people moved out of the missions and settlements of Ernabella, Amata and

Warburton to reoccupy their country; how the *Martu*, with the help of the Strelley mob, moved back to their country in the Great Sandy Desert; how Pintupi people moved westward from the government settlements of Papunya and Haasts Bluff to re-establish themselves in their country in the Gibson Desert; and how the Spinifex people moved back to their country in the Great Victoria Desert. Their stories are all part of the story of the reoccupation of the Western Desert.

The 'homelands movement' is often dated from the election of the Whitlam Labor government in 1972.[1] In many areas, however, the officially recognised movement was a continuation of ongoing efforts to maintain contact with and care for country.

In the early 1970s the well-established government policy of assimilation (which for Aboriginal people living in remote areas had led to the establishment of large settlements and missions) was coming under challenge. The 1967 referendum had drawn the attention of the wider Australian public to the question of rights for Aboriginal people, and a new assertion and calls for self-determination were emerging among Aboriginal activists, exemplified by the establishment of the Aboriginal Tent Embassy on the grounds of Parliament House in Canberra in 1972. Around the same time, land-rights struggles, such as the efforts of the Yolngu of Yirrkala to stop a bauxite mine in their land, as well as the Gurindji cattle-station strike, received national attention.

An influential figure at this time was the economist and advisor to successive governments, H.C. ('Nugget') Coombs. As the chair of the Council of Aboriginal Affairs, he took a close interest in Aboriginal issues and travelled extensively to Aboriginal communities across Australia, including in remote areas where he observed the decentralisation movement then taking place. His advocacy and support for this movement led to a greater recognition of the aspiration for people to establish themselves on their homelands.[2] As a result, the Australian Government started to provide support to assist with the process.

At that time, this was often referred to as the 'outstation movement' and the resulting communities were often referred to as outstations. Over time, the term 'homelands' became more acceptable, although there was some resistance to this term for its the connotation with apartheid in South

Africa, where the Bantustans, or areas set aside for black South Africans under limited and discriminatory self-government, were also referred to as 'homelands'. In remote Aboriginal Australia, however the term 'outstation' implied an ongoing dependence on the central community, whereas the term 'homeland' recognised that people were moving home.

What is not always appreciated is that these communities are not all the same, and some are perhaps more like outstations than homelands. In many areas, people moved out from a large Aboriginal community that may have been a mission or a government settlement and established smaller communities on the country to which they had traditional affiliations. Often they retained a link with the larger community, spending significant amounts of time there. This was particularly true in the tropical north of Australia (for example, in Arnhem Land) and, to some extent, in desert regions. For example, the Western Arrernte people established homeland communities in the country around Ntaria, where the original Hermannsburg Mission was located and which became the site of an outstation resource centre to support the smaller communities. These smaller communities can legitimately be called outstations, but most of the communities we have discussed in the preceding chapters are better thought of as homelands communities.

A recent book on the history of this social movement uses the term 'outstations' to apply to all communities that arose from this decentralising movement. The editors define outstations as follows:

> Outstations are small, decentralised and relatively permanent communities of kin established by Aboriginal people on land that has social, cultural or economic significance to them. Generally speaking, the majority of them have fewer than forty people.[3]

They note that the term 'outstation' comes from the cattle industry where, on the Australian outback's vast cattle properties, an outstation was a small homestead more than a day's ride from the main homestead and which clearly maintained a link to the main homestead. Where Aboriginal outstations retain a link with the hub community, the term 'outstation' seems appropriate. However, in the Western Desert the people with whom I worked were generally explicitly separating themselves from the larger communities where they had been living to form communities that usually had a hundred or more inhabitants.

The Pitjantjatjara people who moved to the homelands communities west of Amata were re-establishing themselves on their own country and, although they retained family and cultural links with the people who remained at Ernabella, this community was not positioned as a resource centre. There were closer linkages with Amata, but I believe many Pitjantjatjara people saw the establishment of Amata in 1961 as merely a stepping-stone for the reoccupation of their own country. The Ngaanyatjarra people who moved out of Warburton Mission also saw themselves as creating new communities on their traditional homelands, not outstations of Warburton.

The *Martu* who moved to Punmu (originally Panaka Panaka) and Kunawarritji, and later Parrngurr, made strategic decisions about how they would reoccupy their homelands, which involved making a clean break from Jigalong. Having left Jigalong, they threw in their lot with the Strelley mob, for reasons discussed in chapter 4, which provided them with the assistance they needed to achieve their long-term aim of reoccupation. Ultimately, their desire for autonomy led to a decisive break from the Strelley mob. They did not see themselves as an outstation of any other community, although they did later re-establish links with Jigalong and the Strelley mob.

The term 'outstation' is perhaps even more inappropriate in the cases of the Pintupi and the Spinifex people. The Pintupi explicitly broke away from Papunya and Haasts Bluff. When I lived in Kintore in 1984 and 1985, not long after the original move westward, the Northern Territory government still categorised Kintore as an outstation of Papunya, meaning that most government funding for community facilities went to the Papunya Council. In an effort to obtain government support for the Pintupi moves westwards, the accepted terminology of 'outstation' was pragmatically followed. Once in Kintore, however, the Pintupi argued forcefully for recognition as an autonomous community: a struggle that they eventually won. They regarded Kintore as their homeland community rather than an outstation—and in fact originally envisaged Kintore as being a hub centre for a number of smaller communities that could have perhaps been called outstations. Their attitude to the idea of Kintore itself being an outstation was exemplified when I was again there in 2012, not long after the Northern Territory government had amalgamated community councils into larger regional shires. Kintore had become part of the MacDonnell Shire (later renamed the MacDonnell Regional Council). When I commented on the somewhat neglected state of the roads around Kintore, my Pintupi friend said, 'We don't have any say any more. Kintore is just an outstation again.'

The Spinifex people in Tjuntjuntjara definitely do not see themselves as living on an outstation. They were moved from Cundeelee to Coonana, and from Coonana they moved to Tjuntjuntjara, leaving behind not a hub community but empty communities: they moved back to their homeland *en masse* and left Coonana for good.

The distinction I make between homelands communities, like those in the Western Desert, and outstations, as smaller communities around a larger hub community, has policy implications. There is a tendency among policy-makers in capital cities to conflate these two categories, wrongly assuming that all such communities are outstations with a 'hub' community. When consideration is given to withdrawing financial support for communities in very remote parts of Australia, there can be insufficient appreciation of the much greater adverse impact on homelands communities without a hub community to which the people may migrate.

The size of Western Desert homeland communities

The communities that arose as a result of the reoccupation of the Western Desert did, in some cases, have small communities nearby that would be more consistent with Myers' and Peterson's definition of outstations, but in many cases these have not been sustained. When I worked for the Pitjantjatjara Homelands Health Service in 1978 to 1981, there were a number of small communities at various sites including Kunamata, Aparatjara, Nyapari, Kanypi, Puta Puta, Kunytjanu, Kata Ala (later Murray Bore), Walypa Pulka and Linton Bore. These small family-based sites were occupied intermittently (some more than others) and used the closest homeland community for shopping and socialising. With the exception of Kanypi and Nyapari, which have been amalgamated into Murputja community, these small communities no longer exist. Since then, some other small communities have come and gone, and some have emerged and remained, such as Patjarr, Tjirrkarli, Warnan and Tjukurrla in Western Australia.

When I lived in Kintore in 1984 and 1985, the Pintupi envisaged it as becoming the hub for a number of smaller family-based communities, such as Muyin, Ininti, Pirnpirr and Nyutjul, which were intermittently occupied for several years, and the Pintupi Homelands Health Service made an effort to support people living in these small communities by providing regular clinic visits. Ultimately, however, for various reasons the people associated with these outstations were absorbed back into the Kintore community. The establishment of Kiwirrkurra in 1985 was more permanent; this involved a larger group of people moving west from Kintore to settle in a community of over 100 people.

The Spinifex people also had plans to extend their reoccupation beyond Tjuntjuntjara. They intended to go deeper into the heart of Spinifex country to Ilkurlka, Tawun, Tjintirrkara and Miramirratjara. However, with the development of facilities at Tjuntjuntjara, and with access to the important sites throughout their country, the *Anangu* were satisfied that this would be their residential base.

There are a number of reasons why these smaller communities either did not persist or did not get established. In some cases, the site chosen had particular significance for an elder; when that elder died it became culturally inappropriate for other people to stay there. The logistical challenges of ensuring access to services, particularly stores, education and health, meant there was a natural tendency for people to stay in communities where these services were available.

Yet another reason was the sociability of Western Desert people: in general, people preferred the company of their peers rather than being dispersed into family groupings. This is not to suggest that the homelands movement was unsuccessful. The reoccupation of the Western Desert, with the dispersal of people from large settlements, was a success. People were back on their country but only a certain degree of dispersion worked well.

It seems that an equilibrium was generally achieved when people lived in communities that were large enough to allow the services and socialisation required but small enough to minimise the interpersonal conflict common in larger settlements.

Most desert homelands communities appeared to stabilise with a population of between 100 and 200 people. The mean average of population estimates for the seventeen currently inhabited homeland communities in the four Western Desert regions I have discussed—the Pitjantjatjara and Ngaanyatjarra homelands, *Martu* country, Pintupi country and Spinifex country—is 135, with a median average of 149. Only one community (Patjarr) has a population below 50; five communities (Kunawarritji, Tjirrkarli, Tjukurla, Kalka and Murputja) have a population between 50 and 100; nine (Pipalyatjara, Marntamaru, Papulankatja, Irrunytju, Warakurna, Warnan, Punmu, Parngurr and Tjuntjuntjara) have a population between 100 and 200; and two (Kiwirrkurra and Kintore) have a population greater than 200.

It is interesting to note that the British evolutionary anthropologist Robin Dunbar, using rigorous scientific methodology, has posited that 150 is the ideal group size for humankind, being the number of individuals with whom one can maintain continuous personal interaction. This has been the size of co-resident groups throughout much of human history.[4] The equilibrium achieved by Western Desert Aboriginal people in the size of their homeland communities seems consistent with this finding.

One place where people did manage to live in smaller, more dispersed communities was not in the Western Desert. In Utopia, as discussed in chapter 1, the traditional owners had a history of living in small groups, and with the support of their own health organisation were able to resist government pressure to centralise. This experience in cattle station country, however, was different from that in the Western Desert.

The move to homelands was always associated with an aspiration for autonomy, which people generally found was increased when they lived in small communities, with the average size of 150 people, on their own country. Sometimes this aspiration led to tensions and fissions within groups after reoccupation.[5] A number of examples of this tendency towards disaggregation has been discussed in the earlier chapters. Ampilatwatja Health

Clinic separated from Urapuntja Health Service in the Utopia area. The Pitjantjatjara Homelands Health Service split to become the Ngaanyatjarra Health Service and the Pitjantjatjara Homelands Health Service, which in turn was eventually absorbed into Nganampa Health Council. The *Martu* at Panaka Panaka (Punmu) and Kunawarritji split away from the Strelley mob. Similarly, in Pintupi country, Kiwirrkurra split from Kintore, and the community administration became part of Ngaanyatjarra Council and the health service needs were met by the Ngaanyatjarra Health Service. In the Great Victoria Desert in South Australia, Oak Valley separated from Yalata so that both the Oak Valley community administration and its health service became new entities. The disaggregating tendency should be seen as a continuation of the aspiration for autonomy that initially motivated the homelands movement.

Health benefits of the homelands movement

A number of the early commentators on the homelands movement have emphasised the social and health benefits of the movement.[6] In 1976 Rod Morice, a senior registrar in psychiatry at Alice Springs Hospital who had developed a relationship with Pintupi people, wrote an article in the *Medical Journal of Australia* about the psycho-social benefits he had observed at the Pintupi outstation of Kungkayunti. He claimed that living in a small, homogenous community in distinct family groups, with no access to alcohol, led to social cohesion and a reintegration of individual and group identity, which he contrasted with the cultural disintegration among the Pintupi he had previously witnessed at Papunya. Jim Downing, a social worker and Uniting Church minister with strong links to the Pitjantjatjara and Ngaanyatjarra people in the 1970s and 80s, noted the following outcomes of the homelands movement: a return to Aboriginal decision-making and control and to a more Aboriginal and unified lifestyle; a strengthening of family and family authority; a recovery of individual and group identity and a growth in confidence; a recovery of useful roles and involvement in the work of the community; an observable improvement in social and general health; and more interest in education with a desire to have control over what their children are taught and to see that they are educated in their own culture. An incidental benefit noted by Downing was that the homelands movement eased pressure on the larger communities from which people were migrating.

The emergence of the counter-narrative

For about a quarter of a century, from the time of the Whitlam government in the early 1970s until the closing years of the twentieth century, these potential benefits of the homelands movement received widespread acceptance and support. In the 1990s, however, a new public narrative emerged. The dysfunctional nature of remote Aboriginal communities was increasingly emphasised and this was often attributed to the homelands movement.

Some of the early critics were associated with two Australian think tanks, the Institute of Public Affairs (IPA) based in Melbourne, and the Centre for Independent Studies (CIS) based in Sydney. Both these think tanks were powerful advocates for a neoliberal approach to political and economic policies, with an emphasis on free markets, deregulation and privatisation.[7] In the neoliberal reconstruction of Aboriginal policy, there was a reassertion of the 'Aboriginal problem' as one of dysfunction, lack of capacity and material disadvantage with a decreased respect for Aboriginal autonomy and increased state intrusion into Aboriginal lives.

Between 2000 and 2004 the IPA published thirty-three articles on Aboriginal affairs, many of them by a former minister in the Keating Labor government, Gary Johns; he was a senior fellow at the IPA from 1997 to 2006. After his departure from the IPA, Johns advocated his perspective on Aboriginal affairs at the Bennelong Society, which had been formed in Melbourne in 2000 by Peter Howson, formerly Minister for Aboriginal Affairs in the McMahon Coalition government and a long-term advocate of assimilation. Its ostensible purpose was to promote debate and analysis of Aboriginal policy in Australia.

The Centre for Independent Studies developed an Indigenous Affairs Research Program in 2005, and published a number of monographs, as well as articles in Murdoch-owned newspapers. An early monograph published in 2005, entitled *A New Deal for Aborigines and Torres Strait Islanders in*

Remote Communities, was co-authored by Helen Hughes, an economist and senior fellow at the CIS (who had previously worked in the Pacific and had no previous experience in Indigenous issues), and Jenness Warin, a nurse who had worked in a number of Aboriginal communities and was a visiting fellow at the CIS. At the time of the monograph's release, Hughes authored an op-ed in Murdoch's flagship newspaper *The Australian*. Sympathetic coverage was given in the same newspaper with an editorial referring to it as a 'seminal article'.

Neoliberal critics of remote Aboriginal communities such as Helen Hughes and Gary Johns frequently referred to the economist and public servant 'Nugget' Coombs as the architect of the homelands movement. They suggested that the movement was a 'socialist Coombsian experiment' in which the Aboriginal people had no agency—an account utterly at odds with my experience of the homelands movement. Neither Hughes nor Johns appeared to have a high regard for Aboriginal capacity to initiate the homelands movements. Alternatively, perhaps, they thought if they could portray Aboriginal people as passive victims of an engineered migration to the homelands, their proposed solution of a forced migration in the other direction may be more acceptable. Tim Rowse, the biographer of Coombs, has said of Hughes's 'odd fixation with Coombs':

> She attributes to Coombs extraordinary executive powers. In fact, Coombs' admiring account (in 1973) of Aborigines' decentralizing movement from settlements and missions to outstations was his response to Indigenous initiatives. In seeking to understand their actions sympathetically, he did not have to move the people about whom he was writing. They were capable of moving themselves.[8]

He also suggested that Hughes was 'not encumbered by evidence'.[9]

Hughes proposed moving people from homelands communities in to larger 'core communities'. Gary Johns went even further in proposing a 'migratory solution', moving people out of remote communities to regional or major cities where they can get work and contribute to the mainstream economy. The theme of the 2006 annual Bennelong Society conference was

'Leaving remote communities'. According to Johns (the Society's president at the time), 'Aborigines living in remote areas are worse off than their compatriots in town and they should therefore be encouraged to leave in search of better opportunities.' In his opening address to the Bennelong Society conference he stated that

> The challenge for government is to stop funding programs that militate against the migratory solution ... The government has begun to stop supporting a recreational lifestyle in the name of preserving a culture. The extent to which aborigines from remote regions will be more akin to refugees and migrants will be a measure of the difficulty of their adjustment to new circumstances ... Fortunately Australia has vast experience of dealing with both.

Commentators such as Johns and Hughes were informed more by prejudicial assumptions than by facts, but their views were given added support by an increasing recognition that all was not well in remote Aboriginal communities. At the turn of the century the Aboriginal lawyer and activist Noel Pearson published *Our Right to Take Responsibility*. He lamented the culture of welfare dependency and addiction in Aboriginal communities, which he blamed on flawed and inappropriate social-welfare policies. His criticism of government welfare policies over the past thirty years was enthusiastically received by neoliberal critics and Pearson became a regular commentator in *The Australian*—a paper that strongly advocates the neoliberal perspective on Aboriginal affairs. (Later Pearson would come to express his regret at the degree of trust he had placed in the conservative side of politics.)[10]

Pearson was critical of the 'progressive left' for placing too much emphasis on the historical causes of Indigenous disadvantage, such as dispossession and racism, which he suggested were inadequate for formulating credible strategies to deal with the current crisis. A selective reading of Pearson's critique led many commentators and government personnel to ascribe the problem in remote communities entirely to cultural and behavioural factors rather than structural inequalities. However, although Pearson emphasised the debilitating effect of passive welfare and the permissive approach to alcohol and other drugs as a fundamental issue demanding immediate action, he did not deny the negative impact of structural influences.

Like Pearson, the anthropologist Peter Sutton criticised the 'liberal consensus', which he claimed had allowed the dysfunction in remote communities to fester. Unlike Pearson, he was willing to lay blame on traditional Aboriginal practices. In his book *The Politics of Suffering: Indigenous Australia and the end of the liberal consensus* published in 2009, Sutton suggested a mismatch between traditional Aboriginal culture and the demands of the wider culture in which contemporary Aboriginal communities are embedded. Sutton accused his fellow anthropologists of wilfully ignoring the violence and suffering in remote Aboriginal communities, leading to soul-searching and debate in the Australian anthropological community. It has also led to the publication of a book of essays edited by Jon Altman and Melinda Hinkson entitled *Culture Crisis: Anthropology and politics in Aboriginal Australia*. Jon Altman, an anthropologist and economist, was the Director of the Centre for Aboriginal Economic and Policy Research at the Australian National University and one of the few voices to publicly defend the homelands movement at this time.

The anthropological critique of the homelands movement was based on more rigorous scholarship and understanding than that of the neoliberal critics such as Johns and Hughes. Peter Sutton had a long association with communities on Cape York since going there as a young anthropologist in the early seventies, and it was his observation of the decline of these communities into severe dysfunction that motivated his writing. In arguing that traditional culture is unsuitable for the contemporary context, he suggested that many Aboriginal affairs policies had ignored the extent to which Aboriginal cultural norms contribute to current problems.[11] This, he suggested, included 'a blindness to the part now played by traditional medical beliefs and practices in blocking certain preventative and curative health measures'. He accused traditional healers of opposing surgery, blood transfusions, injections and rehydration treatment.[12] From my own experience (admittedly in communities different from those where Sutton has mostly worked) traditional healers, *ngangkaris*, were willing to work alongside western medicine without either system interfering with the other.

I have not encountered the opposition to western medical practices that Sutton describes. As many Aboriginal people with an illness express a desire for both medical systems, my experience has been that access to both is often beneficial to recovery from illness. Sutton suggested that the poor health of Aboriginal people is testament to the inefficacy of traditional healing; but of course the same comment could be made about the western medicine used by the same Aboriginal people.

In identifying cultural practices as part of the problem, Sutton de-emphasised the importance of retaining links to country, language and culture. In the same year that Sutton's book appeared, Noel Pearson published an essay arguing that Australian governments had not been sufficiently supportive of Aboriginal peoples' rights to preservation of culture and identity.[13] Pearson expressed the belief that cultural and linguistic continuity must be promoted alongside socio-economic enhancement, and that both these aims require government support. His vision included 'the restoration of culturally and economically sustainable Indigenous homelands'. As he pointed out, the current government was not doing anywhere near enough to support Aboriginal cultural transmission. Pearson recognised the challenges to his vision for a bi-cultural future. It would require, he said 'a significant change of attitude in Aboriginal people, Australian governments and the wider Australian people'.

There was little evidence of the attitudinal change that Pearson called for in government circles. Instead, the numerous, seemingly intractable, problems of remote communities identified by critics such as Pearson, Sutton and others helped to buttress arguments expressed in publications of the IPA, the Bennelong Society and the CIS, and in editorials and opinion pieces in *The Australian* newspaper, that self-determination in remote communities was a failure. The close links between these think tanks and government meant they had a significant influence on policy.

The Northern Territory Intervention

In 2007 the *'Little Children are Sacred': Report of the Northern Territory Board of Enquiry into the Protection of Aboriginal Children from Sexual Abuse* was released. It highlighted problems confronting remote Aboriginal communities in the Northern Territory, including high rates of alcohol abuse and children at risk of sexual abuse. Following this, in June 2007, Prime Minister John Howard announced a 'Northern Territory National Emergency Response' (NTNER), in response to what he described as a 'National Emergency'. The NTNER is usually referred to as the Northern Territory Intervention.

Not long before the Intervention was announced, Helen Hughes published a book on remote Aboriginal communities entitled *Lands of Shame*, which included a number of recommendations. Prior to publication in February, Hughes wrote to the head of the Office of Indigenous Policy Co-ordination in the Australian Government, saying

> I have been defending the Commonwealth Government's Indigenous agenda as the first ever to treat Aborigines and Torres Strait Islanders as Australians. I have given the draft of the book dealing with this theme of homelands to … your department before it is published as I want to ensure that it is supportive of what [Minister for Indigenous Affairs] Mr. Brough is trying to do. I think that the book will attract favourable attention to Commonwealth policies.[14]

Within a few months, most of Hughes's recommendations were implemented as part of the Northern Territory Intervention, while the specific recommendations of the *'Little Children are Sacred'* report were ignored. The similarity between the Intervention measures and what Hughes had proposed in her book was remarkable. Tim Rowse has pointed out many of the contradictions in Hughes's work, and expressed concern about the influence that she wielded on government policy:

> Hughes' critical vagueness about what she is proposing may also be a reason for the vacuum in the social and economic planning of the Australian government (whether Labor or Coalition). *Lands of Shame* may also be a guide not only to the 'philosophy' but also to the intellectual vacuity of Australia's current political elites.[15]

The Intervention was a major milestone in the history of the Australian Government's policies affecting remote Aboriginal communities and was an indication of how much had changed since the Howard government came to power eleven years earlier. It ushered in a new coercive phase of neoliberal Aboriginal policy. Some of the measures included in the Intervention, such as increased policing, were welcomed and in fact reflected long-held community aspirations. Other measures were inappropriate and ill-conceived, often having nothing to do with the ostensible reason for the Intervention. Some critics of the Intervention suggested that the child health checks, at least, were worthy of support. I dispute even this. Most children in remote communities in the Northern Territory had received numerous checks and many had already had repeated hospital admissions. What was needed was a sustainable investment in comprehensive primary healthcare, not more health checks.

The basic problem with the Intervention was the way it was imposed. Melinda Hinkson has argued that,

> at the heart of the government's coercive approach lies a clear intent: to bring to an end the recognition of, and support for, Aboriginal people living in remote communities pursuing culturally distinctive ways of life ... the NT Intervention is aimed at nothing short of the production of a newly oriented, 'normalized' Aboriginal population, one whose concerns with custom, kin and land will give way to the individualistic aspirations of private home ownership, career and self-improvement.[16]

The Aboriginal legal academic Larissa Behrendt saw the Northern Territory Intervention as 'a textbook example of why government policies continue to fail Aboriginal people: the policy approach is ideologically driven rather than making reference to the considerable research on what actually works on the ground'.[17] John Sanderson, a former Chief of the Australian Army and Governor of Western Australia, challenged the neoliberal ideology underpinning the Intervention and stated that, in the Intervention:

> little recognition is given to the much studied and widely understood deleterious effect on physical and mental health of cultural and social

disempowerment. Such an assimilationist approach is most unlikely to work, because it is once again inflicted on Indigenous people rather than generated by them. It is founded on an ideology that may eventually be hotly contested at its source anyway.[18]

In *Lands of Shame* Hughes had made a recommendation for the movement of people from smaller communities into 'core centres'. While this wasn't a stated policy of the Intervention per se, the relocation of people was attempted later by both the Australian and Northern Territory governments. In March 2009 the federal Labor government announced that twenty-nine 'priority remote communities' across the country would be singled out as the only recipients of new development funding, including all new housing projects. Two months later the Northern Territory government announced a 'growth towns' policy, where twenty communities were identified for economic development at the expense of all other remote communities. These policies were clearly aimed at reversing the homelands movement in the hope that people would gravitate to the more privileged and better-resourced communities. Over subsequent years, as so often happens in Indigenous affairs, these policies seem to have been quietly dropped, not because of any change in approach or even because the obvious hardships created by the policies were becoming apparent, but mainly because the predicted migration from other communities to the core centres did not eventuate. The Northern Territory government has, however, amalgamated remote-community councils into regional 'shires' (later re-named regional councils). The policy has effectively removed opportunities for local decision-making through community councils.

Employment and welfare

In the early 2000s the Howard government introduced a number of changes to the mainstream welfare system, which were designed to reduce dependence and to move more people into the labour market. There were also changes made to a specifically Aboriginal program, the Community Development Employment Program (CDEP), which has for many years provided a source of employment and income for Aboriginal people in a variety of settings. The

CDEP was established in 1977, initially in remote communities; during the 1980s and 1990s it was expanded to also provide employment opportunities for Aboriginal people in urban areas. By 2003, 35,000 Aboriginal and Torres Strait Islander people across Australia were employed under the CDEP.

As originally envisaged, the CDEP was a job-creation scheme developed as an alternative to welfare payments. The amount of social-welfare money that would have been available to individual residents in a community was bundled together into a community grant with an added amount as an administrative component to allow a community council to provide local employment for community development projects. Although the scheme had its problems and worked better in some places than others, it was generally well received by Aboriginal people and there were some notable success stories.[19]

By the early 2000s, however, critics including Noel Pearson and neoliberal think-tank commentators were claiming that CDEP was just another form of welfare and that Aboriginal people should be transitioned into the 'real economy'. Helen Hughes called for the outright abolition of CDEP and it was included as a goal of the Northern Territory Intervention. The CDEP was initially wound back in urban areas and in 2014, the Abbott government abolished it altogether. The replacement in remote communities was the Remote Jobs and Communities Program, later changed to the Community Development Program (CDP). The title and acronym was conceivably meant to give an impression to its Aboriginal recipients that it was another form of CDEP but, as the recipients were quite aware, there were significant differences.

CDP is administered by Centrelink, the Australian Government's social-services agency, and delivered by contracted 'providers'. The local autonomy and authority that was a cornerstone of CDEP was removed. Recipients of CDP are required to work five hours per day, five days per week, forty-six weeks per year, in exchange for income-support payments well below the legal minimum wage. The obligations on recipients are more onerous than any other form of social security available to non-Aboriginal Australians, and income penalties (called 'breaching') for non-attendance at appointments and activities are increasingly common, leading to significant financial hardship in remote communities.

Using data from the 2016 Census, Markham and Biddle have shown that from 2011 to 2016, median disposable income for Indigenous people in urban areas rose by $57 per week per person, but over the same period in very remote areas income fell by $12 per person and the Indigenous cash poverty rate increased from 46.9 per cent in 2011 to 53.4 per cent in 2016. Jon Altman has suggested that the CDP contravenes the International Labour Organization's Forced Labour Convention, making it a form of involuntary servitude or slavery, because if people do not present for work or exercise their basic human right to withdraw their labour they are punished with financial penalties.[20] If the Northern Territory Intervention represented a move toward a coercive phase of neoliberal Aboriginal policy, the introduction of CDP could be considered the rise of a punitive phase.

The impoverishment of remote communities caused by the CDP is also contributing to depopulation as some people move to regional centres after they have had other sources of income stopped. This does not mean, however, that movement out of remote communities leads to greater employment opportunities. Nicholas Biddle has shown that Aboriginal people who move to urban areas do not do as well in the labour market as those who already live there and may even do worse than those who stay in remote areas.[21] At an area level, migration from remote communities was associated with a significant and substantial decline in the percentage of the population employed in the destination area. Too often, the move to regional or metropolitan centres leads not to employment and improved livelihood but involvement with alcohol and other drugs and an increase in incarceration, morbidity and mortality.

Despite the evidence of economic hardship it has created in remote communities, the Department of Prime Minister and Cabinet, which oversees the program, maintains that the 'CDP is working'. Whether it is working or not depends on the policy outcome desired. It is not creating more employment, nor improving Aboriginal livelihoods, nor improving the viability of remote Aboriginal communities. It could be argued that if the desired policy outcome is to achieve out-migration from remote communities so that the communities can be eventually closed down, the policy is a success.

Undoubtedly, there are problems such as violence, substance abuse, sexual abuse and poor health in remote Aboriginal communities. There are also challenges in community governance, as well as a sense of social *ennui* or hopelessness about the future, particularly in young people. However, there are some common errors in public-policy discourse that should be corrected. Firstly, I believe the problems of remote communities are not limited to remote communities but should be seen as a reflection of a level of disadvantage common to Aboriginal people in all geographic areas of Australia. Secondly, I do not believe that the homelands movement was the cause of the problems in remote communities; rather, it should be seen as an ongoing part of the solution. Thirdly, the claims of economic non-viability of remote homelands communities should be challenged.

Aboriginal disadvantage is not confined to the homelands

There is a frequent assertion that Aboriginal disadvantage is largely confined to remote communities. The Centre for Independent Studies has a long history of producing misleading claims along these lines. For example, in a 2017 article, Jeremy Sammut stated:

> Nowadays, 80% of Indigenous people who mostly live in metropolitan Australia have the same social outcomes as their non-Indigenous peers. As I have shown in [a previous article] these Indigenous Australians enjoy the full freedoms and opportunities of the Australian Dream as all other Australians regardless of race. The remaining 20% of most disadvantaged Indigenous Australians with appalling social outcomes are excluded from the Australian Dream not due to racism, but due to the continuation of the failed separatist experiments in 'Aboriginal Self-Determination' in rural and remote Indigenous communities.[22]

What Sammut claims to have shown in his previous article in fact relies on concocted data, first invented by Hughes in 2005, and then repeated in various forms in CIS documents since.

In 2007 I published an article in the *Medical Journal of Australia* in which, referencing CIS and Bennelong Society publications, I noted that some commentators blamed the poor health of Aboriginal people on misguided policies that had forced people to live in remote communities, preventing them from benefiting from the mainstream economy. I cited the evidence that the poor health status of Aboriginal people, relative to non-Aboriginal people, is found in all areas where Aboriginal people live. I demonstrated that while some health indicators were better among Aboriginal people living in urban areas, on some other indicators living in very remote areas appeared to have health benefits.[23]

More recent studies confirm that Aboriginal disadvantage is not confined to remote areas and some indicators in fact suggest better outcomes in remote areas. Heather Crawford and Nicholas Biddle have analysed national health and social surveys between 2002 and 2013. They found that during this decade, Aboriginal adults living in remote areas compared with those living in non-remote areas and controlling for the other observable characteristics were significantly more likely to report that their self-assessed health was good to excellent. They were significantly less likely to have high to very high psychological distress, significantly more likely to report that they had been happy most or all of the time, and in the most recent data significantly less likely to report that they had been extremely sad at least some of the time.

In contrast to the CIS claims that social outcomes for 80 per cent of Aboriginal people are not noticeably different from those for non-Aboriginal people, an analysis from the 2011 census by Nicholas Biddle showed that 'there is not a single area where the Indigenous population has better or even relatively equal outcomes compared to the non-Indigenous population'.[24] In his analysis of incomes from the same census, he found that 'for almost every demographic, geographic, educational and employment combination, Indigenous Australians have a lower average income than their non-Indigenous counterparts'.[25] It appears that the CIS commentators have deliberately tried to create a false impression to influence Aboriginal policies. Put simply, they seem to suggest that if homelands communities were closed down and the people moved to towns and cities where they would have 'the same social outcomes as their non-Aboriginal peers', the problem would be solved and there will be no further need to direct government expenditure towards Aboriginal disadvantage. It frames the 'Aboriginal problem' as a problem of the settler-colonial frontier, with the assumption that once Aboriginal land and people are incorporated into the sovereign Australian state, the 'problem' will be extinguished.

Thus, the problems that exist in remote communities reflect Aboriginal disadvantage across all geographic regions of Australia, which in turn is a reflection of the ongoing structure of settler colonialism. It is this that restricts opportunities for Aboriginal autonomy and self-determination, wherever they live. Factors like remoteness, government neglect, lack of services, etc., may add to the problems in these communities, but it is misleading and false to claim that the problems exist merely because people live in homelands communities. The structure of settler colonialism affects Aboriginal people across Australia, not just at the frontier.

Homelands: Problem or solution?

Another frequent assertion is that because the problems of remote communities can be attributed to the homelands movement, the solution is to close the smaller and more remote communities.

The term 'remote communities' includes relatively large communities, most of which pre-dated the homelands movement, as well as the homeland communities that were created when people moved away from the larger communities. In most respects the problems that occur in remote communities are greater in the larger communities. The problems of the larger communities—alcohol, interpersonal violence, high morbidity and mortality rates—were often motivating factors that contributed to the homelands movement. The homelands communities in many cases continue to provide some protection from these problems. Aboriginal people living in homeland communities who have discussed these issues with me express a definite concern that if they were moved back to the larger communities (the Hughesian 'core centres') this would not resolve, and would often exacerbate, the problems.

A study in 1998 by Robyn McDermott and her colleagues showed that people who live in smaller decentralised communities in the Utopia area had more favourable health outcomes with respect to mortality, hospitalisation, hypertension, diabetes and injury, than those living in larger settlements in Central Australia. A follow-up survey ten years later showed that better health outcomes persisted: there was lower overall mortality, cardio-vascular disease mortality, and hospitalisation for cardio-vascular disease compared to the statistics for the Aboriginal population of the Northern Territory as a whole. The authors attributed these benefits to the nature of the Urapuntja Health Service, 'which provided regular outreach to outstation communities, as well as the decentralised mode of outstation living (with its attendant benefits for physical activity, diet and limited access to alcohol), and social factors, including connectedness to culture, family and land, and opportunities for self-determination'.[26]

The evidence, it seems, shows that the problems in remote communities cannot be attributed to the homelands movement. The homelands movement was a process driven by Aboriginal people themselves, as part of their struggle for autonomy. Their aim was to reassert their connection with their country and to leave the conflicts and other problems that existed in large communities. As discussed earlier, most of the homelands communities in the Western Desert have settled to a size consistent with a natural human grouping of around 150 people. It would be counterproductive to remove Aboriginal people in remote Australia from their homelands and once again concentrate them into large communities as was proposed by the social engineers in the neoliberal think tanks. This would increase the problems in remote communities and would be detrimental to health and wellbeing. With appropriate support homelands are part of the solution, not the problem.

Looking after the country

Politicians make frequent reference to 'economic viability' in their discussions of the homelands movement. In 2007 Amanda Vanstone, then Minister for Indigenous Affairs, referred to homelands communities as 'cultural museums' and foreshadowed an end to their funding:

> We need to think about the large numbers of very small settlements or homelands. It is unlikely that many of these homelands will grow to

become viable towns. They raise some important issues for the future such as: how viable are they really? Perhaps we need to explicitly draw a line on the level of service that can be provided to homeland settlements … No more cultural museums that might make some people feel good and leave Indigenous Australians without a viable future.[27]

There are economic opportunities that also have other positive benefits and could be expanded if government genuinely wanted to support the development of homelands communities. One example is the Indigenous art industry, which provides meaningful activity and income for a number of people, especially older people, in remote communities. Another example is the development of environmental-management programs.

The Australian Government supports environmental-management programs under two funding streams. In the Indigenous Protected Areas Program, an area of Aboriginal land is identified and the traditional owners are contracted by the government to manage the environment according to agreed criteria. The Working on Country Indigenous Rangers Program aims to build a skilled workforce to deliver environmental improvements combining modern science and traditional knowledge and skills. These programs aim to improve the health of the ecosystems through protection of biodiversity, reversing environmental degradation and species decline. They also contribute to the control of feral animals and invasive weeds.

In my experience, activities enabled by environmental management are among the most positive innovations in remote communities in recent years. In the early days of the reoccupation of the Western Desert, I witnessed a strong community spirit when people felt empowered to take control of their own lives. Several factors, including recent ill-informed government policies, have diminished this sense of agency and empowerment, and this in turn contributes to the well-publicised problems in contemporary remote communities. Increased levels of despair and depression are reflected in worsening physical and mental health. Land-management programs can help to alleviate many of these problems in remote communities. When people are employed in activities that take them 'out bush', looking after country and undertaking meaningful activities, their attitude to life improves. The changed demeanour and mental outlook in these situations are testament to their efficacy in improving wellbeing. I have noticed direct and indirect impacts on health. As a small but significant example, with a positive outlook on life, people's adherence to medication regimes improves.

There is also empirical evidence of the positive health, economic, socio-cultural, economic and environmental benefits of land-management programs.[28] Paul Burgess and his colleagues have shown that an involvement in caring for country is associated with better nutrition, more frequent physical activity, and fewer chronic-disease risk factors and diagnoses,[29] with consequent cost savings for the health system.[30] A study by Social Ventures Australia of the social, cultural and economic impact of a land management program on *Martu* country calculated that, for every dollar that was invested in the program, approximately three dollars of social value was created.

Darren Farmer (whose mother Joanie was an Aboriginal health worker and board member of Puntukurnu Aboriginal Medical Service when I lived in Jigalong in 1994–95) has said:

> When people go out on country they say, 'I'm here, I know who I am and I know where I come from, and I'm going to take charge of my life,' and in doing so, they're dealing with the dysfunctional aspects of their lives and their families' lives. So you're dealing with the social issues that are going on in town—but you're dealing with them out on country—through a social, cultural and spiritual healing process.[31]

I have seen the benefits of the healing processes to which Darren refers. I believe these activities are, in a way, an extension of the homelands movement. First the people moved back to their homelands, in many cases to get away from some of the more destructive aspects of the post-contact situation in which they had found themselves. Now, instead of forcing them back to these destructive environments, Aboriginal people living on their homelands should be supported to look after their estate. It is good for the country, and it is good for the people.

There are inconsistencies in the government policies regarding remote communities. On the one hand, most programs, such as the so-called

Community Development Program, are paternalistic and imposed from above. They seem to be aimed at coercively integrating people into the capitalist system as quickly as possible, even at the expense of Aboriginal culture and the communities themselves. Even if one believes such integration is desirable, it is clear that these policies are having destructive and costly effects on morbidity, mortality and incarceration rates. They do not encourage self-reliance and they are often actively resisted by the people affected by them.

On the other hand, there are some limited funding streams providing opportunities for cultural reinvigoration through land-management activities with an increase in autonomy and self-esteem. In contrast to the other programs, these are consistent with Aboriginal aspirations. If there is genuine desire to improve the livelihood of the Aboriginal people living in Australia's remotest regions, these funding streams should be supported and augmented. There definitely is room for expansion to allow more remote communities to develop land-management programs and to employ more people within the programs already operating.

There are still those who say that the homelands movement was a failure that must be reversed. As a result of these assertions, the ongoing Aboriginal aspiration for autonomy, self-esteem and connection with country that drove the homelands movement is being undermined by many government policies. I continue to believe that rather than being part of the problem of dysfunction in remote Aboriginal communities, the move to homelands was and remains an appropriate action taken by Aboriginal people themselves that should be supported. After all, the homelands are their homelands.

9

Autonomy in Aboriginal health and the government response

In each of the Western Desert regions where I lived and worked, I was employed by a local community organisation—an Aboriginal community-controlled health service. Just as I was fortunate to find myself involved in the reoccupation of the Western Desert, it has also been a privilege to have been part of the Aboriginal community-controlled health organisation (ACCHO) movement. Unlike the homelands movement, the social movement for control of health services is not confined to remote areas; it is an Australia-wide phenomenon. While the experiences I recount in earlier chapters refer to my involvement in health services in the Western Desert, I have also subsequently worked in such health services in other areas of the country. In this chapter, I will present my personal perspective on this movement and explain why I believe it has achieved a great deal and is deserving of support. I will then examine the level of support received from Australian governments.

In my view there are two broad components of the ACCHO movement that have combined to make it successful. One is the community-controlled component, with the services being a manifestation of the struggle for autonomy and self-determination in the development of Aboriginal civil society. The other component is the distinctive way that ACCHOs provide healthcare. At the heart of the ACCHO sector is a philosophical and practical commitment to comprehensive primary healthcare at the community level.

Aboriginal organisations

Collective organisations of Aboriginal people in Australian settler society have a long history. In the 1940s and 50s, the Australian Government, consistent with its assimilationist policy, supported Aboriginal participation in voluntary organisations, especially if these assisted in delivery of welfare programs. The government was less supportive of collective action to advocate for greater autonomy and Aboriginal rights. One such example is the Pilbara strike and the formation of the North-west (Native) Workers Association in the 1940s (discussed in chapter 4).

In the 1970s, Aboriginal organisations achieved more prominent recognition. When Aboriginal self-determination became the official policy approach to Aboriginal affairs in 1972 under the Whitlam Labor government, the policy shift coincided with a blossoming of Aboriginal organisations, termed by Tim Rowse the 'Indigenous Sector'. The development of these organisations was a significant and resilient manifestation of the policy of self-determination for Australian Aboriginal people.

The policy shift in the 1970s was a response to a movement that was already under way. This movement was cross-generational. Many of the older people involved had a long history of advocating for more rights for their people, including advocating for the constitutional change that was implemented with the 1967 referendum. Some of the younger activists were inspired by contemporary events in other countries, including the civil rights and Black Power movements in North America, as well as the struggle for self-determination that was occurring in many developing countries.

This movement allowed for the emergence of a stronger political voice for Aboriginal people. It also meant that Aboriginal people were organising and developing services for their communities to address the failure of mainstream services to meet their needs. This in turn led to the development of the Aboriginal community-controlled health organisational movement.

Aboriginal community-controlled health organisationss

The Aboriginal community-controlled health organisational movement was initially an urban phenomenon. The first ACCHO was established in the inner-Sydney suburb of Redfern in 1971. At that time Redfern had the largest Aboriginal community in Australia, and the establishment of the health service was a response to financial and discriminatory barriers to accessing mainstream medical institutions at the time.[1] Over the following few years many other Aboriginal communities in metropolitan and provincial cities established their own health services. Services were established in Adelaide around the same time as Redfern was being established, in Fitzroy in inner Melbourne in 1973 and in Perth in 1974. The Central Australian Aboriginal Congress opened a community-controlled health service in Alice Springs in 1974. The establishment of ACCHOs in remote Aboriginal communities came later in the same decade, as discussed in previous chapters. With the support of the Central Australian Aboriginal Congress, the Urapuntja (originally Angarappa) Health Service at Utopia started in December 1977, and the Pitjantjatjara Homelands Health Service and the Lyappa Medical Service at Papunya both started in 1978.

In the early years many ACCHOs relied on local-community volunteers and donations from aid organisations, but eventually funding from the Commonwealth Department of Aboriginal Affairs (established in 1972) became available. As ACCHOs were established, they often supported the aspirations of other communities to obtain control of their own health services. Staff from an established health service would sometimes be released to spend time with a newer organisation to assist with its development. This mutual support was formalised by the creation of the National Aboriginal and Islander Health Organisation (NAIHO), which became a vibrant and politically active organisation under the leadership of some notable Aboriginal activists. These leaders were dedicated to the concept of community control and ensured that the national organisation retained strong links with the community-based organisations. To avoid being a peak body that made decisions on behalf of the members, NAIHO made a conscious effort to support decision-making at the community level. As the NAIHO leaders had themselves been involved in the establishment of early ACCHOs, they understood the commitment to autonomy within community organisations constituting its membership.

Over the years, NAIHO became more dependent on government funding, and in the late 1980s, disagreements within the organisation itself, as well as between the Australian Government and NAIHO, led to a cessation of funding and the demise of NAIHO. A national organisation of ACCHOs re-emerged a few years later, now named the National Aboriginal Community Controlled Health Organisation (NACCHO). NACCHO continues as the national peak body representing the interests of ACCHOs across Australia. At the state and territory level, peak bodies also formed to support and represent the interests of ACCHOs within each jurisdiction.

Nearly half a century after the first ACCHO was opened in Redfern, there are over 140 ACCHOs across Australia providing comprehensive primary-healthcare services to local Aboriginal communities. These ACCHOs are incorporated community-based organisations, with membership from the local Aboriginal community, and boards of directors elected from the membership.

In 2017 Megan Campbell and her colleagues published the results of a structured review of the literature relating to the effectiveness of ACCHOs. The literature demonstrated that ACCHOs make a major contribution to improving Aboriginal health by increasing knowledge and expertise, as employers and trainers, by improving access to primary healthcare and by providing best practice in comprehensive primary healthcare. The authors also observed that ACCHOs are notable within the Australian health system for the emphasis on addressing the socio-economic determinants of health, which have been estimated to account for around 50 per cent of the health deficit at a population level.

ACCHOs as Aboriginal organisations

Aboriginal organisations are an outcome of the Aboriginal struggle for autonomy that has been an essential component of Aboriginal social movements. The struggle for self-determination and autonomy is worthy of support from a social-justice and human-rights perspective, but also because it is a powerful contributor to improved health. In the words of Sir Michael Marmot: 'autonomy is closely linked with self-esteem and the earning of respect ... Low levels of autonomy and low self-esteem are likely to be related to worse health'.

Marmot and others have also shown that a sense of agency is an important determinant of health. The loss of control associated with the destruction of Aboriginal society and an ongoing denigration of Aboriginal culture is one of the major impacts of settler colonialism on Aboriginal people and their health. The emergence of Aboriginal organisations, including ACCHOs, is one attempt to regain control. Aboriginal organisations in Newcastle, for example, have been described as 'not simply a sector or a service provider. Rather, they symbolise autonomy and control and are at the heart of, and central to, urban Aboriginal community-building and development.'[2]

Patrick Sullivan has argued that Aboriginal organisations like ACCHOs, insofar as they emerge from and represent the interests of Aboriginal communities, constitute Aboriginal civil society. He has suggested at least three reasons why the importance of Aboriginal organisations should be recognised: 'They are the critical ingredient in Aboriginal people's material security, an expression of Aboriginal political identity and an appropriate modernisation strategy with the evolution of Aboriginal civil society.'[3]

Sullivan explains how the Aboriginal-organisation sector provides the institutional framework for Aboriginal civil society and the principal means of Aboriginal civic engagement with the rest of Australian society. Aboriginal organisations, he says, 'are both the drivers of positive change and the social manifestation of such social change'.[4] The role of Aboriginal organisations, including ACCHOs, in developing civil society, the sphere between individuals and families on the one hand and the state and large corporate institutions on the other, is not always sufficiently recognised.

Aboriginal organisations such as ACCHOs are also an expression of the localised nature of Aboriginal politics, allowing decisions about priorities to be made at the local community level, by people who are aware of the local issues. This is the principle of subsidiarity, which means that decisions made as close as possible to the people affected by the decisions are likely to be better decisions than those made more remotely. In a paper outlining their aspirations for an improved health policy for Australia, health economist Ian McAuley and policy analyst John Menadue proposed that the principle of subsidiarity should be a key policy driver. The best example of subsidiarity in the Australian health system at present is the Aboriginal community-controlled health organisational sector. The struggle for autonomy entailed a struggle to ensure that decisions affecting the health and wellbeing of Aboriginal people are made by the people with the most knowledge of the actual problems needing resolution.[5]

Aboriginal organisations clearly increase the opportunities for cultural security in service delivery, including healthcare. The Australian Health Ministers' Advisory Council (AHMAC) has developed a 'Cultural Respect Framework for Aboriginal and Torres Strait Islander Health', which states that 'cultural respect is achieved when the health system is a safe environment for Aboriginal and Torres Strait Islander peoples and where cultural differences are respected … (Some barriers to healthcare access) are clearly cultural. These include health service provider attitudes and practice, communication issues, mistrust of the system, poor cultural understanding and racism.'

In his unpublished PhD thesis, Shane Houston provided an account of cultural security in the provision of healthcare for Aboriginal people in Australia. Mainstream health services, he asserted, are based on non-Aboriginal culture, with insufficient consideration given to the cultural security of Aboriginal people. He showed that Aboriginal people commonly demonstrate a preference for accessing community-controlled services because they are delivered in ways that are considered culturally secure. In this situation, it is the quality (or cultural appropriateness) of service and not geographic proximity that is most important to consider. Houston questioned the assumption that geographic proximity to a service equates to equality of access:

> Such problems can also apply, perhaps in varying ways, to Aboriginal and Torres Strait Islander communities in urban, rural and remote settings, a point often overlooked, particularly in respect of urban communities. The assumption there is generally that, if you live in close geographic proximity

to a service, then access is often considered equal. Such simplistic thinking overlooks the substantial unfreedoms suffered by Aboriginal and Torres Strait Islander communities especially in settings where they are a minority either as a proportion of the total population or as a proportion of the service users.[6]

Aboriginal organisations allow the creation of public spaces where Aboriginal people can comfortably interact with their peers. The waiting room of an Aboriginal community-controlled health service is a space in which all, or at least most, people (including those on the other side of the reception desk) are Aboriginal, and the 'yarning' that occurs in this space contributes to a sense of community solidarity. This is a particularly important feature in urban centres where such spaces are otherwise limited.

Aboriginal organisations are a major employer of Aboriginal people. They also provide further training for their staff, which increases employability and self-esteem. These features of Aboriginal organisations in themselves contribute to improved health and wellbeing for Aboriginal people.

There is another feature of Aboriginal organisations relating to employment that has received less attention. For non-Aboriginal professionals like myself, Aboriginal organisations create opportunities to work within a system that is culturally secure for the clients and is less likely to reproduce the settler-colonial power structures. I have always had the impression that when I am accountable to the community in which I work, I am able to be much more effective than would otherwise be the case. This important feature of Aboriginal organisations, as enablers for non-Aboriginal professionals to work in partnership with Aboriginal colleagues in helping to achieve Aboriginal aspirations, and to learn from their Aboriginal colleagues, is not sufficiently recognised.

ACCHOs as community health services

When the ACCHO social movement began in the 1970s, it happened alongside international movements for improved healthcare delivery, especially in developing nations and among disadvantaged and minority groups within the industrialised world. Two interrelated movements—the community-health movement and the comprehensive primary-healthcare movement—influenced the thinking of early ACCHO activists, who adapted some of the ideas behind these international movements.

The concept of 'community health' developed in the mid-twentieth century (as did the related concept of community development). It recognised that healthcare provision should be relevant to the needs of the community, that it should be socially and culturally appropriate, and that it should involve the active participation of the community. This approach also involved recognition that many health problems are related to the social, economic and political environment in which people live, and action at a community level is often required to manage the problems.

The concept of community health developed a following in many countries, including Australia. In 1973 the Whitlam government established a Community Health Program with three stated objectives: to shift the emphasis from treatment to prevention of disease; to provide an alternative to traditional general practice in the delivery of primary healthcare; and to reduce dependence on the institutional health system.

Funding was to be provided to state governments (which under the Australian Constitution have responsibility for healthcare delivery) on a cost-sharing basis, to establish community health centres. The implementation of the program varied between states. In subsequent years government support for the Community Health Program declined and, over time, the initial concept of community health centres with links to the community was largely lost, as boards of management were disbanded and government took over. The community health centres that have survived in some identifiable form are in Victoria, where funding went directly to community groups rather than to the state government, and in New South Wales, where women's health centres had strong community support. A community health centre in Inala in Queensland has continued to operate and since the early 2000s—thanks to the work of the Aboriginal general practitioner Noel Hayman—has become a notable example of a community-health centre meeting the needs of the local Aboriginal population. The adopted approach is very similar to that of the ACCHO.

Twenty years ago, when community health centres in South Australia were still functioning, a study conducted by Megan Warin and her colleagues investigated community perspectives towards two models of primary healthcare: the fee-for-service general practice model and the model of publicly funded community health services. The role of ACCHOs was not mentioned, but these might be considered Aboriginal-specific publicly funded community health services. Ninety-five per cent of respondents preferred the community health service model to the alternative. The main positive features reported were having more time with the doctor, being treated as a 'whole person', having more choice and control, focus on health promotion and disease prevention, access to other services and greater opportunities for community participation. This study demonstrated that community health centres had strong community support, but this did not halt the decline in funding.

There is one sector in the Australian health system, however, where the original ideals of the community health movement have been maintained—the ACCHO sector. The Aboriginal activists who were involved in the struggle for improved healthcare in the 1970s found the community health concept applicable to their situation. With the collective aspiration for autonomy and cultural identity characteristic of the Aboriginal organisational movement, the activists placed emphasis on the need for the community to be in control. While the community health concept has largely disappeared from the rest of the Australian health system, it continues to underlie the approach to healthcare within ACCHOs and this approach is, I believe, a contributor to the success of the ACCHO model.[7]

In traditional western medical practice, a consultation is very much an individual affair, between a doctor and a patient. In traditional Aboriginal medical care, a consultation is a social event, with a small crowd of people being present as a *ngangkari* attends to a patient, contributing to a validation of the patient's illness and allowing a group expression of sympathy. While such public consultations are clearly not always appropriate in the contemporary setting, community-health practice borrows something from this approach. From the practitioner's perspective the attitude is generally that of being part of a healthcare team. From the patient's perspective, community health practice appreciates that the patient lives in a social world, and the consultation will consider how the social environment may contribute to the desired outcome.[8]

Looking beyond the individual consultation, part of the work of a community health practitioner includes what is sometimes called clinical governance. Many ACCHOs have well-developed clinical governance; in particular, they have implemented systems that make the best use of electronic medical records and multi-disciplinary team members to ensure that there are consistent pathways of care for people with common health and wellbeing issues, with resulting better outcomes. This aspect of ACCHOs is not always recognised, although in a review of clinical governance in primary healthcare in Australia Christine Phillips and her colleagues noted that 'the Aboriginal community-controlled sector is in the vanguard of clinical governance in Australia … input from the [ACCHO] sector should be sought from others in Australia to inform the implementation of clinical governance across all primary healthcare'.

Concurrent with, and related to, the development of the community health movement in the mid-twentieth century was the Primary Health Care (PHC) movement, which was also reflected in the development of ACCHOs. In 1978 the WHO and UNICEF sponsored the International Conference on Primary Health Care at Alma Ata in the USSR (now Almaty in Kazakhstan). The Alma Ata Declaration defined primary healthcare as essential healthcare universally accessible to individuals and families in the community by means acceptable to them, through their full participation and at a cost the community and country can afford, in the spirit of self-reliance and self-determination. There was an emphasis on community participation and, recognising the importance of the social and economic environment, on inter-sectoral collaboration. The declaration framed primary healthcare in the context of social justice, human rights and emancipatory development.

When I became involved in the ACCHO sector, there was recognition that the Alma Ata declaration articulated the aspirations of the activists who were responsible for the development of the ACCHOs and reflected what was already happening in Aboriginal communities within Australia. The fact that the WHO supported this approach was a cause for optimism.

However, in the years following the Alma Ata conference, the more comprehensive aspects of primary healthcare were downplayed as more technical aspects were emphasised. Walsh and Warren published an article in 1979 suggesting that the aspirations of the Alma Ata declaration were impractical and over-optimistic. They proposed an alternative approach that they called Selective Primary Health Care (SPHC), which involved specific interventions for certain priority diseases. This provoked a debate; supporters of Comprehensive Primary Health Care (CPHC) suggesting that the new approach destroyed the spirit of Alma Ata and was less likely to have a sustainable impact on health improvement. They argued that a comprehensive method, with its bottom-up approach, was more likely to have an impact on overall health and wellbeing than the top-down programs advocated by supporters of SPHC. Funding agencies, however, liked the fact that SPHC offered the possibility of easily replicable programs designed to address a particular disease or condition with clear objectives and with a limited time frame, compared to the more open-ended funding requirements that were needed to support Comprehensive Primary Health Care.

The debate between SPHC and CPHC was mirrored by the debate between vertical programs and horizontal programs. Vertical programs like SPHC are designed to be delivered from a centralised agency across various localities, whereas horizontal programs aim to improve health through service integration at the PHC level according to local circumstances. While governments and funding agencies tend to prefer SPHC and vertical programs, the ACCHO movement is based very much on a comprehensive model of primary healthcare favouring horizontal programs.

The comprehensiveness of CPHC in the ACCHO movement can be represented on three axes. On the first axis, CPHC means that, as much as possible, a range of services is available to meet the diverse health and wellbeing needs of the community. This means that an ACCHO provides more than just the services of a general medical practitioner. Programs dealing with such issues as dental health, alcohol and drug issues, mental health and domestic violence are also provided where possible, either on-site within the ACCHO premises or through partnerships and facilitated referral pathways.

The second axis means that any health problem is viewed through the prism of an understanding of the social determinants of health. That is, as well as dealing with the immediate health problem, as much as possible the organisation will investigate ways to alleviate the problem within the community by addressing its determinants. The third axis involves ensuring access to healthcare for sub-populations who might have particular barriers to access, such as young people or homeless people.

The concept of 'community health' has become less visible in Australia today. Primary Health Care has a narrower definition than it once did, and support for a comprehensive approach has declined. However, both community health and comprehensive primary healthcare concepts were adapted and maintained in the ACCHO sector. This has allowed the development of a unique model of primary healthcare provision that thus far has been maintained despite external pressures to adopt a narrower approach to healthcare.

Barriers to primary healthcare access by Aboriginal people have been framed as being related to factors that are locational, economic and/or sociocultural.[9] In other words, there are barriers of availability, affordability and acceptability, all of which ACCHOs have been shown to overcome. To these three barriers, another, which I call appropriateness, could be added.

The appropriateness of the healthcare provided by ACCHOs is partly due to their culturally secure environment. However, it is also due to ACCHOs' comprehensive primary healthcare approach. This is a major factor in improving access to primary healthcare for Aboriginal people. The fact that ACCHOs provide an appropriate model of healthcare has not always been recognised by recent governments, which have frequently promoted mainstream general practice in preference to ACCHOs. This will be discussed in the next sections.

Government and ACCHOs

In 1967 a national referendum led to constitutional amendments that granted federal involvement in Indigenous affairs; prior to this, the states had sole responsibility for policies regarding their respective Aboriginal populations.

As Aboriginal communities started organising to develop their own health services, the new constitutional powers arising from the 1967 referendum meant that the Australian Government was able to respond by providing funding to the burgeoning ACCHO movement.

There was often opposition to this from the state governments, which by the 1970s had begun to develop some programs to deliver healthcare to Aboriginal communities. The Commonwealth Department of Aboriginal Affairs provided funding directly to community organisations like ACCHOs, bypassing state and territory administrations, which led to accusations of interference and duplication of services. According to Patrick Sullivan, citing Nugget Coombs, the Australian Government encouraged Aboriginal organisations to incorporate '... explicitly to circumvent state governments and [allow the Australian Government] to directly fund the delivery of community development programs'.[10] I have discussed my experience in previous chapters of the resistance from the state and territory health departments to the establishment of the early ACCHOs, sometimes leading to less than adequate interagency cooperation.

As a result, community organisations frequently struggled to be recognised and heard as the voice of Aboriginal communities. The states and territories, maintaining a role in service delivery alongside Commonwealth-funded Indigenous organisations, often ended up in a competitive and uncooperative relationship with Aboriginal organisations. As was noted by Steve Kunitz and Maggie Brady in 1995, in contrast to the Federal Bureau of Indian Affairs in the US, which funded a comprehensive national Indigenous healthcare system, in Australia there was never a serious commitment by the federal government to be the sole administering agency for Aboriginal health programs. State and territory government departments continued to provide services and, instead of working with Aboriginal organisations as a legitimate voice of the community, they often deliberately bypassed them. In addition, the lack of clarity between the federal government on the one hand, and state and territory responsibilities on the other, often resulted in 'passing the buck' between the two levels of government.

As the ACCHO sector became more established, the resistance from state and territory health departments gradually waned (more so in some jurisdictions than others). Yet, health funding for ACCHOs continued to be piecemeal, short-term and with little coordination. In the 1980s the need for a National Aboriginal Health Strategy was promoted by the ACCHO sector, and this was supported by federal, state and territory health departments. A comprehensive consultation process ensued, which culminated in the Report of the National Aboriginal Health Strategy Working Party, usually known as the NAHS Report. A major strength of the NAHS report was its wide acceptance by Aboriginal people, and by the ACCHO sector in particular, due to the sense of ownership over the strategy that developed during the consultation process. The release of the report was seen as a major event in the struggle to achieve better healthcare for Aboriginal people.

Another report of significance was released two years after the NAHS report. The Royal Commission into Aboriginal Deaths in Custody was established by the Australian Government in 1987 in response to some well-publicised custodial deaths. The royal commission undertook a comprehensive process of investigating the underlying issues leading to high rates of Aboriginal incarceration and its report was released in 1991. It was a lengthy document containing many recommendations, some of which were of direct relevance to Aboriginal organisations. Recommendation 192 stated that preference should be given to these organisations in the delivery of services to Aboriginal people, along with other recommendations about how Aboriginal organisations could be better supported.

In 1990 the Australian Government established the Aboriginal and Torres Strait Islander Commission (ATSIC) as a means of increasing Aboriginal self-determination in the national and regional administration of Indigenous Affairs. Funding for Aboriginal organisations including ACCHOs was transferred from the DAA to ATSIC. ATSIC consisted of elected regional councils across Australia, tasked with making decisions about disbursement of funding earmarked for their region. Thus, ATSIC was seen by some as a mechanism adopted by government to absolve itself of responsibility for making the politically difficult decisions about the distribution of scarce resources to meet the significant needs of Aboriginal communities.

In many regions, particularly the Northern Territory, ACCHOs felt that their regional councils were not equipped to make appropriate decisions about how much funding should be directed towards primary healthcare delivery and questioned whether ATSIC was the most appropriate structure for funding Aboriginal healthcare. The argument was made that funding responsibility should be transferred to the federal health department as it not only had a responsibility to fund health services for Aboriginal citizens of Australia, but also had the expertise to make appropriate funding decisions. While there was some opposition from the ATSIC leadership, Noel Pearson was among the Aboriginal leaders who gave their support to the arguments for transferring funding responsibility for ACCHOs. In 1994 the Office of Aboriginal and Torres Strait Islander Health Services (OATSIHS) was established as part of the federal Department of Health.

By the mid-1990s there was a degree of optimism within the ACCHO sector. ACCHOs were now an established part of the health system in Australia and had recognition and support from the Australian Government. State and territory governments had, at least to an extent, overcome the resistance to their federal funding as they saw that ACCHOs were addressing health with minimal cost to their own budget; in fact, they were saving money by reducing hospitalisations.

The need for coordination at different levels of government was recognised and in 1995, a tripartite forum was established in each state and territory, consisting of representatives from the federal health department, the state or territory health department and the ACCHO sector. By this time ACCHOs had peak bodies in each state and territory that represented the ACCHO sector on the tripartite forums. The formation of tripartite forums was a significant development, amounting to recognition that the Aboriginal organisational sector was effectively another level of government for Aboriginal communities.

This developing productive partnership between governments and the ACCHO sector stalled with the election of the Howard government in 1996, heralding a major shift in Aboriginal-affairs policy. We have seen in chapter 8 how this shift affected remote communities, but it also had an impact on Aboriginal healthcare. The Howard government claimed that persisting health and other social inequalities between Aboriginal and non-Aboriginal Australians were due to previous governments placing too much emphasis on 'symbolic' issues such as Aboriginal rights and the question of an apology for past iniquitous policies.

In response, the Howard government shifted the policy emphasis to what was termed 'practical reconciliation' which, it claimed, would concentrate more on ensuring that services were provided to address Aboriginal disadvantage. This led to a policy agenda of sidelining engagement with Aboriginal organisations and instead emphasising socio-economic need and so-called dysfunction. This shift in emphasis was called by the government a 'new arrangement in Indigenous affairs'.

Like many neoliberal governments around the world, the Howard government proclaimed the need for welfare reform. A major component of the government's approach to Aboriginal welfare policy was the concept of 'mutual obligation'. In 2004 this concept was applied to Indigenous policy with the introduction of Shared Responsibility Agreements, or SRAs, where services provided to Aboriginal communities became dependent on the achievement of goals determined by government. Among the many problems with SRAs, the way they were negotiated led to an undermining of community strengths and organisation. The network of Aboriginal community-controlled organisations, with roots in Aboriginal communities, could have provided the political organisation required to engage with governments to determine the terms of SRAs. However, the government deliberately avoided engaging with representative community organisations, insisting that they would engage directly with 'the community'; the concept of 'community' remained undefined.

In 2004 the Commonwealth minister with responsibility for Aboriginal affairs, Amanda Vanstone, stated that 'we have assumed the bodies we speak to have the authority to speak on behalf of the community. That's not an assumption we can make. Really, the only people who can authorise others to speak on their behalf are the individual, the family unit, or the community.'[11] Speaking on ABC radio in 2005, Vanstone described the new arrangement in Indigenous affairs as a 'new conversation, going directly to communities'. Ignoring the history of the development of the Aboriginal organisational sector, she then went on to say that 'for many, this is the first time they've been given the opportunity to express where they want to go and how they see government can play a role'.[12]

By circumventing the role of established Aboriginal community-based organisations, the Australian Government ensured that the real power in any negotiations resided with itself. Ultimately, such arrangements were unlikely to be truly mutual or shared. Properly conceived, a strategic approach involving mutual obligation that allowed genuine sharing of rights and responsibilities, while showing respect for community structures and organisations, could have provided the basis for transformative policy development. In fact, a truly mutual obligation agreement at the national level would involve the negotiation of a treaty—a concept that the Howard government strenuously resisted, even though Indigenous peoples in New Zealand and North America attribute their comparatively better health outcomes at least partly to the fact that they have been able to negotiate treaties with their governments. In 2004, in its response to a report of the Council of Aboriginal Reconciliation in which a treaty had been mooted, the Australian Government stated that 'such a legally enforceable instrument as between sovereign states would be divisive, would undermine the concept of a single Australian nation and would create legal uncertainty and future disputation'.[13]

As most knowledgeable commentators predicted, the Howard government's approach to SRAs did not lead to any improvement in Aboriginal health. With such a blatant power disparity between the negotiating parties, many communities were wary of entering into agreements. This wariness was portrayed by government officials as a problem of community dysfunction and incapacity.

This government narrative of Aboriginal community dysfunction was consistent with the reassertion of the 'Aboriginal problem' that was being promoted at the time by commentators working for the neoliberal think tanks, as discussed in the previous chapter. This narrative now dominated government policy, with a tendency to blame Aboriginal people, communities and organisations for their own plight. Rather than accepting that government had a responsibility to ensure adequacy of services, the emphasis was placed on deficiencies within the Aboriginal community. This was exemplified by John Howard himself, who in 2004 made the following statement:

I am very unhappy—as most Australians are—at the health standards of Aboriginal people. They still lag way behind the rest of the community and it is not just a question of money, because a lot more money has been put into Aboriginal health. It is a question of culture. It is a question of practice. It is a question of attitude. It is a question of community responsibility.[14]

This concentration on individual, family, community and organisational dysfunction ignored the structural context that contributes to health and other social problems. It also gave the government an excuse for the lack of progress towards the reduction of inequalities. Coalition senators stated in 2004 that 'no government can help a community that is not committed to helping itself'. Commenting on the policy environment at the time, the Dean of the Faculty of Law at the University of New South Wales, Hal Wootten, wrote: 'The emerging conservative narrative is little more than a return to assimilation ... Essentially it regards Aboriginality as a deficiency, a burden that handicaps Aboriginals in the modern world and should be shed.'

ATSIC, in the meantime, was coming under increased pressure. Problems at the senior management levels were leading to criticism, and a comprehensive review called for reform of the ATSIC structure. The Howard government, however, with its narrative of the failure of self-determination, decided that it was better to discard ATSIC altogether rather than reform it. In 2004 ATSIC was abolished.

A 'whole-of-government' approach was pursued after the abolition of ATSIC. Under this approach, there was to be no Australian Government department with dedicated responsibility for Aboriginal affairs. Aboriginal programs were now to be subsumed under other portfolios. An Office of Indigenous Policy Coordination (OIPC)—designed to have more of a coordinating role, rather than directly providing or funding services for Aboriginal programs—was created in 2004. The OIPC was initially in the Department of Prime Minister and Cabinet, then moved to the Department of Immigration and Multicultural Affairs and subsequently to the Department of Family and Community Services. Each move contributed to the general policy confusion.

At the regional level, this coordinating role was to be carried out through the Indigenous Coordinating Centres (ICCs). However, there was little evidence of effective coordination between different government departments with responsibilities for service delivery to Aboriginal people. In fact, the evidence showed that there was less co-ordination than was occurring prior to the policy change and the abolition of ATSIC. The overall impact on those affected by these policies, Aboriginal people and their organisations, was further stress and uncertainty and severe constraints on long-term planning.

Mainstreaming

The other component of the 'new arrangement in Indigenous affairs', which had an even greater impact on ACCHOs, was the emphasis on 'mainstreaming' of service delivery. In other words, there was a shift away from funding Aboriginal-specific programs, towards an expectation that mainstream service providers would take on the responsibility for providing services to both Aboriginal and non-Aboriginal people.

In one sense, mainstreaming might be interpreted as all government departments accepting their responsibility to Aboriginal people, which could in turn mean developing Aboriginal-specific programs to supplement general services. This change from one Aboriginal department with overall responsibility for service delivery to a situation where all relevant departments take responsibility for all services, including Aboriginal-specific services, was basically equivalent to the 'whole-of-government' approach, which in turn could be interpreted as being consistent with a degree of self-determination. It was in fact what many Aboriginal community-controlled health organisations argued for in the mid-1990s when they successfully proposed that funding for Aboriginal health services be transferred from ATSIC to the federal Department of Health.

The way that 'mainstreaming' emerged, however, indicated that there was now an expectation that Aboriginal people should access the same services as non-Aboriginal people, rather than Aboriginal-specific services, which amounted to an attack on the network of Aboriginal organisations already delivering services to Aboriginal people. Aboriginal-specific services, and particularly those under community control, were now often denounced as practising 'separatism'. These changes applied across all aspects of Aboriginal affairs, including health. When funding for Aboriginal community-controlled health organisations was transferred from ATSIC to the federal Department of Health in 1994, the section within the department responsible for funding ACCHOs was initially called the Office of Aboriginal and Torres Strait Islander Health Services (OATSIHS). This name was changed during the term of the Howard government to the Office of Aboriginal and Torres Strait Islander Health (OATSIH).

This change indicated that it was now not specifically concerned with funding ACCHOs. With the official government strategy of mainstreaming, OATSIH started directing funds to mainstream organisations as well as, and often in preference to, ACCHOs, so that ACCHOs were often regarded as just one group of providers of medical services among others. Increasingly, large non-Aboriginal private sector and not-for-profit organisations, in competition with Aboriginal community-controlled organisations, were the beneficiaries of government tendering and contracting processes.

The need to 'mainstream' health service was particularly emphasised in urban areas, even though it was in urban areas where the failure of mainstream health services had led to the beginning of the ACCHO movement in the 1970s. In December 2006 the then Minister for Indigenous Affairs, Mal Brough, made the following statement:

> Setting up parallel services ... often with lower standards and expectations, has not produced the results that organisations like ATSIC sought to deliver. Indeed sometimes these parallel services have alienated people from the broader community and from opportunities. Our approach will be to facilitate access to all services, rather than establish alternatives ... In urban areas where most Indigenous Australians live, the aim is to improve the functioning of mainstream services for Indigenous Australians and improve access to jobs in the mainstream economy.

The mainstreaming approach was not based on evidence. During the term of the Howard government, the Commonwealth Grants Commission undertook an inquiry into Aboriginal funding. As noted by Jon Altman, this important report never received the attention it deserved. The findings of the CGC report included evidence that mainstream services do not meet the needs of Aboriginal people to the same extent that they meet the needs of non-Aboriginal people. It also showed that Aboriginal Australians in all regions access mainstream services at a much lower rate than non-Aboriginal people, and that mainstream programs do not adequately meet the needs of Aboriginal people because of barriers to access.

In primary healthcare, the policy of mainstreaming tended toward a privileging of mainstream general practice over ACCHOs, which was unsupported by evidence. Work published by Katherine Ong and colleagues in 2012 showed that there are higher rates of utilisation and adherence to treatments delivered by ACCHOs compared to mainstream general practice. Theo Vos and colleagues in 2010 showed that the health impact of interventions delivered by ACCHOs appears to be 50 per cent greater than if these same interventions are delivered by mainstream health services, primarily due to improved Aboriginal access. Other studies (for example by Katie Panaretto and her colleagues and David Peiris and his colleagues) have shown that ACCHOs do at least as well, and on many indicators better, in the systematic management of chronic diseases, which are a major contributor to the Aboriginal health burden.

One of the few studies to investigate Aboriginal people's access to mainstream general practice was a two-year project conducted by Pippa Craig in the south-western Sydney region. In the first phase, receptionists working in GP surgeries in the region were interviewed about their usual practices in dealing with Aboriginal people face-to-face or over the telephone. It is appropriate to ascertain the attitudes and practices of receptionists, as they are the first-contact personnel in surgeries and can have a significant effect on access.

According to the report, most receptionists acted in an indirectly discriminatory way, unintentionally disadvantaging Aboriginal patients by not recognising their special needs. Most receptionists had little cultural awareness of the differences between Aboriginal and non-Aboriginal people, but while the report suggested they would benefit from some training, only half of those interviewed expressed interest in attending training. In ACCHOs, the receptionists are usually local Aboriginal staff, contributing to the more culturally secure environment.

Craig also interviewed ten GPs who saw a significant number of Aboriginal patients, to identify any difficulties or issues they encountered. A common concern was 'losing track of Aboriginal clients', with difficulties in following-up treatments and ensuring compliance given irregular attendance. This 'losing track' is much less of a problem in ACCHOs that employ staff from the local Aboriginal community who usually have knowledge of people's movements. The difficulty in promoting lifestyle changes such as regular exercise or dietary improvements was also mentioned as a problem for fee-for-service GPs, as was the difficulty in establishing confidentiality and trust. The report's author suggested that developing trust required long appointments, but 'the system was against it'.

The 'system' that did not work well was fee-for-service general practice, whereas the healthcare model developed in ACCHOs is more effective at meeting the needs of Aboriginal patients. Some of the mainstream GPs interviewed stated that they avoided getting involved in mental health or drug and alcohol issues. The fact that these are such important aspects of primary healthcare for Aboriginal people raises further questions about the appropriateness of mainstream general practice as the preferred providers of primary healthcare for Aboriginal people.

Aboriginal people who attend a GP, in an ACCHO or elsewhere, are more likely to have complex health issues compared to non-Aboriginal Australians. The *Bettering the Evaluation and Care of Health* (BEACH) study for many years provided insights into the patient demographics, reasons for encounter, problems managed, treatment and referrals in general practice across Australia. The 2003 BEACH report showed that 1.4 per cent of general practice consultations involved patients identified as Aboriginal and Torres Strait Islander people. The nature of problems managed for Aboriginal patients differed somewhat from the non-Aboriginal consultations, but the number of problems managed per encounter was the same. Two studies have used similar methodology to the BEACH study to investigate consultations in urban ACCHOs: in the first study, data were analysed from all consultations at Danila Dilba Aboriginal Medical Service in Darwin by David Thomas and his colleagues. In the second study data collected from consultations at the Townsville Aboriginal and Islander Health Service were analysed by Sarah Larkins and her colleagues. Both of these studies showed that significantly more problems were managed in each consultation in ACCHOs compared to consultations with Aboriginal patients in mainstream general practice. This suggests that ACCHOs are better able to manage the more complex health problems in Aboriginal patients compared to fee-for-service general practice.

As well as the evidence that Aboriginal people achieve better outcomes when services are provided by an ACCHO, there is also evidence that Aboriginal people prefer to get healthcare from Aboriginal-specific health services. An Aboriginal health survey in South Australia, conducted by the University of Adelaide for the South Australian Department of Health, found that a majority of the Aboriginal respondents preferred an Aboriginal specific health service, while only 9.6 per cent preferred a non-specific service.

The alacrity with which many politicians and bureaucrats appeared to accept the policy shift away from self-determination and towards mainstreaming despite the lack of supporting evidence suggested that support for genuine Aboriginal self-determination within the bureaucracy had always been fragile.

The New Public Management

The impact of the 'new arrangement in Indigenous affairs' introduced by the Howard government was exacerbated by a change in the way the Commonwealth public service functioned. The change was based on a theory of public administration called the New Public Management. Developed in the 1980s, the New Public Management is based on the assumption that market-oriented policies and practices lead to greater cost-efficiency, competitive performance and leadership.[15] This approach increased the control of ministers over the public service and led to a more centralised, managerialist approach to Aboriginal affairs, including Aboriginal health. As described by Patrick Sullivan, 'fake markets are created within the bureaucracy, and by the bureaucracy for its dependent organisations, in order to introduce the magic of capitalism to its fundamentally different order of social activity'.[16]

This new approach to public administration deprived community organisations and civil society of decision-making powers. Under the New Public Management, the values that are inherent in Aboriginal organisations, such as community solidarity, importance of culture and local decision-making were replaced by formal managerialist procedures linked to key performance indicators and externally imposed targets. Sullivan claimed that this approach 'fundamentally re-imagined Aboriginal people as subjects of governance' with an 'increasing pressure on Aboriginal organisations to conform to the remote control of their activities in a field where multiple non-Aboriginal actors pursue incommensurate interests, often with very short time-lines'.[17] In a paper published in 2018, Janet Hunt provided a case study of how the services provided by a successful Aboriginal organisation, with well-established links to the community, were undermined by the New Public Management approach.

Increasingly, Aboriginal health-policy decisions were made in the offices of the Canberra bureaucracy—often with no apparent basis in evidence—and far removed from the day-to-day reality of Aboriginal people. A more effective response would have been to devolve decision-making and resources to organisations who were dealing with these realities on a daily basis. Instead, bureaucracies appeared to want to get more information by requesting more and more data from local organisations, further constraining their ability to provide quality primary healthcare. According to Patrick Sullivan,

> contemporary public management has facilitated the destruction of the Aboriginal community-controlled sector ... through the Australian public sector's inability to appreciate Aboriginal forms of management; its inability to take into account the value provided by culturally informed local third-sector organisations; and its inability to hear local competence expressed in a dialect and idiom foreign to dominant public sector discourse.[18]

In a study on the impact of the New Public Management on Aboriginal organisations in Newcastle, Howard-Wagner found that

Aboriginal organisations, which formerly operated like community co-operatives and had a far more societal function in relation to community-development and self-determination, now operate in a competitive social service market, competing with mainstream not-for-profits, and each other, for funding.[19]

Research showed that under this new form of management, ACCHOs were being increasingly over-burdened with reporting requirements.[20] The government responded with statements that they would reduce the reporting burden but, in fact, reporting requirements only continued to increase. In Sullivan's words,

> the Indigenous sector is paradoxically under-acknowledged and over-regulated ... [Government funding contracts] impose more onerous reporting requirements and more intrusive interventions in the affairs of the sector ... the Indigenous sector is particularly vulnerable to inefficiency and inappropriate service delivery because of its reliance on government funding, and consequently to remotely conceived policies and remotely administered regimes of regulation and accountability.[21]

Reflecting the 'audit culture' of the New Public Management, the Commonwealth health department made a major investment in establishing a system of national key performance indicators (called nKPIs) against which ACCHOs were required to report as part of their funding agreements. The nKPIs included indicators of health risk (e.g. smoking rates) and health-system performance (e.g. numbers of health checks performed). While initially it was stated that nKPIs would not be used to determine funding levels, there are now strong suggestions that this is likely to happen.

With electronic medical records used by most ACCHOs, the actual reporting of nKPIs is quite straightforward, but there are, nonetheless, problems with this approach. In particular, the heavy government investment in nKPIs has led to anxiety in many health services about ensuring that they score well against the indicators. This can lead to the activities of the health service becoming distracted by efforts to increase the nKPI scores, at the expense of other comprehensive primary healthcare activities that are not covered by the nKPIs. In addition, the ever-increasing use of nKPIs is leading to ACCHO activity being increasingly determined by the federal health department bureaucracy rather than by health priorities identified at the local community level.

Government funding of ACCHOs

Over time, difficulties with funding, especially the short-term fragmented nature of contracts from multiple funding sources, have limited the effectiveness of the services provided. ACCHOs have often found that performance criteria imposed on them are more onerous compared to other sectors within the health system. As an example, Derbal Yerrigan in Perth had its funding cut when an increasing service demand led to an 'overspend' whereas, at the same time, the Perth teaching hospitals, which had an overspend 120 times greater than that of Derbal Yerrigan, were given an extra $100 million to cover the difference.[22]

In April 2007, forty of Australia's leading Aboriginal, health and human-rights organisations launched a campaign to 'Close the Gap' in health inequality between Aboriginal and non-Aboriginal Australians. The campaign called on all levels of Australian government to put in place firm targets, funding and timeframes to address these inequalities, including providing equal access to primary healthcare for Aboriginal people within ten years.

With the election of Kevin Rudd later that year, there was hope that his new Labor government would respond to the campaign and implement better health policies. This hope was reinforced when, in March 2008, he signed a Statement of Intent that committed to developing a comprehensive, long-term plan of action, which would be targeted to need, evidence-based and capable of addressing the existing inequalities in health services in order to significantly lift Aboriginal health and life expectancy by 2030. It also stated its aim to ensure the full participation of Aboriginal and Torres Strait Islander peoples and their representative bodies in all aspects of addressing their health needs, and to supporting and developing Aboriginal and Torres

Strait Islander community-controlled health services in urban, rural and remote areas.

Unfortunately, the Labor government—first under Kevin Rudd, then Julia Gillard—failed to deliver on these commitments. The proposed 'partnership' with Aboriginal peoples and their organisations, and the support for Aboriginal community-controlled health services, did not materialise. On the contrary, the government's approach to Aboriginal health policy was characterised by a failure to engage with Aboriginal partners. The main funding commitment was the Indigenous Health National Partnership, introduced by the Council of Australian Governments (COAG). This partnership, however, was only between the federal government on the one hand, and state and territory governments on the other. Aboriginal organisations and communities were conspicuously excluded from the policy process as well as, for the most part, from COAG funding. Most of the funds were directed to government bureaucracies and to mainstream health organisations such as Divisions of General Practice.[23] Community-controlled health organisations and their state, territory and federal representative bodies continued to be sidelined and under-funded.

The initiatives funded through the Indigenous Health National Partnership were pre-determined centrally in Canberra, with little opportunity for local Aboriginal health organisations to address their locally identified priorities. Instead, these organisations ended up with siloed funding streams for issues decided upon within the Canberra bureaucracy, with stringent reporting requirements and performance indicators attached to the funding. This was indicative of a government preference for a selective primary healthcare model and a vertical approach to funding, in contrast to the emphasis on comprehensive primary health care and horizontal programs that was a hallmark of the ACCHO approach to improving health outcomes.

The Labor government did nothing to ameliorate the mainstreaming agenda of its predecessor. In 2009, when Kevin Rudd announced a funding increase through the Closing the Gap (CTG) program, he said that government strategy would focus on 'the mainstream health system, because that is where 70 per cent of Indigenous people are treated'. This figure, it turned out, was based on flawed data,[24] but it continued to be repeated by health department bureaucrats long after this inaccuracy had been demonstrated. Most of the CTG funding continued to be directed to mainstream organisations. A colleague who worked for a company contracted to evaluate components of the CTG health funding reported to me that when the report showed improved results for funding going to ACCHOs rather than mainstream general practice, the health department requested a rewrite of the report. They wanted evidence to support their policy, but not evidence that might challenge it.[25]

In 2011 with the Labor party still in power, Sullivan stated that 'Aboriginal groups tend to embrace whole-of-government and reject mainstreaming'. Under the Labor government, he suggested, 'whole-of-government remain[ed] an aspirational goal while the policy environment of mainstreaming continu[ed] apace'.[26]

Any hope of improved policies with the 2013 election of the Coalition government were quickly crushed. Abbott moved the Aboriginal affairs portfolio to the Department of Prime Minister and Cabinet (PM&C) and, although the Department of Health retained responsibility for most Aboriginal health funding, the sections with responsibility for substance abuse and social and emotional wellbeing were transferred to PM&C. These are significant and complex health issues, which ACCHOs attempt to address as part of the comprehensive primary healthcare approach and having the funding for these issues in a separate department added to their difficulties.

Funding for all aspects of Aboriginal policy that fell under PM&C was administered through a program called the Indigenous Advancement Strategy (IAS). Aboriginal organisations hoped that this program would fund some comprehensive primary healthcare, particularly related to substance abuse and social and emotional wellbeing. Many ACCHOs and other organisations put considerable investment into preparing submissions for funding from the IAS, but most of these were rejected, with the bulk of IAS funding going to non-Aboriginal organisations. The Australian National Audit Office subsequently found that the department did not effectively implement the strategy and that the department's grants administration processes fell short of the standard required.

As frequently happens with a change of government, the Abbott government restructured the health department. The OATSIH was abolished and subsumed under a new division called the Indigenous and Rural Health Division. Within a few years another restructuring led to an Indigenous Health Division with a section called the Indigenous Australians' Health Program (IAHP), which had the responsibility for funding ACCHOs. The IAHP indicated that direct funding for ACCHOs would be capped at $360 million per year.

IAHP subsequently developed a formula to determine how funding is to be distributed among existing ACCHOs. The ACCHO sector has long supported the concept of developing a needs-based funding formula for comprehensive primary healthcare for Aboriginal people to ensure that the greater health needs of Aboriginal people are able to be met. However, the IAHP formula is not strictly speaking needs based. When it appeared that many health services were likely to receive less funding, which would in turn mean cutting services, the ACCHO sector advocated for 'grandfathering', meaning that health services receiving funding above that which was calculated by the formula should have their funding remain at the current level. The government has agreed to this and increased the allocation for ACCHOs over the following three years. Whether the funding will then be capped at this level remains to be seen.

Commonwealth funding for Aboriginal health is currently defective in two ways: first, the funding is insufficient; and second, the funding that is available is not spent well. In 2013–14, Commonwealth health funding for Aboriginal people was $1.21 for every $1 spent on every non-Aboriginal person; at state and territory level, it was $2 for every $1 spent on non-Aboriginal Australians.[27] The reason for the relatively higher expenditure at state and territory level is that these governments have responsibility for hospital expenditure, and Aboriginal people are far more likely to be hospitalised than non-Aboriginal Australians. Hospital expenditure for Aboriginal people was 1.9 times higher than that for non-Aboriginal Australians in 2013–14.[28]

There is a pervasive myth, promulgated by some politicians, that too much money is spent on Aboriginal health (recall John Howard: 'it is not just a question of money, because a lot more money has been put into

Aboriginal health'). If there is more spending on Aboriginal health, this is not because the government decides to spend more on improving health for Aboriginal people; it is largely because Aboriginal people are sicker and require more hospitalisation.

Access to primary healthcare is an effective way to reduce hospitalisations. If the Australian Government increased funding for primary healthcare and ensured that the funding went to where it was most effective (the ACCHO sector), rates of hospitalisation—and so hospital expenditure—for Aboriginal people could be expected to decrease. Currently, the government is failing on both these counts.

Medicare funding

Since the 1990s ACCHOs have had another source of income. The national health-insurance program Medicare provides reimbursement to medical practitioners for consultations on a fee-for-service basis. Previously, GPs employed by ACCHOs (which received funding including a budgetary component for GPs' salaries) were not allowed to claim Medicare reimbursement, as this was seen as 'double-dipping'.

In the 1990s it was shown that per capita Medicare payments for medical services to Aboriginal people were significantly less than the per capita payment for services to non-Aboriginal people. Part of the reason for this, of course, was that Aboriginal people receive healthcare from services with salaried GPs (particularly ACCHOs, but also some state- and territory-managed community health services). However, the government decided that this was a gap that should be closed. Consequently, an exemption under subsection 19(2) of the *Health Insurance Act 1973* was legislated that enabled ACCHOs and some remote state- and territory-funded Aboriginal-specific health services to bulk-bill Medicare for services provided, even though their GPs were salaried. In most cases arrangements were made for Medicare reimbursement to be paid to the ACCHO that employed the GP and paid the salary.

This has had the effect of allowing an extra source of funding for ACCHOS. It has, however, also had adverse effects. The Department of Health has used access to Medicare as an excuse not to provide much needed extra funding when requested by ACCHOs; a common response is that they should increase their Medicare income. Medicare was designed to reimburse GPs and other medical practitioners in fee-for-service settings. There is less compatibility between Medicare funding and ACCHOs with the community-health model of providing comprehensive primary healthcare, with salaried multi-disciplinary teams. Increasing reliance on Medicare funding has the effect of shifting ACCHOs away from the community-health model towards a model with a more central role for a GP working on a fee-for-service basis. While policy-makers with a mainstreaming agenda may see this as a good thing, making ACCHOs more like mainstream general practice is destructive of the community-health approach that is so essential to the ACCHO sector.

ACCHOs into the future

The ACCHO sector has now been part of the Australian health system for nearly fifty years. In that time, it has shown itself to be an appropriate and effective way of delivering healthcare to Aboriginal people. Inevitably, there are times when any organisation may experience problems with management and delivery of services; Aboriginal organisations, including ACCHOs, are not immune from this.

ACCHOs may experience problems with organisational and clinical governance. In the case of problems with organisational governance, this may involve excessive interference from the community-elected board of directors. More commonly perhaps, the chief executive officer may make unilateral and inappropriate decisions without sufficient oversight and accountability. Clinical governance problems arise when systems and structures are not sufficiently robust to ensure optimal primary healthcare. This is often a particular problem when there is a high turnover of clinical staff (which itself may be reflection of organisational governance failings).

A paradoxical feature of the ACCHO sector is that the high level of community engagement and employment of local Aboriginal people, while generally beneficial, can also be problematic. It can lead, for example, to concerns among some patients about confidentiality. Most ACCHOs adhere to strict confidentiality principles so, in my experience, the concern is more often based on perception rather than reality, but it is a challenge that ACCHOs must address.

These occasional problems reflect the fact that the autonomy of ACCHOs, which is their strength, can also be a source of vulnerability. The problems can be resolved, however, particularly with early identification and appropriate intervention. The ACCHO sector itself is best placed to do this, particularly through its state-based peak bodies, but there is an understandable tension between respecting the autonomy of local organisations and intervening to assist with managing problems.

A factor contributing to organisational problems is the diminished support from government in the past two decades. The resultant vulnerability of the ACCHO sector within the Australian health system has sometimes led to a defensiveness, which in turn decreases the likelihood of addressing problems. Also, as Morgan Brigg and Jodie Curth-Bibb suggest, the pressure on ACCHOs to adapt to a type of corporate governance has contributed to unrepresentative management structures with ACCHOs. There are inevitably challenges in governance for ACCHOs in negotiating the intercultural space between the Aboriginal community and the settler-colonial state.

ACCHOs are subject to 'long-standing ... prejudices that the settler-state and its agents are purveyors of good governance while Aboriginal people are in need of government's tutelage'.[29] An over-emphasis on corporate governance at the expense of community organisation and participation can lead to overwhelming pressures on ACCHOs. Not only does this situation tend towards a transfer of control from the community to government; corporate governance can also undermine transparency and accountability at the community level. Therefore, ACCHOs are at risk of

> becoming either a) quasi government-controlled health services, limiting the possibilities for effective healthcare and innovation informed by indigenous terms of reference or, b), organisational vehicles through which a small and arguably unrepresentative number of Aboriginal people come to control ACCHSs through a perversion of the corporate model. Both dynamics undermine ACCHSs governance and delivery of health services.[30]

This dynamic is a threat at all levels of the ACCHO sector, including the peak bodies. The national peak body NACCHO, which often deals directly with the federal government, is particularly vulnerable in this regard. It must negotiate the space between, on the one hand, its relationship with and accountability to government, and on the other hand its accountability to its constituent members, the ACCHOs. The philosophy of community control implies that (perhaps more so than for other peak bodies) NACCHO is expected to be guided by decisions made at the community level—at the level of the ACCHOs themselves. This clearly presents difficulties, and NACCHO sometimes attracts criticism from within its membership that it is too close to government.

Overall, however, the Aboriginal organisational sector has managed to negotiate the intercultural space and survive. Today, most organisations function at least adequately, and often remarkably well. The discourse of Aboriginal dysfunction has exaggerated the problems that do exist, giving a false image of the sector. The ACCHO movement emerged as a social movement within the Aboriginal struggle for autonomy and self-determination and has been a remarkable innovation in Australian healthcare. It is deserving of celebration and support, which has not always been forthcoming.

Since the turn of the century health policy has been too often based on an antipathy to the Aboriginal organisational sector. It appears that, in the neoliberal phase of Australian settler colonialism, government resistance to Aboriginal autonomy, exemplified by the ACCHO movement, has led to successive governments ignoring the evidence for the most cost-effective investment in improving Aboriginal health and wellbeing. This risks undermining Aboriginal autonomy and Aboriginal civil society. Whether this is a policy goal, or an unintended consequence of misguided policies, is debatable.

There are some tentative signs of a change in attitude within the Australian Government. Very early in the Covid-19 pandemic, there was an effective collaboration between the Australian Government and the ACCHO sector. This contributed to the low rates of morbidity and mortality in Aboriginal communities, at least during 2020. That the government performed so poorly with regard to other areas—such as aged care, quarantine and the vaccine rollout—makes its engagement with the ACCHO sector even more remarkable. It is perhaps an indication that the federal Department of Health has regained a greater understanding of the important role that ACCHOs play. I am unsure that there would have been the same level of engagement from the Australian Government ten or twenty years earlier.

Another positive sign suggesting a change in direction at the federal level occurred in late 2019 when the Australian Government agreed that the Aboriginal organisational sector should be included at meetings of the Council of Australian Governments (COAG) when Aboriginal affairs are on the table. Unfortunately, not long afterwards the pandemic overtook events and COAG was superseded by the National Cabinet.

Whether in the post-Covid era there will be greater government support for the ACCHO sector remains to be seen. What we can expect is that Aboriginal people and their communities and organisations will continue to struggle for autonomy and self-determination. The Aboriginal community-controlled health organisational sector, in all areas of Australia including in remote areas, has not only proved to be effective, it has also been remarkably resilient. I consider myself privileged to have been involved with it.

Conclusion

Dignity is more important than penicillin or toilets.
Dr Trevor Cutter, 1978

In this book I have described my experiences working with different Western Desert peoples and given some details about the trajectories of two social movements—the homelands movement and the Aboriginal community-controlled health service movement. By the term 'social movement' I mean collective political actions which develop to address specific issues and which demand that bureaucratic systems enable, rather than constrain, local decision-making. Iris Marion Young identified three categories of social movements: firstly, those that challenge decision-making structures and the right of the powerful to exert their will; secondly, those organising autonomous services; and thirdly, movements of cultural identity. These categories apply to both of the social movements discussed in this book. The first category applies equally to both the Aboriginal community-controlled health organisational movement and the homelands movement; the second category is more dominant in the Aboriginal community-controlled health organisational movement, and the third more dominant in the homelands movement.

Social movements are agents of social autonomy, which emerge from and expand the sphere of civil society—that is, the sphere between individuals and families on the one hand and the state and large corporate institutions on the other. Some commentators suggest that social movements act at the interface between civil society and the state, and this could well apply to the social movements under consideration here. Colonisation of Australia led to major disruptions in Aboriginal society, and the social movements such as the ones described here can be seen as an autonomous struggle by Aboriginal peoples to develop their civil society within the Australian settler-colonial state and the economy in which they are now embedded.

The bureaucratic state, however, tends to absorb or destroy social movements, particularly in situations like settler colonialism where authority and sovereignty is contested. This tendency has certainly been occurring in Australia but so far these social movements have been able to resist complete absorption or destruction. In the 1970s, when the social movements were developing, government policy reflected the social-democratic approach of the time and, after some initial resistance, it became supportive of the movements, to an extent. There were always limits to government support but, in general, it persisted for about a quarter of a century, regardless of which party was in power in Canberra. Around the turn of the twenty-first century, coinciding with the developing hegemony of neoliberalism, there was another policy shift, heralding a return to policies reminiscent of the so-called assimilation era. By then, however, both the homelands movement and the ACCHO movement had made significant gains and were able to maintain themselves in a more hostile, or at best ambiguous, policy context.

From a neoliberal perspective, the role of the government is to either get out of the way of the market or facilitate, subsidise and provide security for free-market mechanisms. Civil society, as a sphere of action with relative autonomy from both the state and the market, is viewed from this perspective as an obstacle to these mechanisms. There is little consideration for social justice in this perspective; according to Hayek, the guru of neoliberalism, social justice is a 'mirage'.

The social engineering solutions to the 'Aboriginal problem' proposed by neoliberal commentators are far removed from any connection with community and cultural fit. It may appear paradoxical that neoliberal institutions, despite the advocacy of 'small government', have encouraged and supported increased government intervention in Aboriginal lives but, in neoliberal ideology, if a group of people seem intransigent to absorption into the free market it is seen as a government responsibility to apply disciplinary measures to facilitate this absorption. In the settler-colonial context in remote Aboriginal communities, this may have the added attraction to free-market fundamentalists of freeing up large areas of land for extractive capitalist profits.

The unwillingness to support Aboriginal aspirations for autonomy demonstrates that more is at play than just the obvious and continuing failure of bureaucracies to understand and utilise the local knowledge needed for successful Aboriginal programs. More significantly, the neoliberal narrative has contributed to a new phase in the structure of settler colonialism in Australia, which has profound consequences for the future wellbeing of Aboriginal people. Under neoliberalism and the extension of market relations into the social sphere,

> the state itself has become morally authoritative and entitled. It makes demands of citizens—that they pay their dues, minimise their risk to society and mitigate their burden on the state through self-reliance. In this task the neoliberal state ... offers assistance through capacity-building, but always with the threat of coercion if this capacity is not forthcoming.[1]

It appears that it is the confluence of neoliberalism and the ongoing settler-colonial project that is particularly damaging to Aboriginal civil society. Patrick Wolfe has suggested that settler colonialism is driven by a 'logic of elimination' that works to relocate Aboriginal people from their land and culture. In my time working in the Western Desert, particularly in more recent years, I have seen this logic of elimination at work in two different ways. Too often punitive policies enacted in response to the homelands movement and the continual threats of community closures have appeared as examples of the desire to remove Aboriginal people from their land. Recent Aboriginal health policies often appear to be another instance of the 'logic of elimination' at work, aiming to bypass or undermine Aboriginal organisations, to eliminate Aboriginal efforts to develop their own civil society and forms of citizenship.

The Canadian First Nations scholar Glenn Sean Coulthard argues that, despite changes in the governance structure of settler colonisation over the last fifty years, Canadian settler colonialism remains structurally oriented around achieving the same effect: 'the dispossession of Indigenous peoples of their land and self-determining authority'. He further argues that

Conclusion

> In settler-colonial contexts such as Canada ... state-sanctioned approaches to reconciliation tend to ideologically fabricate such a transition by narrowly situating the abuses of settler colonization firmly in the past. In these situations, reconciliation itself becomes temporally framed as the process of individually and collectively overcoming the harmful 'legacy' left in the wake of past abuse, while *leaving the present structure of colonial rule largely unscathed.*[2]

The same arguments may be applied in Australia. The academic Sarah Maddison has analysed the reasons for the ongoing failure of Australian governments to adequately address the consequences of settler colonialism on Aboriginal peoples. She concludes that 'answers to the dilemmas of settler colonialism cannot be found *within* the settler state. If there are answers to these seemingly entrenched issues—and I believe there are—they can only be located outside of settler control in the hands of Aboriginal and Torres Strait Islander people themselves.'[3]

The longer I have worked in the area of Aboriginal health, the more I have become convinced of the fundamental importance of First Nations' autonomy and self-determination as a necessary pre-condition for Aboriginal people achieving the standard of health to which they are entitled. This is a significant challenge in the contemporary context, and whilst I do not have a great deal of confidence in our current major political parties to lead the way, I do have some confidence that the Australian people can urge governments in the right direction, as they have with other areas of social policy in recent years.

Settler colonialism is not something confined to the past. For Patrick Wolfe, in an oft-repeated quotation, 'invasion is a structure, not an event'. The Aboriginal struggle for autonomy is ongoing, and at the time of writing this book, justice and autonomy for the Aboriginal people of the Western Desert is as remote as it ever has been during the forty years I have known them.

Notes

Introduction
1 Tonkinson, 1974, p. 41.
2 Macoun, p. 95.

1 Alice Springs and out bush: A time of Utopian idealism
1 The early history of Congress can be found in Rosewarne, Vaarzon-Morel, Bell, et al.
2 Tracker, who passed away in 2015, is the subject of a Stella Prize–winning biography by Alexis Wright.
3 The question of why Aboriginal people should have their own health services is an ongoing one. In 1985 I had a letter published in the *Medical Journal of Australia* responding to a previous letter asking that very question. The reasons I believe there is a need for Aboriginal health services are outlined in chapter 9.
4 Bowman, p. 77.
5 McDermott, O'Dea, Rowley, et al.
6 Rowley, O'Dea, Anderson, et al.

2 The Pitjantjatjara and Ngaanyatjarra homelands
1 Gara, 2003a.
2 Ibid.
3 Elkin, 1931, p. 49.
4 Elkin, 1934.
5 Kerin, p. 28.
6 Ibid.
7 Brooks and Plant, p. 124.
8 Quoted in Tynan, p. 75.
9 Quoted in Morton, p. 71.
10 Quoted in Morton, p. 72.
11 Ibid.
12 Milliken, p. 206.
13 Ibid., p. 94.
14 Quoted in Morton, p. 85.

15 Tynan, p. 188.
16 Milliken, p. 106.
17 Ibid., p. 258.
18 Grayden, p. 41.
19 Ibid., p. 68.
20 Haebich, p. 1040.
21 Grayden, p. 174.
22 Royal Commission into the British Nuclear Tests, paras 1322–1324.
23 Ibid., para 1335.
24 Edwards, 2016, p. 26.
25 Verburgt, p. 20.

3   The Pitjantjatjara home-made health service

1 Intra-peritoneal infusion is rarely used nowadays; if intravenous access is not achieved, inter-osseous infusion (a needle into the bone marrow) is used. This technique was not used at the time I was employed by the PHHS.
2 https://www.youtube.com/watch?v=Y761eAKOUMI
3 *Malpa* means friend; in referring to the '*malpa* system' Ushma meant the system that developed whereby a non-Aboriginal worker often had a friend or mate to work with as cultural guide and mentor. In my case, my *malpa* was Bobby Daniels.
4 The Radford Report was a government-commissioned evaluation of the three remote Aboriginal community-controlled health services which had commenced in 1977–78 (PHHS, Urapuntja Health Service and Lyappa Medical Service). The evaluation was completed in 1981, after my departure from the PHHS.

4   The Strelley mob and the *Martu*

1 Tonkinson, 1974, p. 32.
2 A comprehensive history of the pastoral workers' struggle and Don McLeod's involvement can be found in A. Scrimgeour, 2015. See also Wilson, McLeod and Noakes.
3 Clancy's story can be found in Palmer and McKenna.
4 A. Scrimgeour, 2014, p. 96.
5 Ibid., p. 100.
6 The story of the impact of Cold War on the *Martu* can be found in the official history of the Woomera Rocket Establishment (Morton) and, from a *Martu* perspective, in Davenport, Johnson and Yuwali.

7 Tonkinson, 1977, p. 71.
8 I believe this was due to the term *Panaka* becoming *nyaparu*, meaning that the word was to be avoided as it resembled the name of somebody who had died.
9 This point was conveyed to me by Robyn Withnell in a personal communication.
10 McLeod, p. 123.
11 Hale and Scrimgeour, p. 127.
12 The reason the homestead was given this name is contested. One story has it that during WWII the station manager's wife, Christina Gordon, known as 'the Missus', ran the station single-handedly, living in the homestead. Another story is that another station manager's wife in the pre-war years rarely left the homestead, back in the days when *Marrngu* worked there under the old regime.
13 Noakes.
14 Wright, p. 405.
15 I experienced an example of Don McLeod's antipathy towards the national Aboriginal leadership when (or just after) I was living at Strelley. I had encouraged the affiliation of SRAMS with the National Aboriginal and Islander Health Organisation (NAIHO), as I believed this would assist with supporting the developing health service and I attended a NAIHO meeting with Snowy Jittermarra. After I left Strelley, Don accused me of being a 'NAIHO mole', an accusation he subsequently withdrew after I discussed it with him. However, Don's disapproval of my attempts at an alliance with NAIHO was an indication of his suspicion of alliances with other Aboriginal activist organisations. He was not a man for alliances.

5   Pintupi country, Pintupi health

1 Giles, p. 27.
2 Kimber, p. 3.
3 See Holcombe.
4 Long, p. 33.
5 Nathan and Leichleitner, p. 36.
6 F. Myers, personal communication.
7 Kimber, p. 29.
8 Myers, 2016, p. 85.
9 Myers, 1986, p. 41.
10 Rob Amery, personal communication.
11 Stead, Kimber, Hempel and Styles, p. 15.

6 The Spinifex people

1. 'Spinifex' or hummock grass is a widespread ground cover throughout much of Central Australia including the Great Victoria Desert. The term is used for a number of different species of hummock grass, particularly of the genus *Triodia*, and is not actually true spinifex (genus *Spinifex*) which occurs only on coastal dunes (Shephard, p. 41).
2. Sources for early contact history of the Spinifex people include Brady; Cane, 2002; Gara, 2017 and Townley.
3. Gara, 2017, p. 357.
4. All Carlisle's citations are from Townley, pp. 92–5.
5. Gara, 2017, p. 362.
6. As discussed in chapter 2, the 'major trials' were conducted in 1956–57, and the so-called 'minor trials' continued until 1963.
7. Tynan, p. 193.
8. Cane, 1994.
9. Ibid.
10. Ibid.
11. The name of the program was later changed to Medical Outreach—Indigenous Chronic Disease Program (MOICDP).

7 First contact, last contact

1. For example, Bird-David et al., Kaplan.
2. For example, Gammage, Pascoe.
3. Dunbar, p. 305.
4. Brody, p. 150.
5. Quoted in Kirk, p. 171.
6. Kirk, p. 173.
7. Kimber, p. 26.
8. Toohey, p. 34.
9. The surname Richter was chosen for the family because the old man had two brothers living at Irrunytju who had been given the English surname Richter.
10. Trusswell; Trusswell and Hansen.
11. Littlejohn, Davies et al.
12. Elphinstone and Drummond.

8 The reoccupation of the Western Desert and the counter-attack

1. See Peterson and Myers, p. 9. Just as the election of the Whitlam Labor government may be seen as a watershed in Aboriginal affairs, so may be the election of the Howard Coalition government in 1998—albeit of a very different kind. While it may be noted that it was a Labor government which was responsible for the initial reforms in 1972, and a conservative government which introduced a change of direction a quarter of a century later, it should also be noted that in both cases, once these changes were introduced, they subsequently had bipartisan support from both major political parties.
2. Coombs, 1978; Coombs, 1994; Rowse, 2000.
3. Peterson and Myers, p. 2. While I suggest below that this definition is too limited, and that this has policy implications, it should be noted that the book edited by Peterson and Myers presents a much wider range of social arrangements of 'outstations'. Indeed, the title of their book, *Experiments in Self-determination*, reflects what I argue here: that this social movement was an assertion of autonomy in which people experimented with new living arrangements.
4. R. Dunbar, 2003; Earl et al.
5. This tendency is discussed in Myers, 2016.
6. See, inter alia, Coombs, 1978; Nathan and Leichleitner.
7. According to Elizabeth Strakosch, neoliberalism 'celebrates the self-reliant individual and denounces the regulation of such individuals as unproductive. However it simultaneously allows increased coercion by the state where individuals or groups are deemed to lack appropriate capacities'. See Strakosch.
8. Rowse, 2012, p. 130.
9. Ibid., p. 132.
10. Pearson, 2017.
11. It should be noted that Sutton's critique was not unchallenged by his anthropological colleagues, as, for example, in many of the articles in Altman and Hinkson.
12. Sutton, 2009, pp. 85, 141.
13. Pearson, 2009.
14. Gibson.
15. Rowse, 2012, p. 139.
16. Hinkson, p. 6.

17   Behrendt, p. 18.
18   Sanderson, p. 35.
19   See Jordan.
20   Altman, 2017.
21   Biddle, 2009.
22   Sammut, p. 9.
23   I did not express the view that people in the homelands are 'generally much better than those in the towns'. This misreading was made by a Melbourne-based anthropologist in an attempt to attribute some of the problems existing in remote Aboriginal communities on confused thinking by 'White anti-racists', among whom, presumably, she included me (Kowal, 2010, footnote 10).
24   Biddle, 2013b, p. 19.
25   Biddle, 2013a, p. 14.
26   Rowley, O'Dea, Anderson, et al.
27   Vanstone, 2007, p. 45.
28   van Beuren, Worland, Svanberg and Lassen.
29   Burgess, Johnston, et al.
30   Campbell, Burgess, et al.
31   Social Ventures Australia, p. 4.

9   Autonomy in Aboriginal health and the government response

1   See Foley.
2   Howard-Wagner, p. 225.
3   Sullivan p. 55.
4   Ibid., p. 50.
5   In the Australian settler-colonial context, however, it is possible that the principle of subsidiarity may be used against the interests of Aboriginal communities. An example can be seen with the establishment by the Australian Government in recent years of regional primary healthcare organisations (originally called General Practice Divisions, then Medicare Locals, then Primary Health Networks). These were designed to make decisions about funding primary healthcare activities at the regional level, exemplifying the principle of subsidiarity (see J. Dunbar). Primary Health Networks, when given primary healthcare funding responsibility at a regional level, do not necessarily direct funds specifically identified for Aboriginal health to Aboriginal organisations, even though ACCHOs

will usually be the most cost-effective way of delivering services. Regional non-Aboriginal structures may be more likely to demonstrate prejudice and racial discrimination in their decision-making than more distant entities. Consequently, for the principle of subsidiarity to be appropriate for Aboriginal policy, there must also be respect for Aboriginal autonomy and cultural security.

6   Houston, p. 166.

7   On a personal level, I consider my work in ACCHOs as community health practice. When I started working in Aboriginal health, I was employed as a general practitioner but over time realised that by working in a community organisation my role went beyond individual healthcare. I subsequently obtained qualifications in public health, the health of populations, which I operationalise at the community level. I consider that the combination of general practice and public health I apply in my practice makes me a community health practitioner.

8   The advantages of a more social approach to medical consultations are obvious and there is an increasing recognition within the Australian general practice community that such an approach is desirable. However, fee-for-service, and the funding system for general practice involving Medicare reimbursements, continues to encourage an individual rather than a social approach. There have been some recent efforts to introduce changes to Medicare funding which takes a more social approach but at the same time the community healthcare model which has existed in ACCHOs is being forced towards a more individualised approach (see below).

9   See for example Otim.

10   Sullivan, 2011, p. 51.

11   Quoted in Strakosch, 2015, p. 124.

12   Vanstone, 2005.

13   Quoted in Strakosch, 2015, p. 115.

14   Reported by AAP.

15   Walker, et al., p. 5.

16   Sullivan, 2018, p. 203.

17   Sullivan, 2011, pp. 67, 70.

18   Ibid., p. 205.

19   Howard-Wagner, p. 230.

20   Dwyer, et al.

21   Sullivan, 2011, p. 62.

22   Henry, Houston and Mooney.

23 Divisions of General Practice (also known as GP Divisions) were created by the Commonwealth health department in 1992, to develop better co-ordination of primary healthcare services in a particular region. In 2010 the Labor government replaced the Divisions by a new form of primary healthcare organisation confusingly named 'Medicare Locals'. In 2015 the Coalition government replaced and consolidated the 62 Medicare Locals with 32 Primary Health Networks, each covering a larger area. PHNs continue to receive funding which might be better directed to ACCHOs.
24 Couzos and Delaney-Thiele.
25 In a letter to *Quarterly Essay* responding to a critique of neoliberalism, the former head of the Australian Public Service Michael Keating admitted that 'too often the use of a commercial consultancy firm results in the government getting the sort of analysis and advice that it wants to receive rather than frank and fearless advice, as the consultant wants to please in order to gain another contract' (Keating, 2018, p. 122).
26 Sullivan, 2011, pp. 47, 33.
27 AHMAC, 2017.
28 Ibid.
29 Brigg and Curth-Bibb, p. 202.
30 Ibid., p. 200.

Conclusion

1 Strakosch, p. 25.
2 Coulthard, loc. 591, my italics.
3 Maddison, p. 234.

Bibliography

AAP (10 December 2004), 'Howard "unhappy" with Aboriginal health', *The Age*.
AHMAC (2004), *Cultural Respect Framework for Aboriginal and Torres Strait Islander Health*, Canberra, ACT.
AHMAC (2017), *Aboriginal and Torres Strait Islander Health Performance Framework 2017 Report*, Canberra, ACT.
Altman, J. (2017), 'Modern slavery in remote Australia?' *Arena*, 150: 12–15.
Altman, J. and Hinkson, M. (eds) (2007), *Coercive Reconciliation: Stabilise, Normalise, Exit Aboriginal Australia*, North Carlton, Vic.: Arena Publications.
Altman, J. and Hinkson, M. (eds) (2010), *Culture Crisis: Anthropology and Politics in Aboriginal Australia*, Sydney, NSW: University of New South Wales Press.
Anderson, H. and Kowal, E. (2007), 'Culture, history and health in an Australian Aboriginal community: The case of Utopia', *Medical Anthropology*, 31(5): 438–57.
Australian National Audit Office (2017), *Indigenous Advancement Strategy*, Canberra, ACT.
Batty, P. (ed.) (2006), *Colliding Worlds: First Contact in the Western Desert 1932–1984*, Melbourne, Vic.: Museum Victoria.
Behrendt, L. (2007), 'The emergency we had to have', in J. Altman and M. Hinkson (eds), *Coercive Reconciliation: Stabilise, Normalise, Exit Aboriginal Australia*, North Carlton, Vic.: Arena Publications, pp. 15–20.
Berndt, R. (1959), 'The concept of "The Tribe" in the Western Desert of Australia', *Oceania*, 30(2): 81–107.
Berndt, R. and Berndt, C. (1942), 'A preliminary report of field work in the Ooldea region, western South Australia', *Oceania*, 12(4): 305–30.
Biddle, N. (2009), *The Geography and Demography of Indigenous Migration: Insights for Policy and Planning*, Canberra, ACT: Australian National University, Centre for Aboriginal Economic Policy Research.
Biddle, N. (2013a), *CAEPR Indigenous Population Project: Income*. Canberra, ACT: Australian National University, Centre for Aboriginal Economic Policy Research.
Biddle, N. (2013b), *CAEPR Indigenous Population Project: Socioeconomic Outcomes*. Canberra, ACT: Australian National University, Centre for Aboriginal Economic Policy Research.
Bird, D., Bird, R.B. and Parker, C. (2005), 'Aboriginal burning regimes and hunting strategies in Australia's Western Desert', *Human Ecology*, 33(4): 443–65.

Bird-David, N., et al. (1992), 'Beyond "the original affluent society": A culturalist reformulation', *Current Anthropology*, 33(1): 25–47.

Bowman, M. (2015), *Every Hill Got a Story*, Richmond, Vic.: Hardie Grant Books.

Brigg, M. and Curth-Bibb, J. (2017), 'Recalibrating intercultural governance in Australian Indigenous organisations: The case of Aboriginal community-controlled health', *Australian Journal of Political Science*, 52(2): 199–217.

Britt, H., et al. (2003), *General Practice Activity in Australia 2002–2003*, Canberra, ACT: Australian Institute of Health and Welfare.

Brady, M. (1986), 'Leaving the spinifex: The impact of rations, missions, and the atomic tests on the southern Pitjantjatjara', *Records of the South Australian Museum*, 20: 35–45.

Brody, H. (2000), *The Other Side of Eden: Hunters, Farmers, and the Shaping of the World*, New York, NY: North Point Press.

Brooks, D. and Plant, V. (2016), 'Out of sight, out of mind, but making the best of it: How outstaions have worked on the Ngaanyatjarra Lands', in N. Peterson and F. Myers, *Experiments in Self-determination: Histories of the Outstation Movement in Australia*, Canberra, ACT: ANU Press, pp. 121–34.

Brough, M. (2006), *Blueprint for Action in Indigenous Affairs* (speech).

Burgess, C. and Johnston, F., et al. (2009), 'Healthy country, healthy people: The relationship between Indigenous health status and "caring for country"', *Medical Journal of Australia*, 190(10): 567–72.

Campbell, D., Burgess, C., et al. (2011), 'Potential primary healthcare savings for chronic disease care associated with Australian Aboriginal involvement in land management', *Health Policy*, 99(1): 83–9.

Campbell, M., et al. (2017), 'Contribution of Aboriginal community-controlled health services to improving Aboriginal health: An evidence review', *Australian Health Review*, 42(2): 218–16.

Cane, S. (1994), *The Spinifex People: Community Development at Tjuntjuntjara, Ilkurlka and Tuwan*, Kalgoorlie, WA.

Cane, S. (2002), *Pila Nguru: The Spinifex People*, North Fermantle, WA: Fremantle Arts Centre Press.

Commonwealth Grants Commission (2001), *The Indigenous Funding Inquiry*, Canberra, ACT: ATSIC.

Coombs, H.C. (1978), *Kulinma*, Canberra, ACT: ANU Press.

Coombs, H.C. (1994), *Aboriginal Autonomy: Issues and Strategies*, Cambridge UK: Cambridge University Press.

Coulthard, G. (2014), *Red Skins, White Masks: Rejecting the Colonial Politics of Recognition*, Minneapolis, MN: University of Minnesota Press.

Couzos, S. and Delaney-Thiele, D. (2009), 'Closing the gap depends on ACCHSs', *Medical Journal of Australia*, 190(10): 541.

Craig, P. (2002), *Access of Urban Indigenous Populations into Local Primary Healthcare Services*, Sydney, NSW: University of New South Wales, Centre for Health Equity Research and Evaluation.

Crawford, H. and Biddle, N. (2017), *Changing Associations of Selected Social Determinants with Aboriginal and Torres Strait Islander Health and Wellbeing, 2002 to 2012–13*, Canberra, ACT: Australian National University, Centre for Aboriginal Economic Policy Research.

Cutter, T. (1976), *Report on Community Health Model: Health by the People*, Alice Springs, NT: Central Australian Aboriginal Congress.

Davenport, S., Johnson, P. and Yuwali (2005), *Cleared Out: First Contact in the Western Desert*, Canberra, ACT: Aboriginal Studies Press.

Downing, J. (1988), *Ngurra Walytja: Country of My Spirit*, Darwin, NT: ANU North Australia Research Unit.

Duguid, C. (1972), *Doctor and the Aborigines*, Adelaide, SA: Rigby.

Dunbar, J. (2011), 'When big isn't beautiful: Lessons from England and Scotland on primary healthcare organizations', *Medical Journal of Australia*, 195(4): 219–21.

Dunbar, R. (2003), 'The social brain: Mind, language and society in evolutionary perspective', *Annual Review of Anthropology*, 32: 163–81.

Dunbar, R. (2014), *Human Evolution*, London, UK: Penguin Books.

Dwyer, J., O'Donnell, K., Lavoie, J., Marlina, U. and Sullivan, P. (2009), *The Overburden Report: Contracting for Indigenous Health Services*, Darwin, NT: Cooperative Research Centre for Aboriginal Health.

Earl, T., Gamble, C. and Poinar, H. (2011), 'Migration', in A. Shryock and D. Lord Smail (eds), *Deep History: The Architecture of the Past and Present*, Berkeley, CA: University of California Press, pp. 191–218.

Edwards, W. (1992), 'Patterns of Aboriginal residence in the north-west of South Australia', *Journal of the Anthropological Society of South Australia*, 30(1): 2–32.

Edwards, W. (2016), 'From Coombes to Coombs: Reflections on the Pitjantjatjara outstation movement', in N. Peterson and F. Myers, *Experiments in Self-determination: Histories of the Outstation Movement in Australia*, Acton, ACT: ANU Press.

Elkin, A.P. (1931), 'The social organization of South Australian tribes', *Oceania*, 2(1): 44–73.

Elkin, A.P. (1934), *Missionary Policy for Primitive Peoples*, Morpeth, NSW: St John's College Press.

Elphinstone, J. and A. Drummond (1964), 'Health of natives in the Sandy Desert of Western Australia', *Report of Commissioner of Public Health Western Australia, Appendix XV*, Perth, WA: Government Printer.

Foley, G. (1982), 'Aboriginal community-controlled health services: A short history', *Aboriginal Health Project Information Bulletin*, 2: 13–15.

Gammage, B. (2011), *The Biggest Estate on Earth: How Aborigines Made Australia*, Sydney, Melbourne, Auckland and London: Allen & Unwin.

Gara, T. (2003a), 'Desert myths: Caves of gold and lost reefs', Brock Memorial Lecture, Royal Geographical Society of South Australia (unpublished).

Gara, T. (2003b), 'Explorers and prospectors', *Trust*, Warburton, WA: Warburton Arts Project (WAP Press), pp. 15–23.

Gara, T. (2017), 'Ooldea, the Spinifex people and the bomb', in P. Brock and T. Gara (eds), *Colonialism and its Aftermath: A History of Aboriginal South Australia*, Adelaide, SA: Wakefield Press.

Gibson, J. (22 November 2007), 'Book sent to department to match Brough's policy', *Sydney Morning Herald*.

Giles, E. (1889), *Australia Twice Traversed: The Romance of Exploration* (vol. 2), London, UK: Sampson Low, Marson, Searle & Rivington.

Grayden, W. (1957), *Adam and Atoms*, Perth, WA: Frank Daniels Pty Ltd.

Greaber, D. and Wengrow, D. (2021), *The Dawn of Everything: A New History of Humanity*, London, UK: Allen Lane.

Hackett, C. (1936), *Boomerang Leg and Yaws in Australian Aborigines*, London, UK: Royal Society of Tropical Medicine and Hygiene.

Hale, M. and Scrimgeour, A. (2012), *Kurlumarniny: We Come from the Desert*, Canberra, ACT: Aboriginal Studies Press.

Hamilton, A. (1971), 'Socio-cultural factors in health among the Pitjantjatjara: A preliminary report' (mimeograph).

Henry, B., Houston, S. and Mooney, G. (2004), 'Institutional racism in Australian healthcare: A plea for decency', *Medical Journal of Australia*, 180(10): 517–20.

Hinkson, M. (2007), 'Introduction: In the name of the child', in J. Altman and M. Hinkson (eds), *Coercive Reconciliation: Stabilise, Normalise, Exit Aboriginal Australia*, North Carlton, Vic.: Arena Publications, pp. 1–14.

Holcombe, S. (2004), 'The politico-historical construction of the Pintupi-Luritja and the concept of tribe', *Oceania*, 74: 257–75.

Houston, S. (2004), 'The past, the present and the future of Aboriginal health policy', Perth, WA: Curtin University, Department of Economics (PhD thesis).

Howard-Wagner, D. (2018), 'Aboriginal organisations, self-determination and the neoliberal age: A case study of how "the game has changed" for Aboriginal organisations in Newcastle', in D. Howard-Wagner, M. Bargh and I. Altamirano-Jimenez (eds), *The Neoliberal State, Recognition and Indigenous Rights: New Paternalism to New Imaginings*, Canberra, ACT: ANU Press, pp. 217–37.

Hughes, H. (2007), *Lands of Shame*, Sydney: Centre for Independent Studies.

Hughes, H. and Warin, J. (2005), *A New Deal for Aborigines and Torres Strait Islanders in Remote Communities*, Sydney, NSW: Centre for Independent Studies.

Hunt, J. (2018), *'Normalising' Aboriginal Housing in the Kimberley: Challenges at the Interface of New Public Management Approaches*, Working Paper No. 123/2018, Canberra, ACT: Australian National University, Centre for Aboriginal Economic Policy Research.

Johns, G. (2006), 'Social stability and structural adjustment', Paper presented at the Bennelong Society Sixth Annual Conference: Leaving Remote Communities, Melbourne, Vic.

Jordan, K. (ed.) (2016), *Better Than Welfare? Work and Livelihoods for Indigenous Australians after CDEP*, Acton, ACT: ANU Press.

Kaplan, D. (2000), 'The darker side of the "original affluent society"', *Journal of Anthropological Research*, 56(3): 301–24.

Keating, M. (2018), *Quarterly Essay*, vol. 71, Carlton, Vic.: Black Inc., pp. 119–26 (correspondence).

Kerin, R. (2011), *Doctor Do-good: Charles Duguid and Aboriginal Advancement 1930s–1970s*, North Melbourne, Vic.: Australian Scholarly Publishing.

Kimber, R.G. (1982), *The Pintubi of the Kintore Ranges 1982: Historical Survey*, Alice Springs, NT.

Kirk, R. (1983), *Aboriginal Man Adapting*, Melbourne, Vic.: Oxford University Press.

Kowal, E. (2010), 'Is culture the problem or the solution?', in J. Altman and M. Hinkson (eds), *Culture Crisis: Anthropology and Politics in Aboriginal Australia*, Randwick, NSW: UNSW Press.

Kunitz, S. and Brady, M. (1995), 'Health care policy for Aboriginal Australians: The relevance of the American experience', *Australian Journal of Public Health*, 19(6): 549–58.

Larkins, S., et al. (2006), 'Consultations in general practice and at an Aboriginal community-controlled health service: Do they differ?' *Rural Remote Health*, 560: 1–12.

Lavoie, J. (2004), 'Governed by contracts: The development of Indigenous primary healthcare', *Journal of Aboriginal Health*, 1: 6–24.

Lea, T. (2020), *Wild Policy: Indigeneity and the Unruly Logics of Intervention*, Stanford, Ca: Stanford University Press.

Lee, R. and DeVore, I. (eds) (1968), *Man the Hunter*, Chicago, Ill: Aldine Publishing Company.

Littlejohn, M., et al. (2014), 'Molecular virology of hepatitis B virus, sub-genotype C4 in Northern Australian Indigenous populations', *Journal of Medical Virology*, 86(4): 695–706.

Long, J. (2006), 'Meetings with strangers', in P. Batty (ed.), *Colliding Worlds: First Contact in the Western Desert 1932–1984*, Melbourne, Vic.: Museum Victoria, pp. 30–36.

McAuley, I. and Menadue, J. (2007), *A Health Policy for Australia: Reclaiming Universal Healthcare*, Sydney, NSW: Centre for Policy Development.

McDermott, R., O'Dea, K. and Rowley, K., et al. (1998), 'Beneficial impact of Homelands Movement on health outcomes in Central Australian Aborigines', *Australian and New Zealand Journal of Public Health*, 22(6): 653–8.

McLelland, J.R. (1985), *The Report of the Royal Commission into the British Nuclear Tests in Australia: Aboriginal Coalition*, Canberra, ACT: Australian Government Publishing Service.

McLeod, D. (1984), *How the West Was Lost*, Port Hedland, WA: self-published.

Macoun, A. (2016), 'Colonising white innocence: Complicity and critical encounters', chapter 6 in S. Maddison, et al., *The Limits of Settler Colonial Reconciliation*, Singapore: Springer, pp. 85–102.

Maddison, S. (2019), *The Colonial Fantasy: Why Australia Can't Solve Black Problems*, Crows Nest, NSW: Allen & Unwin.

Markham, F. and Biddle, N. (2018), *Income, Poverty and Inequality*, Canberra, ACT: Australian National University, Centre for Aboriginal Economic Policy Research.

Marmot, M. (2003), 'Self-esteem and health: Autonomy, self-esteem and health are linked together', *British Medical Journal*, 327: 574–5.

Milliken, R. (1986), *No Conceivable Injury: The Story of Britain and Australia's Atomic Cover-up*, Ringwood, Vic.: Penguin Books Australia.

Morice, R. (1976), 'Women Dancing Dreaming', *Medical Journal of Australia*, 76(2): 939–41.

Morton, P. (1989), *Fire Across the Desert: Woomera and the Anglo-Australian Joint Project 1946–1980*, Canberra, ACT: Australian Government Publishing Service.

Myers, F. (1986), *Pintupi Country, Pintupi Self: Sentiment, Place and Politics Among Western Desert Aborigines*, Washington, DC: Smithsonian Institute Press.

Myers, F. (2016), 'History, memory and the politics of self-determination at an early outstation', in N. Peterson and F. Myers (eds), *Experiments in Self-determination: Histories of the Outstation Movement in Australia*, Canberra, ACT: ANU Press, pp. 81–104.

Nathan, P. and Leichleitner, D. (1983), *Settle Down Country: Pmere Arlaltyewele*, Melbourne, Vic.: Kibble Books.

National Aboriginal Health Strategy Working Party (1989), *Report of the National Aboriginal Health Strategy Working Party*, Canberra, ACT.

Noakes, D. (1987), *How the West Was Lost: The Story of the 1946 Aboriginal Pastoral Workers' Strike*, Mitchell, ACT: Ronin Films (film).

Northern Territory Board of Inquiry into the Protection of Aboriginal Children from Sexual Abuse (2007), *Ampe Akelyernemane Meke Mekarle: "Little Children are Sacred": Report of the Northern Territory Board of Inquiry into the Protection of Aboriginal Children from Sexual Abuse*, Northern Territory Government.

O'Brien, G. and Plooij, D. (1973), *Culture Training Manual for Medical Workers in Aboriginal Communities*, Adelaide, SA: Flinders University, School of Social Sciences.

Ong, K., et al. (2012), 'Differences in primary healthcare delivery to Australia's Indigenous population: A template for use in economic evaluations', *BMC Health Services Research*, 12: 307.

Otim, M. (2001), *Indigenous Health Economics and Policy Research*, Discussion Paper No. 4. Melbourne, Vic.: University of Melbourne, VicHealth Koori Health Research and Community Development Unit.

Palmer, K. and McKenna, C. (1978), *Somewhere Between Black and White*, Melbourne, Vic.: Macmillan.

Panaretto, K., et al. (2014), 'Aboriginal community-controlled health services: Leading the way in primary care', *Medical Journal of Australia*, 200(11).

Parkinson, A. (2007), *Maralinga: Australia's Nuclear Waste Cover-up*, Sydney, NSW: ABC Books.

Pascoe, B. (2018), *Dark Emu: Aboriginal Australia and the Birth of Agriculture.* Melbourne, Vic.: Scribe Publications.

Pearson, N. (2000), *Our Right to Take Responsibility*, Cairns, Qld: Noel Pearson & Associates.

Pearson, N. (2009), *Radical Hope: Education and Equality in Australia*, Melbourne, Vic.: Black Inc.

Pearson, N. (2017), 'Betrayal', *The Monthly*, December/January: 24–34.

Peiris D., et al. (2012), 'The Treatment of cardiovascular Risk in Primary care using Electronic Decision suppOrt (TORPEDO) study: Intervention development and protocol for a cluster randomised, controlled trial of an electronic decision support and quality improvement intervention in Australian primary healthcare', *BMJ Open*, 2(6).

Peterson, N. and Myers, F. (2016), 'The origins and history of outstations as Aboriginal life projects', in N. Peterson and F. Myers (eds), *Experiments in Self-determination: Histories of the Outstation Movement in Australia*, Canberra, ACT: ANU Press, pp. 1–24.

Phillips, C., et al. (2010), 'Can clinical governance deliver quality improvement in Australian general practice and primary care? A systematic review of the evidence', *Medical Journal of Australia*, 193(10): 602–7.

Rosewarne, C., Vaarzon-Morel, P., Bell, S., et al. (2007), 'The historical context of developing an Aboriginal community-controlled health service: A social history of the first ten years of the Central Australian Aboriginal Congress', *Aboriginal Health & History*, 9(2): 114–43.

Rowley, K., O'Dea, K. and Anderson, I., et al. (2008), 'Lower than expected mortality for an Australian Aboriginal population: 10-year follow-up in a decentralised community', *Medical Journal of Australia*, 188(5): 283–7.

Rowse, T. (2000), *Obliged to be Different: Nugget Coombs' Legacy in Indigenous Affairs*, Port Melbourne, Vic.: Cambridge University Press.

Rowse, T. (2002), *Indigenous Futures: Choice and Development for Aboriginal and Islander Australia*, Randwick, NSW: UNSW Press.

Rowse, T. (2005), 'The Indigenous sector', in D. Austin-Broos and G. Macdonald, *Culture, Economy and Governance in Aboriginal Australia*, Sydney, NSW: Sydney University Press, pp. 213–30.

Rowse, T. (2012), *Rethinking Social Justice: From 'Peoples' to 'Populations'*, Canberra, ACT: Aboriginal Studies Press.

Sahlins, M. (1972), *Stone Age Economics*, London, UK: Routledge.

Sammut, J. (2016), 'Not so black and white: Stan Grant's nostalgia for injustice', *Quadrant*, June: 20.

Sammut, J. (2017), *The History Wars Matter*, Sydney, NSW: Centre for Independent Studies.

Sanderson, J. (2007), 'Reconciliation and the failure of neo-liberal globalisation', in J. Altman and M. Hinkson (eds), *Coercive Reconciliation: Stabilise, Normalise, Exit Aboriginal Australia*, North Carlton, Vic.: Arena Publications, pp. 31–36.

Schrader, G. (2016), 'The Pipalyatjara Store' (unpublished document).

Scrimgeour, A. (2014), '"We only want our rights and freedom": The Pilbara pastoral workers strike, 1946–49', *History Australia*, 11(2): 79–102.

Scrimgeour, A. (2018), *On Red Earth Walking: The Pilbara Aboriginal Strike 1946–1949*, Clayton, Vic.: Monash University Publishing.

Scrimgeour, D. (1985), 'Aboriginal health services in Western Australia', *Medical Journal of Australia*, 143(12–13): 634 (letter).

Scrimgeour, D. (2007), 'Town or country: Which is best for Australia's Indigenous peoples?' *Medical Journal of Australia*, 186(10): 532–3.

Shephard, M. (1995), *The Great Victoria Desert*, Chatswood, NSW: Reed Books.

Stead, J., Kimber, R., Hempel, R. and Styles, R. (1982), *A Review of the Pintubi Move to Kintore Ranges*. Alice Springs, NT.

Strakosch, E. (2015), *Neoliberal Indigenous Policy: Settler Colonialism and the 'Post-welfare' State*, Hampshire, UK: Palgrave Macmillan.

Sullivan, P. (2011), *Belonging Together: Dealing with the Politics of Disenchantment in Australian Indigenous Policy*, Acton, ACT: Aboriginal Studies Press.

Sullivan, P. (2018), 'The tyranny of neoliberal public management and the challenge for Aboriginal community organisations', in D. Howard-Wagner, M. Bargh and I. Altamirano-Jimenez (eds), *The Neoliberal State, Recognition and Indigenous Rights: New Paternalism to New Imagings*, Canberra, ACT: ANU Press, pp. 201–15.

Sutton, P. (1990), 'The pulsating heart: Large scale cultural and demographic processes in Aboriginal Australia', in B. Meehan and N. White (eds), *Hunter-gatherer Demography, Past and Present, Oceania Monograph 39*, University of Sydney, Oceania Publications, pp. 74–7.

Sutton, P. (2009), *The Politics of Suffering: Indigenous Australia and the End of the Liberal Consensus*, Carlton, Vic.: Melbourne University Publishing.

SVA Consulting (2014), *Evaluative Social Return on Investment Report: Social, Economic and Cultural Impact of Kanyirninpa Jukurrpa On-Country Programs*, Melbourne, Vic.: Social Ventures Australia.

Taylor, A., et al. (2012), *South Australian Aboriginal Health Survey*, Adelaide, SA: University of Adelaide, Population Research and Outcome Studies.

Thomas, D., et al. (1998), 'Clinical consultations in an Aboriginal community-controlled health service: How are they different to consultations with Australian general practice?' *Australian and New Zealand Journal of Public Health*, 22: 86–91.

Tonkinson, R. (1974), *The Jigalong Mob: Aboriginal Victors of the Desert Crusade*, Menlo Park, Ca: Cummings Publishing Company.

Tonkinson, R. (1977), 'Aboriginal self-regulation and the new regime: Jigalong, Western Australia', in R.M. Berndt (ed.), *Aborigines and Change: Australia in the '70s*, Atlantic Highlands, NJ: Humanities Press, pp. 65–73.

Toohey, P. (4 May 2004), 'The last nomads', *The Bulletin*, pp. 28–35.

Townley, G. (2001), 'Missionaries, mercenaries and misfits: Service relations in the administration of remote Aboriginal communities in the Western Desert region of Australia', Perth, WA: University of Western Australia (PhD thesis).

Trott, P. (27 July 1982), 'Stand-off on the edge of the desert', *West Australian*.
Truswell, S. (1979), 'Diet and nutrition in hunter-gatherers', in *Health and Disease in Tribal Societies*, Amsterdam, New York: Excerpta Medica, Ciba Foundation Symposium 49.
Truswell, S. and Hansen, J. (1968), 'Serum lipids in bushmen', *Lancet* 2: 684.
Tynan, E. (2016), *Atomic Thunder: The Maralinga Story*, Sydney, NSW: UNSW Press.
van Beuren, M., Worland, T., Svanberg, A. and Lassen, J. (2015), *Working for Our Country: A Review of the Economic and Social Benefits of Indigenous Land and Sea Management*, Philadelphia, PA: The Pew Charitable Trusts.
Vanstone, A. (31 May 2005), 'Vanstone snubbed by Aboriginal leaders', *The World Today*, ABC Radio National.
Vanstone, A. (2007), 'Beyond conspicuous compassion: Indigenous Australians deserve more than good intentions', in J. Wanna (ed.), *A Passion for Policy: Essays on Public Sector Reform*, Canberra, ACT: ANU E-Press, pp. 39–46.
Verburgt, B. (1999), *They Called Me Tjampu-tjilpi (Old Left-hand)*, Victoria Park, WA: Hesperian Press.
von Hayek, F. (1982), *Law, Legislation, and Liberty: A New Statement of the Liberal Principles of Justice and Political Economy*, London, UK: Routledge and Kegan Paul.
Vos, T., et al. (2010), *Assessing Cost-effectiveness in Prevention: ACE–Prevention September 2010 Final Report*, Brisbane, Qld: University of Queensland.
Walker, B., Porter, D. and Marsh, I. (2012), *Fixing the Hole in Australia's Heartland: How Government Needs to Work in Remote Australia*, Alice Springs, NT: Desert Knowledge Australia.
Walter, M. (2010), 'Market forces and Indigenous resistance paradigms', *Social Movement Studies*, 9(2): 121–37.
Wilson, J. (1961), *Authority and Leadership in a 'New-style' Aboriginal Community: Pindan, Western Australia*, Perth, WA: University of Western Australia (MA thesis).
Wilson, J. (1980), 'The Pilbara Aboriginal movement', in R. Berndt and C. Berndt (eds), *Aborigines of the West: Their Past and Present*, Perth, WA: University of Western Australia Press, pp. 151–67.
Wolfe, P. (1999), *Settler Colonialism and the Transformation of Anthropology*, London, UK: Cassell.
Wootten, H. (2003), 'Self-determination after ATSIC', *Academy of Social Sciences: Dialogue*, 23(2): 16–25.
Wright, A. (2017), *Tracker: Stories of Tracker Tilmouth*. Artamon, NSW: Giramondo Publishing Co.

Index

Note: DS denotes author

Abbott, Kathy 5–6
Abbott Coalition government 199, 235, 236
Aboriginal and Torres Strait Islander Commission (ATSIC)
  abolition by Howard government 158, 225
  attempts to centralise services at Utopia (1990) 13
  funding responsibilities 221–2, 227
  Regional Council 13, 158
Aboriginal community-controlled health organisations (ACCHOs) 56–7, 208, 210–11, 211–14
  clinical governance 217
  collaboration with government during COVID-19 240–1
  community health services provision 214–19
  government funding 233–7
  factors undermining 240, 243–5
  impact of Howard government welfare reforms 223–6
  impact of mainstreaming of service delivery 226–30
  Medicare funding and implications 237–8
  models underpinning 216–17, 218–19
  organisational and clinical governance challenges 238–41
  principle of subsidiary 213
  reporting burden 230–3
  tripartite forum 222
  See also Aboriginal community-controlled health services; National Aboriginal community-controlled health organisation (NACCHO); National Aboriginal and Islander Health Organisation (NAIHO)
Aboriginal community-controlled health services 104, 242
  cultural safety and security 213–14
  peak bodies 154, 211, 240
  See also Aboriginal community-controlled health organisations (ACCHOs)
Aboriginal disadvantage 201–3
Aboriginal Health Council of South Australia 152, 159
  DS as public health medical officer (2007) 153–4
  DS resigns (2015) 163
Aboriginal Health Organisation (South Australia) 70
Aboriginal health workers 6, 55
  Jamieson (Mantamaru) community 48
  Kintore community 121, 124–5, 127
  Kiwirrkurra community 137
  pay structure in Pitjantjatjara Homelands Health Service 57, 58
  Pipalyatjara community 45
  Strelley Regional Aboriginal Medical Service 95–6
Aboriginal pastoral strikes 75, 77–83, 102
Aboriginal peoples
  barriers to primary healthcare access 219
  desert skills 176
  endemic health conditions 179–80
  impact of disease on 170
  land-management practices 168
  median disposable income 200
  organisations advocating for rights 26
Aboriginal reserves 18–19 *See also* Central Australian Aboriginal Reserve
Aboriginal significant sites 28, 29, 149
  Pintupi people 112, 120
  Pitjantjatjara people 37, 38, 45
  Spinifex people 142, 148, 151, 176, 181
  See also individual Dreaming sites
Aboriginal Tent Embassy 184
Aboriginal-owned cattle stations *See* Utopia Station, Strelley mob
Aborigines Advancement League of South Australia 25
Aborigines' Inland Mission 39, 48
Adams, Joan 135
Adelaide News 33
Advertiser 24
Agricultural Revolution 167, 168, 183
Albrecht, Pastor 111–12
alcohol bans 83, 85, 123
alcohol rehabilitation 6 *See also* 'Congress Farm'
alcohol-related diseases 62–3
Alice Springs and surrounds 17–18, 109
Alice Springs Hospital 1, 125–6
Alice Springs Hospital Pharmacy 59
Altman, John 194, 200, 228
Alyawarr people 9
Amata 38, 47, 186
Amery, Rob 118
Ampilatwatja Health Centre 13, 189–90
A$\underline{n}$angu 17, 18
  effects of atomic bomb tests 27, 147
  land title rights around Uluru 44
  move to Kalka 65–6
  movement in and out of Western Desert 19
  resettlements 148–50
  use of Pitjantjatjara language 52
Anangu Pitjantjatjaraku Yankunytjatjaraku (APY) Lands 71–2
Anderson, Bob 145
Anderson, Helen 9
Angarappa Health Service 13, 210 *See also* Urapuntja Health Service
Anmatjerre people 9
Aparatjara community 48
Apostolic Church of Australia 77, 85 *See also* Jigalong Mission
atmospheric nuclear-weapons testing moratorium 31
atomic bomb testing 25 *See also* Cold War; Maralinga; Woomera Rocket Range

INDEX

ATSIC *see* Aboriginal and Torres Strait Islander Commission
The Australian 192, 193
Australian Aborigines' Evangelical Mission (AAEM) 145
Australian Antigen 133
Australian Freedom from Hunger 64
Australian Government
 assimilationist policies 184, 209, 243
 collaboration with ACCHOs during COVID-19 pandemic 240–1
 cost-sharing with states for healthcare 215
 environmental-management programs 205–6
 failure to engage with Aboriginal partners 233–4
 Guided Projectiles Committee 26
 involvement with ACCHOs 219–26, 233–7
 Labor's reversal of homelands movements 198
 parliamentary select committee 32–4
 problematic funding models 236–7
 royal commissions 27, 150, 221
 social-democratic approach (1970s) 243
 state and territories opposition to federal funding 220
 See also Department of Aboriginal Affairs (DAA); Office of Aboriginal and Torres Strait Islander Health (OATSIH); Office of Aboriginal and Torres Strait Islander Health Services (OATSIHS)
Australian Health Ministers' Advisory Council (AHMAC) 213
Australian Inland Mission (AIM) 21
Australian National Audit Office 235
autonomy
 factors undermining 191, 199, 203, 240, 243–4
 Martu 98, 99–100, 186
 Pintupi people 88, 173, 182, 186–7
 struggle for 189–90, 204, 212, 245

through ACCHOs 208–19, 240–3
See also Strelley mob

Baird, Ian 149, 152, 164, 176, 177
Baker, Ivan 49, 55–6, 64
Balfour, Lewis J. 21
Balgo Mission 113
Barr, Andy 40, 59
Bates, Daisy 27, 142–3
Beadell, Len 24, 27, 30, 113, 116
Beale, Howard 147
Beazley, Kim 114
Bega Garnbirringu Aboriginal Health Service 151–2, 157
Behrendt, Larissa 197
Belair, Sol 56
Bell, Neil 11
Bennelong Society 191, 192–3, 195
Benson, Jill 153–4, 158, 159
Berndt, Catherine 33, 143
Berndt, Ronald 33, 143
Bettering the Evaluation and Care of Health (BEACH) study 229–30
Bewley, Ken 100
Biddle, Nicholas 200, 202
Bidu, Neil 95
Bin Bin, Dooley 78–9
Bird, Doug 168
Bird, Rebecca Bligh 168
Blackstone mining camp 35
Brady, Maggie 220
Bridger, Margaret
Brigg, Morgan 239
British Atomic Weapons Research Establishment 28
Brody, Hugh 169
Brokensha, Peter 37
Broome Regional Aboriginal Medical Service 95
Brough, Mal 227
Brown, Sarah 137
Bryce, Suzanne 64, 65, 67
Bucknall, Gwen 82, 93
Bucknall, John 82, 93, 94, 98
Burgess, Paul 206
bush medicine 53
bush repairs 131
Butement, Alan 29
Butler, Ray 92, 102
Butler, Roma (nee Peterman) 45, 47
Buynder, Paul van 104

Camp 61 93, 97–8
Campbell, Megan 211

Canadian settler colonialism 244–5
Cane, Scott 149, 151–2
Canning Stock Route 76–7
Carlisle, Anthony 144, 145
Cartwright, Gary 127, 135
Central Australian Aboriginal Alcohol Programs Unit (CAAAPU) 6
Central Australian Aboriginal Congress 3, 4, 127, 175, 210
 Board of Management 5
 DS as general practice trainee 6–8
 DS resigns 50
 health-service development study 7–8
 NT health department's views 7
 provision of healthcare support for Kintore 119
 transfer of administration to Utopia 13
Central Australian Aboriginal Reserve 18–19
Central Australian Exploring and Prospecting Association Expedition 111
Central Land Council 175
centralised health services, Utopia's residents oppose 10
Centre for Aboriginal Economic and Policy Research 194
Centre for Independent Studies (CIS) 195
 claims about Aboriginal disadvantage 201, 202–3
 Indigenous Affairs Research Program (2005) 191
Centrelink 199
CGC Report 228
Chalmers, Mac 10
Chalmers, Rose 10
Chambers, Mark 104
Chapman, Leon 138
Chibawe, Robby 108
chlamydia 63
Claire (John Holliday's partner) 135–6
Clarke, Bette 175
clinical governance 217, 238–41
'Close the Gap' campaign 233–5
Cold War
 Anglo-Australian atomic weapons partnership 23–34
 effect on Aboriginal people 83–5, 146
 space race programs 84
Common Cause (social reform group) 25–6

INDEX

Commonwealth Grants Commission 227–8
Communicare 108
communication
  medical consultations using radio 59–60, 96, 126–7
  schooling support using radio 97–8
Communist Party of Australia 25–6
Community Aid Abroad 64
Community Development Employment Program (CDEP) 58, 198–9
Community Development Program (CDP) 199, 206–7
community health centres 215–16
community-controlled health service model, positive factors 52, 211–19
community-health movement 215, 216, 219
Comprehensive Primary Health Care (CPHC) 218
comprehensive primary-healthcare movement 215
'Congress Farm' 6
Coombes, Victor 36
Coombs, H.C. (Nugget) 184, 192, 220
Coonana Station 149
Cooper, Ikuta 65–6
Cooper, Tjapalyi 65–6
Coppin, Peter (Kangkushot) 81, 82, 98–9
Cosmo Newberry Mission 34
Coulthard, Glenn Sean 244
Council of Aboriginal Affairs 184
Council of Aboriginal Reconciliation 224
Council of Australian Governments (COAG) 234, 241 *See also* National Cabinet
Council of Ngangkaris 117
Crack, Geoff 73
Craig, Pippa 228–9
Crawford, Heather 202
Cultural Respect Framework for Aboriginal and Torres Strait Islander Health 213
cultural safety and security 213–14, 228–9
Culture Crisis: Anthropology and politics in Aboriginal Australia (Altman & Hinkson) 194
Cundeelee Mission 28, 145, 147–8
Curth-Bibb, Jodie 239

Cutter, Trevor 3, 4, 6, 70–1, 175
health service feasibility study 7–8
Cutter Report (1976) 8, 41, 117
Cutter-Tregenza Report (1982) 70–1
Cyclone Tracy 1

Daniels, Bobby Jakamarra 55
Daniels, Rosie 54
Danila Dilba Aboriginal Medical Service 230
Davidson, Belle 48
Davidson, W.S. 33
Davies, Tony (El Punj/Watiwara) 11, 65, 67
Davis, Annie 45, 50, 55, 67
Davis, Bill 45, 50, 55, 64, 67
de Voy, Kate (Brian Kelly's partner) 97
decentralised services, benefits to outstation communities 15
Dent, Amanda 164
dental care services 160
Department of Aboriginal Affairs (DAA)
  funding 8, 89
  funding for ACCHOs 210, 220–1
  funding for Pitjantjatjara Homelands Health Service 55
  funding for Pintupi Homelands Health Service 119
  funding for single-engine plane hire 129–30, 175
  transfer of funding responsibilities to ATSIC 221–2
Department of Family and Community Services 225
Department of Health and Ageing (DoHA) 154, 157–8
Department of Immigration and Multicultural Affairs 225
Department of Prime Minister and Cabinet 200, 225, 235
Derbal Yerrigan 233–7
'Desert Meeting' (1982) 88–9
diabetes 133–4
diarrhoea in babies 125–6
dingo scalp trades 18–19, 23, 38
Divisions of General Practice 234
Dixon, Annie 13, 121, 122, 127, 129, 131, 135, 138
Docker River community 44
Doctor George 53, 103, 128, 130, 181
donovanosis 63

Dooley, Jim 123, 130
Dowling, Graham 139
Downing, Jim 190, 191
drought
  Central Australia (1950s) 33–4
  effect on movement of peoples 19, 113
D'Sousa, Nigel 121, 122, 127, 128
Duguid, Charles 19–22, 34, 112
  advocacy for rights of Aboriginal people 19, 21
  aims of Ernabella Mission 35–6
  DS and Schrader visit 50–1
  opposition to atomic bomb tests 24–5, 26, 29
Dunbar, Robin 189
Duncan, Pip 13
Dunn, David 151
Dunstan, Brian 108

Earle, William 18
Eckert, Paul 38, 45
education
  bilingual and bicultural 82–3, 86
  one-teacher schools 39, 93
Edwards, Bill 36, 143
electronic health information systems (medical records) 107–8, 163–4, 217, 232–3
Elkin, A.P. 19, 20, 143
Elsie (health worker) 95
employment and welfare changes 198–201
Emu Field atomic tests 27
Endean, Colin 160
epidemic diseases following Agricultural Revolution 169
Ernabella Community Council Inc. 36
Ernabella Mission 18–22, 35–6
  infant deaths 34, 35
  Pan-Pitjantjatjara meeting (1975) 39
  resists assimilationist policies 23
European Launcher Development Organisation (ELDO) 84

Family Medicine Program 135
Farmer, Darren 206
fee-for-service general practice model 216, 238
  cultural safety and security concerns 228–9
Finke River Mission 111, 112
Flynn, John 21
Foley, Gary 56, 57

INDEX

Forrest, John 17–18
Forrester, Vince 5
Foster, Wilton 44
Fox, Albert 66
Fraser, Donald 71
Fraser Coalition government 41, 42, 92

Gallegos, Roxanne (Colin Endean's partner) 160
Gara, Tom 143
Geraldton Regional Aboriginal Medical Service 95
Gibbs, Ned 88–9
Gibbs, Nyaparu (Billy) 86
Gibbs, Yala Yala 122
Gibson, Alfred 109, 111
Gibson Desert 17, 109–10
last hunter-gatherers 171–5
Giles, Ernest 17, 37, 109, 111, 142
Giles Weather Station 28, 29–30, 34–5
Gillard Labor government 234
Girgiba, Cheryl 97
Glastonbury, Mercy 45
Glastonbury, Ray 45
Golding, Judith 48, 104
gonorrhoea 62
Gosse, William 17, 37
Graeber, David 168
Grayden, Bill 32–4
Great Sandy Desert 75
Europa trial rocket firings (1964/65) 84–5
movement of people 76–7
Great Victoria Desert 141–2
early contact history 142–8
hunter-gatherer families 171, 175–8
movement of Spinifex people in 143–4
See also Spinifex country
Green, Harrie 143, 145–6
Green, H.E. 34
Green, Jenny 11
Grogan, Glenis 49, 51–2, 54, 55, 58, 67
Guided Projectiles Committee 29
Gurindji Strike 75,184

Haasts Bluff 111–13, 115, 117, 173, 186
Hale, Monty (Minyjun) 99
Hallett, Brian 164
Hambour, Rick 2
Hamilton, Annette 50
Hammond, Roger 65, 67
Hansen, Debbie 149

Hansen, Ken 115
Hansen, Leslie 115
Hargraves, John 173–4
Harold, John 97, 98
Harold, Trish 97
Hawke Labor government 150
Hayman, Noel 215
Health Information Systems 163
challenges with homelands community 58
inadequacies of hand-written notes 126
Puntukurnu Aboriginal Medical Service (PAMS) 107–8
See also electronic Health Information Systems
Health Insurance Act 1973 237
health surveys 15, 33, 133, 204, 230
Hearn, Artie 68
Henry, Alec 65, 67
hepatitis B 133, 179
Hermannsburg 111
Hermannsburg Mission 114, 185
Hetzel, Basil 4
high-frequency radio consultations 59–60
Hill, John 6
Hinkson, Melinda 194, 197
Holcombe, Jeff 123
Holding, Clyde 173
Holliday, John 135, 137
Hollows, Fred 40
homelands 184–5, 187
homelands communities 39–41, 183–7
government policies undermining 207
health outcomes 203–4
indigenous art industry 205
intermittent occupation 187–8
population equilibrium 189, 204
Vanstone's 'cultural museums' 204–5
Western Desert 187–90
homelands movement 39, 184, 242
anthropological critique 194
health benefits 190–1
neoliberal counter narratives 191–5
policies to reverse 198
horizontal programs *See* Comprehensive Primary Health Care (CPHC)
Horner, Cusha 11
Horner, Rod 11
Houston, Shane 213

Howard Coalition government
assimilationist policies 198
changes to mainstream welfare system 198–9, 222
closure of ATSIC 158
closure of CDEP 58
Northern Territory National Emergency Response (NTNER) 196
views towards Aboriginal funding 236–7
See also OATSIH
Howell, Herbert 53
Howson, Peter 191
Hughes, Helen 191–2, 193, 196–7, 199, 201
Hunt, Janet 231
hunter-gatherers 167–8, 171
health condition and healthcare 177, 178–81
immunisations 180
impact of disease on 170
post-contact health risks 172–3, 180–1
reintegration into communities 181–2

ili tjukurrpa (wild fig dreaming) site 38
Imanpa community 43
immunisations 180
Indigenous Advancement Strategy (IAS) 235
Indigenous Affairs Research Program (2005) 191
Indigenous and Rural Health Division 236
Indigenous Australians' Health Program (IAHP) 236
Indigenous Coordinating Centre (ICCs) 226
Indigenous Health Partnership 234
Indigenous National Land-care Award 164
Indigenous Protected Areas 205
Industrial Revolution 169, 183
infant health problems 61–2, 125–6
Institute of Aboriginal Development (IAD) 65
Institute of Public Affairs (IPA) 191, 195
International Conference on Primary Health Care (Alma Ata Declaration) 217–18
International Labour Organization's Forced Labour Convention 200

INDEX

Irrunytju community 38, 39, 44
  community advisors 47, 116
  health services 48, 72

Jamieson 49 *see also* Marntamaru community
Jigalong Mission 75, 77, 85
Jigalong mob 85–6, 88–9
Jittermarra, Snowy 93, 95, 102
Johns, Gary 191, 192, 193
Johnson, Clay 93
Johnson, David 159–60, 162, 163
Johnson, Luana 93, 94
Johnson, Messina 93
Johnson, Ross 93, 94
Jones, Rosalie 135–6
Jula, Caroline 79, 80

Kakarrara Wilurrara Health Alliance (KWHA) 156–9, 160
Kakarrara Wilurrara Regional Council 158
Kalka 50, 51, 54–5
  accommodation and administrative set up 64–70
  population 52
Karonie 145
Kartujarra people 77, 86
Kass, Bob 125–6
Keane, John 135
Kelly, Brian 87, 97
Kerin, Rani 20
Kerrie (Steve Patman's partner) 122, 123
kidney disease 133–4, 137
Kilgarriff, David 153
Kimber, Dick 170
King Edward Memorial Hospital 135, 136
Kintore 88, 121–8
  Aboriginal health workers 121, 127
  alcohol bans 123
  birthing 131–2
  establishment of dialysis unit in 137
  DS leaves for Perth (1985) 134–6
  infant and child health problems 125
  intermittent occupancy of communities 188
  language spoken in 113
  lobbies for funding for community health service 119
  medical officer role interview 120–1
  outstation versus homelands 186–7

population 117
  trips made in light aircraft 129–31
  Western Desert art movement 123
  See also Pintupi country
Kintore School 123
kipara tjurkurrpa (bush turkey dreaming) 151, 176, 181
Kiwirrkurra community 72, 124, 125, 128–31, 136–8, 188
  Aboriginal health workers 129, 137
Kunamata community 48
Kowal, Emma 9
Kukatja language 113
Kunawarritji community 130, 168, 186, 190
  outreach services 104, 105, 106, 108
  population 189
  reoccupation 88, 95, 97, 98
Kunitz, Steve 220
Kunti Kunti, Jack 116, 122
Kunytjanu community 48

Lalla Rookh School 93
Land Councils 103, 130
land rights meeting 49
Lands of Shame (Hughes) 196, 198
Lane, Debra 95
Lark, Jon 149, 152
Larkins, Sarah 230
Layton, Janet 4
Lester, Yami 27, 71, 117
Liddle, John 5
'Little Children are Sacred': Report of the Northern Territory Board of Enquiry into the Protection of Aboriginal Children from Sexual Abuse (2007) 195–6
Locke, Annie 143
Long, Jeremy 113, 114–15, 171
Love, J.R.B. 20–1
Lungkata, Shorty 122
Luritja language 113
Lutheran missions 111, 145–6, 153 *See also* Yalata Mission
Lyappa Congress 117
Lyappa Medical Service 117–18, 210
lympho-granuloma venereum (donovanosis) 63

MacAdam, Elliot 70–1
Macaulay, Robert 30, 32, 35, 84, 147, 148
Macdonnell Regional Council 138

MacDonnell Regional Council 187
MacDougall, Walter 114, 146, 147
  advocacy for rights of Aboriginal people 29, 32
  'Protector of Aborigines' role 29, 84
Mackenzie, Ray 108
Macumba, John 6
Maddison, Sarah 245
Madin, Simon 138
mainstreaming of service delivery 226–30, 234–5
  cultural safety and security 228–9
  studies 229–30
Major, Riley Tjangala 128
malu tjukurrpa (kangaroo dreaming) site 37, 38, 45
Manning, Peter 89
Manyjilyjarra people 75, 77, 86, 88 *See also* Martu
Maralinga 26–34
  public relations exercise to stop public criticism 30–1
  radioactive contamination 31, 32
Maralinga Prohibited Area 146–7, 150
Marmot, Michael 212
Marntamaru community 39, 48, 53 *See also* Jamieson
Marrngu 76, 78
  collective action and organising power 80
  relationship with McLeod 81–2, 99
  split between *Martu* and (1983) 98–100
  See also Pindan mob (movement)
Marshall, Barry 97
Marshall, Chris 55
Martu 75, 83, 95, 186
  cultural and linguistic ties with Pintupi 88
  effect of rocket firings on 83–4
  impact of Canning Stock Route on 76–7
  joins Strelley mob 186
  reconciliation between desert and Jigalong communities 103
  split between *Marrngu* and (1983) 98–100, 190
McAuley, Ian 213
McCall, Chris 48
McCaul, Peter 119

McDermott, Robyn 203–4
McGlew, Peter 100
McGuinness, Bruce 56
McKenna, Clancy 78–9
McLean, Thelma 48
McLeay, Lizzie 13, 108
McLeay, Toby 13, 108
McLeod, Don 25, 87, 101
  establishment of Nomads Pty Ltd 82, 89–90, 92
  involvement with pastoral strikes 77–9, 80
  relationship with *Marrngu* 81–2, 99
  See also Pindan mob (movement)
McMahon Coalition government 191
McMahon, Charlie 128–9
media
  exaggeration of tension between Strelley and Jigalong mobs 89
  influence on Aboriginal policies 33, 34, 192, 193, 195
  intrusion on Pintupi hunter-gatherer reunion 173
Medibank bulk billing 92
medical consultations using two-way radio 59, 96, 106, 126–7
Medical Journal of Australia 190, 201–2
Medical Specialists Outreach Assistance Program - Indigenous Chronic Disease (MSOAP-ICD) 158–9
Medicare funding 237–8
Menadue, John 213
Menzies, Robert 26
Menzies government 31
Menzies School of Health Research 104
metformin usage 133–4
Meyers, Naomi 56
Mick, Ginger 47, 48
Mick, Nelly (Josephine) 45, 47
Middleton, S.G. 145
Mijijimaya community 101
Milpuddie family 146–7
mining operations
  community-operated 37–8, 45
  use of 'yandy' 76, 80
Minyintiri, Dickie 53
minyma tjuta tjukurrpa (Seven Sisters dreaming) site 148
missionaries' reasons for entering reserves 18–19
Mitchell, Ernie 53, 81, 82, 98–9
Monash University 4

Monte Bello Islands 27, 28
Morgan, Marie 45
Morgan, Patrick 45
Morice, Rod 190
Mount Ebenezer Station 43
Mount Margaret Mission 22
Mr Yates 53
Mugarinya Pastoral Company 82
Munoz, Estrella 121, 122, 127
Murdoch, Rupert 33, 34
Murray, Giselle 124
Murray, Julia 10, 11
Murray, Neil 123–4
Myers, Fred 66, 115, 118, 175

Nampitjinpa, Kawayi 121, 124, 127
Nampitjinpa, Marlene 121, 124, 127, 129, 132
Nancy (health worker) 95
Nangala, Mantuwa 124, 127, 129
National Aboriginal and Islander Health Organisation (NAIHO) 56–7, 119, 210–11
National Aboriginal Community-Controlled Health Organisation (NACCHO) 211, 240
National Aboriginal Health Strategy 221
National Cabinet 241
national key performance indicators (nKPIs) 232–3
native patrol officers 26, 29, 30
Nelson, Hugh 4, 6
Nelson, Jock 9
Nelson, Peg 9
neoliberal approach
  counter narrative to Aboriginal policies 191–5
  impact on Aboriginal policies 222–5, 243–4
  influence on Aboriginal policies 196–7, 200, 207
Neville, A.O. 144
A New Deal for Aborigines and Torres Strait Islanders in Remote Communities (Hughes & Warin) 191–2
New Public Management 230–3
Ngaanyatjarra Council 72, 137, 190
Ngaanyatjarra Health Service (NHS) 72, 157, 190
  health provision to Kiwirrkurra 137–8, 139
  hepatitis B control program 133
Ngaanyatjarra homelands 17–18, 22–3, 42

excision of land for Giles Weather Station 28–9
Hollows' trachoma team visit 40
Ngaanyatjarra language 53
Ngaanyatjarra people 16, 17–19, 39
  formation of Ngaanyatjarra Council 71–2
  land rights struggle 90
  loss of language 52–3
  reoccupation of homelands 34–9, 186
  significant sites 29
  See also Yarnangu
Nganampa Health Council 71, 120, 124, 127, 190
  DS as medical advisor (1983) 129–30
ngangkari (traditional healers) 53–4, 96, 127, 181–2
  Sutton's views on 194–5
  ways of practice 216–17
  working alongside western medicine 54, 103
ngintaka tjukurrpa (perentie lizard dreaming) 120
Ngurlipatu people 76
Ngwarraye, Kutadji 12
Ngwarraye, Michael 12, 16
1967 referendum 184, 209, 219–20
Nomads Health Service 100
Nomads Pty Ltd 82–3, 89–91
non-specific urethritis 62 *See also* chlamydia
Northern Development and Mining Company 81
Northern Territory
  Aboriginal health worker training program 57
  amalgamation of community councils 138, 187, 198
  creation of Aboriginal reserves 18
  establishment of small communities 38
  funding for outstations 115
  tourism development around Uluru 44
Northern Territory Administration 10
Northern Territory health department
  health services to Kintore and Papunya 118–19
  medical records 126
  views towards Congress 7
Northern Territory Intervention 195–8, 199

INDEX

Northern Territory Labor Party 5
Northern Territory National Emergency Response (NTNER) 196 *See also* Northern Territory Intervention
Northern Transport 59
North-west (Native) Workers Association 80, 209
North-West Aboriginal Reserve (South Australia) 36
Novak, Robert 122, 123
nutritional-health programs 64
Nyamal people 76
Nyangumarta people 76
Nyapari community 48
Nyiapali people 77
nyinyi tjukurrpa (zebra finch dreaming) site 38

Oak Valley community 150, 190
Oak Valley Maralinga Health Service 154, 157
Oberdoo, Jacob 82, 93
Office of Aboriginal and Torres Strait Islander Health (OATSIH) 152, 154, 155, 222, 227, 236 *See also* Indigenous and Rural Health Division
Office of Aboriginal and Torres Strait Islander Health Services (OATSIHS) 227
Office of Indigenous Policy Co-ordination (OIPC) 196, 225
Office of the Registrar of Aboriginal Corporations (ORIC) 139
O'Flynn, Tom 37, 38
one-teacher schools 39, 93
Ooldea 142
Ooldea Mission 27, 28, 145
otitis media 62, 180
Our Right to take Responsibility (Pearson) 193
outstation movement 184
outstations 115, 185–7
   health outcomes 204
   outreach services 15
   See also homelands
Overland Telegraph Line 2, 17

Pan-Pitjantjatjara meeting (1975) 39
Panaka Panaka 87, 97
   Martu and *Marrngu* split (1983) 98–100
   See also Punmu
Papulangkatja (Blackstone) community 39, 48

Papunya 112, 113–15
   funding for health service (1978) 117, 210
   health service feasibility study 7
   Western Desert art movement 123
Papunya Council 117–18, 186
Papunya School 123
Papunya Tula artists cooperative 123
Parker, Paul 116
Parker, Tilau 116
Parrngurr 106
Partial Test Ban Treaty 31
Paru (Spinifex) 87
pastoral industry 76
   improved conditions for Aboriginal workers 80
   strikes 77–83
Patman, Steve 122, 123
Paupiyala Tjarutja Aboriginal Corporation (PTAC) 150–1, 152–3, 154, 164
Pearson, Noel 193–4, 195, 199, 222
Pennington, Katie 156
Perkins, Charlie 3, 173, 174
Perkins, Neville 3, 4, 5
petrol-sniffing 62–3
Phillips, Christine 217
Pijikarli people 76
pila nguru 141
Pila Nguru Aboriginal Corporation (PNAC) 164
Pilbara, early contact history 76–7
Pilbara strike (1940s) 75, 209
Pindan mob (movement) 81–2
Pintupi country *110*
   early contact history 109–15
   hunter-gatherer families 171
   reoccupation of Kintore Range 116–21
Pintupi Homelands Health Service 72, 103, 173, 188
   Aboriginal health workers 124–5
   board of directors 124
   early years 121–8
   DS joins as non-voting independent director 139
   governance structure 139
   health services to Kiwirrkurra 136–7
   incorporation of *ngangkari* into health team 128
   progress report 132–3
   receives DAA funding 119
   request for light aircraft for outreach services 129–30

short-term locum stints 138
Pintupi people
   cultural and linguistic ties with *Martu* 88
   deaths from infectious diseases 170
   endemic health conditions 179–80
   fight for autonomy 186–7
   impact of Cold War 114
   last hunter-gatherers 171–5
   reoccupation of Kintore 88
   tensions between Papunya Council and 117–18
Pintupi-Luritja 113
Pipalyatjara community 37–8, 39, 40, 45, 48
The Pitjantjatjara and their Crafts (Brokensha) 37
Pitjantjatjara Council 8, 13, 39, 41, 120
   funds administration for Pitjantiatjara Homelands Health Services 55
   health service delivery report (1981) 69–70
   meeting at Jamieson 49
Pitjantjatjara homelands 17–18, *42*
   bush trip into (1978) 43–9
   Hollows' trachoma team visit 40
Pitjantjatjara Homelands Health Service 22, 72–3, 190, 210
   acute conditions 96
   funding and grants 55, 64
   DS resigns (1981) 69–70, 91
   location for residential base 50, 64–70
   medical and pharmaceutical supplies 58–9
   medical officer (1978–1981) 49, 187
   mobile clinic challenges 60–1
   model of healthcare 57
   outreach services 51–2
   problems with service delivery report (1981) 69–70
   reduction in areas covered 124
   support of *ngangkari* consultations 54
   See also Nganampa Health Council; Pitjantjatjara-Ngaanyatjarra Health Service (PNHS)
Pitjantjatjara language 21–2, 50, 52, 65, 68
   meetings conducted in 56
   preventative health campaigns in 64

Pitjantjatjara people 16, 17–19, 39
   reoccupation of homelands 34–9, 186
   See also A*n*angu
Pitjantjatjara-Ngaanyatjarra Health Service (PNHS) 70, 124
   as locum medical officer (1981/82) 91
Pitjara, Gloria 12
Piyirti 130, 136
The Politics of Suffering: Indigenous Australia and the end of the liberal consensus (Sutton) 194
Porter, Molly 48
Porter, Teddy 51
Potter, Katie 11–12, 13
Potter, Roy 11–12, 13
power relations disparity 9, 77, 224
Preece, Richard 55
Presbyterian Church 19–21, 36
   See also Ernabella Mission
Primary Health Care (PHC) movement 217–18, 219, 228
Punmu 87, 103, 106 See also Panaka Panaka, Rawa Soak
Puntukurnu Aboriginal Medical Service (PAMS) 103–8, 206
   Community Health Board 107
   outreach services 105–8
   role as medical officer (1993) 105–8
Purple House 137
Puta Puta community 37, 38, 45–6, 48
Puwarka (*ngangkari*) 95, 96

Rainow, Stephan (Stephi) 46, 64, 65, 67
ration depots 112, 144, 145
Rawa Soak (Roha's Soak) 87 See also Panaka Panaka, Punmu
rehabilitation camps 87
rehabilitation programs 6
remote communities 95
   acknowledgement of challenges 200–1, 203
   chronic diseases prevalence 133–4, 137
   claims about Aboriginal disadvantage in 201, 202–3
   effect of CDP on 200
   effects of government policies 66–7, 243–4
   environmental-management programs 206–7

   funding considerations 187
   health problems 61–4
   healthcare support via two-way radio 59, 96, 100, 106, 126–7
   rescue mission in aircraft 131
Remote Jobs and Communities Program 199 See also Community Development Program (CDP)
Report of the National Aboriginal Health Strategy Working Party (NAHS Report) 221
Richards, Arthur 45
Richter, Ian 177, 181
Rivalland, Paul 137
Robinson, Barb 123
Robinson, Danay 123
Robinson, Nabi 95
Ross, Sally 127, 135
Rowse, Tim 80, 192, 196, 209
Royal Australian College of General Practitioners 58
Royal Commission into Aboriginal Deaths in Custody (1987) 221
Royal Commission into British Nuclear Tests in Australia (1985) 27, 150
Royal Darwin Hospital 1
Royal Flying Doctor Service (RFDS) 21, 152
   Alice Springs 59, 126
   Eastern Goldfields 72
   Kalgoorlie 39, 40, 48, 162–3
   Port Hedland 96, 103, 106
Rudd Labor government, Statement of Intent 233–4
Rural Doctors Workforce Agency (RDWA) 159
Rural Health West (RHW) 159
Ryan, Ben 122

Sadler, Howard 91
Sahlins, Marshall 167
Sambo, Mary 95
Sammut, Jeremy 201
Sanderson, John 197–8
Sawenko, Toly 10, 13
Sawenko, Valentine 11, 12
Scales, Eva 46
Scales, Ushma 46, 64, 65, 67–8
Schrader, Glendle 13, 37, 44, 67, 71
   as community advisor at Pipalyatjara 38, 40, 59
   request for community-controlled health service 40–1, 49
   visits Duguid with DS 50–1

Scrimgeour, Anne 80, 91, 93, 94
Scrimgeour, Callum 108
Scrimgeour, Laura 105
Scrimgeour (nee Bridger), Margaret 98, 100, 105, 120
Scrimgeour, Sophie 105
Selective Primary Health Care (SPHC) 218, 234
self-determination 4, 7, 208, 212, 240
   factors undermining 174–5
   government policies 14, 41, 182, 209
settler colonialism 2, 166
   Canadian 244–5
   impact on Western Desert region 179–80, 183
   ongoing effects 203, 212, 243–5
sexually transmitted diseases (STIs) 62–3
Shared Responsibility Agreements (SRAs) 222
Sharp, Janet 87
Shaw, Geoff 5, 9 See also Tangentyerre Council
Sherwood, John 98
'Shower-block Song' 64
Sister Pat 44
Sleigh, Adrian 118
social determinants of health 4, 219
social movements 242
Social Ventures Australia 206
Sofer, Albert 145
South Australia
   assimilationist policies 23
   creation of Aboriginal reserves 18
   establishment of small communities 38
   first Aboriginal health director 70–1
   funding for Nganampa Health Council 71
   one-teacher schools 39
   'Protector of Aborigines' 29
   small homelands communities 48
South Australian Aborigines' Protection Board 27, 36, 143, 145
South Australian atomic bomb test site See Maralinga
southern Pitjantjatjara language 141
Spinifex Arts 164
Spinifex country 17, 141, *140*, 149

INDEX

hunter-gatherer families 171, 175–8
nuclear testing sites 27
reoccupation 150–1
significant sites 160
Spinifex Health Service 159–65
  dental care provision 160
  DS as medical director (2015–2019) 163
  review report (2011) 160–2
  social, cultural and economic development 164–5
Spinifex people 141
  reoccupation of Tjuntjuntjara 150–1, 187, 188
  resettlements 147–8, 148–50, 176
  royal commission compensation 150
  See also pila nguru
Spinifex Ranger Program 164
Stevens, Anne 151
Stewart, Bob 145
Strelley Community School 82–3, 87, 91, 93
Strelley mob 75, 85–6, 102
  co-operative set up 89–91
  Martu joins 186
  Pintupi decline offer to join 88
  split (1960) 100
  tensions between government departments and 101
  tensions between Jigalong and 88–9
Strelley mob stations *74*
Strelley Regional Aboriginal Medical Service 91–8
  Aboriginal health workers 95–6
  administration and operational structures 92–3
  desert clinical trips 94–5
  DS resigns (1983) 100, 120
  See also Nomads Health Service
Strelley Station
  alcohol ban 83, 85
  expansion of desert communities 82, 87–9
  Strelley mob leaves for Warralong Station 101
subsidiary principle 213
Sudan refugee camp 136, 177
Sullivan, Patrick 212, 220, 230–1, 232, 235
Sunday Times 33
Sutherland, Gregor 2
Sutton, Peter 19, 194–5
syphilis 63

Tait, Peter 120, 121
Tait, Wendy 121
Talgarno Prohibited Area 83
Tangentyerre Council 5
Thomas, David 230
Thomas, Kathy 95
Thomas, Mark 163
Thomas, Pit Pit 101
Thompson (nee Hayes), Maria 65
Thompson, Simon 47, 51, 65, 67
Thomson, Donald 26, 29
Tietkens, William Harry 111, 120
Tilmouth, Tracker 5, 102
Tindale, Norman 32, 143, 147
tjala tjukurrpa (honey-ant dreaming) 112
Tjangala, Uta Uta 122
Tjapaltjarri, Benny 121, 124, 127, 129
Tjapaltjarri, George Nyunmul (Doctor George) 53, 103, 128, 130, 181
Tjapaltjarri, George Tjampu Martin 124, 127, 129, 137, 168, 172
Tjapananka, Pinta Pinta 172
Tjilari, Andy 53
Tjungurrayi, Victor 128
Tjungurrayi, Willy 122
Tjuntjuntjara Aboriginal Health Service 151–6 *See also* Spinifex Health Service
Tjuntjuntjara Community Council *See* Paupiyala Tjarutja Aboriginal Corporation (PTAC)
Tjuntjuntjara review report (2009) 154–5, 156–7
Tjupurulla, Nosepeg 122
Tjutjupayi 45
Tom, Helen 4, 6, 8, 10–11, 13
Tonkinson, Myrna 50
Tonkinson, Robert 86, 183
Townley, Graham 155–6
Townsville Aboriginal and Islander Health Service 230
trachoma 35, 40, 180
traditional Aboriginal medical care 216
traditional healers *See* ngangkari (traditional healers)
traditional law 16
Trans-Australian Railway 27, 28, 142, 144
Trees, Janelle 163
Tregenza, Bronnie 47, 51
Tregenza, John 'Tungku' 51, 64, 67, 149

administrator and community advisor roles 38, 47 49, 55, 59, 116
Cutter–Tregenza Report (1982) 71
Tregenza, Julian 47, 51
Tregenza, Yolonde 47, 51
Tullawon Health Service 154, 157
DS as part-time medical director (2000) 153

UNICEF 217
United Aborigines Mission (UAM) 19, 22, 28
  establishment of Ooldea Mission 143
  rivalry with Lutheran missionaries 145–6
United Kingdom nuclear programs 23–6, 28–9, 32, 83, 84
United States of America
  funding for national Indigenous healthcare system 220
  McMahon Act 26
Urapuntja Health Service 13, 108, 127, 190, 210
  advocacy for community needs 13
  organisational structure 14–15
  outreach services to outstation communities 204
urban communities
  ACCHO movement 210
  mainstreaming of funding towards 227–8
Utopia Station 8, 9–15, 189, 210
  DS as locum GP 10–13
  See also Angarappa Health Service; Urapuntja Health Service

Vanstone, Amanda 204–5, 222
Verburgt, Bob 30, 36–7
vertical programs *See* Selective Primary Health Care (SPHC)

Wade, Bill (*Aliluya-nya*) 19, 22
  See also United Aborigines Mission (UAM)
Walker, Dennis 56
Walumpirr (Walumpirrnga) 130, 136
Walungurru Community Incorporated 116 *See also* Kintore
Walytitjata community 48

INDEX

Warakurna community 39, 47–8
Warburton Ranges Mission 22–3, 34, 72, 175
  assimilationist policies 52
  establishment of health-record system 58
  permanent settlement (post 1960s) 38
Warin, Jenness 191–2
Warin, Megan 216
Warnmun people 76
Warralong School 93, 101
Warren, Robin 97
Warumpi Band 124
Watama, Charlie 122
Watarru 31–2
Wave Hill cattle station 75
Weapons Research Establishment (WRE) 24, 84
welfare colonialism 2
West Australian 89, 177
West Australian Central Reserve 51, 72
Western Australia
  assimilationist policies 23
  community-health nurse outreach visits 39
  creation of Aboriginal reserves 18, 144
  discovery of goldfields 18, 142
  DS's trip with Schrader and Porter 51
  health department's transfer of community control 105, 107
  hostility towards Warburton Ranges Mission 22–3
  mining camps 34–5, 36–7
  one-teacher schools 39
  Pitjantjatjara homelands communities 47–8
  ways to weaken activities of strikers 81
Western Australia Department of Native Affairs 78, 79, 85, 144
Western Desert
  hunter-gatherer families 171, 175–8
  network of roads 113, 116, 148
  reoccupation movement 184, 187–90
Western Desert art movement 123
Western Desert languages 17, 112–13
Western Desert Nganampa Walytja Palyantjaku Aboriginal Corporation (the 'Purple House') 137
Western Desert Outstations Council 117, 119
Western Desert Puntukurnuparna Aboriginal Corporation (WDPAC) 103, 130
  DS's consultancy services 104–5
White Springs Mission 81
Whitlam Labor government 92, 184
  Community Health Program (1973) 215
  self-determination policies 209
WHO 217
Wicks, Chris 93
Wicks, Glenda 93
Williams, Carol 108
Williams, Daphne 123
Williams, Ditch 86, 87
Williams, Jack 92, 102
Williams, Leo 43, 44, 47
Wilson, John 81
wiltjas (traditional shelters) 37, 123
Wingellina 38 *See also* Irrunytju community
Wingrow, David 168
Withnell, Robyn 89
Wolfe, Patrick 244, 245
Woomera Prohibited Area 24, 27
Woomera Rocket Range 30, 83, 84, 114
Wootten, Hal 224
Working on Country Indigenous Rangers Program 205
Wozencroft, Belinda 106
Wright, Alexis 102
Wynter, Jo 6

Yakatunya 149
Yalata Community Council 153
Yalata Health Service 150, 160
Yalata Mission 28, 145–6
Yalata-Maralinga Health Service 150, 153 *See also* Tullawon Health Service
Yandeyarra Station 81, 82, 99, 100
Yankunytjatjara homelands 20, 21, 27
Yankunytjatjara people 17–19, 39 *See also* A<u>n</u>angu
Yarnangu 17, 22, 38
yaws (treponemal infection) 179
Yayayi community 115
Yougala, Crow 93
Young, Frank 65
Young, Iris Marion 242

Zimran, Smithy 119, 122